Life, Death and Decisions:

Doctors and Nurses Reflect on Neonatal Practice

Hazel E. McHaffie

Peter W. Fowlie

Hochland & Hochland Limited

Throughout this report, for convenience and to avoid cumbersome alternatives, the pronoun *he* is used for the baby unless a specific baby girl is alluded to; *she* is used for a midwife or neonatal nurse, and *he* for a doctor.

Published by Hochland & Hochland Limited, 174a Ashley Road, Hale, Cheshire, WA15 9SF, England

First edition

ISBN 1-898507-55-4

British Library Cataloguing in Publication Data
A catalogue record for this book is available from the British Library

Printed in Great Britain

Contents

List of Tables and Figures

Tables

Figures

Acknowledgements

As much as we should like to acknowledge every respondent and Neonatal Unit by name, an undertaking has been given to safeguard both individual and institutional anonymity. We can therefore do no more than express profound gratitude to all those doctors and nurses who gave so generously and often courageously of themselves. They shared not only their experience, but their pain and doubts. It was an enormous privilege to be allowed into their thoughts and feelings.

The consultants deserve a special mention. Not only did they consent to their Units being involved, but they personally contributed important insights into the whole issue of withdrawing treatment which substantially strengthened the value of the findings. Theirs is the burden of the final decision and it was particularly encouraging to have them individually giving hours of their time to this enquiry.

Other people in the Neonatal Units also contributed by freeing up colleagues to talk about these issues, making space available for private interviews, and creating a welcoming and supportive environment which positively influenced the whole experience of fieldwork. We thank the managers in each hospital for granting permission for this sensitive study to be carried out in their place of work.

The Scottish Office Home and Health Department funded this research in its entirety. Throughout the study period, PWF held an MRC Training Fellowship. We are grateful for the backing of these two organizations as well as that of our parent institutions, the University of Edinburgh Department of Medicine (HEMcH) and University of Dundee Department of Child Health (PWF).

Many individuals also supported and encouraged us throughout the course of this study. Professor Alex Campbell gave generously of his friendship and wise counsel, carefully checked manuscripts and offered helpful suggestions. Professor Sandy McCall Smith lent his authority to our consideration of the legal aspects. Computing experts in Edinburgh and in Surrey ensured we retained our sanity when software packages and machines threatened it. Members of the Institute of Medical Ethics Working Party on Prolonging Life and Assisting Death were enthusiastic about both the planning and execution of this research.

Special thanks go to Institute staff who offered on-going support through all stages of the work. Dr Kenneth Boyd maintained an unfailing level of interest and encouragement, critiqued every document we produced and periodically discussed the ethical issues with us. Rosalyn McHaffie spent endless hours typing quotes, searching the literature and assisting with computing difficulties. She transformed tables of raw data into meaningful graphs. We valued their constant good humour, and belief in the importance of this venture.

Our families too contributed by tolerating long absences from home, periods of preoccupation with these profound issues and the effects of emotional overload. We are grateful for their unconditional support and for all the hours of unpaid proof reading.

Foreword

Hundreds, if not thousands, of articles and books have been written about the difficult ethical questions surrounding the withholding and withdrawal of life prolonging treatment. Many have focused on the poignant problems posed by infants severely impaired by congenital abnormality or damaged by the complications of premature birth. Clinicians have been joined in vigorous debate by academics of all kinds – mainly theologians, philosophers and lawyers – and the view that it is sometimes right to stop aggressive treatment and allow certain infants to die has provoked strong reaction from 'pro-life' lobbyists. As a result, the policies and practices of neonatal units have been closely scrutinized, sometimes they have been applauded or condemned, and occasionally they have been subjected to administrative, legal or governmental harassment.

Neonatologists, while justifiably basking in the dramatic successes of neonatal intensive care, are only too aware of the tragedy that can result for both the infant and his or her family when survival is compromised by major disability involving the brain. At one time or another, most have agonised over this treatment dilemma and, with the family, have sought what they sincerely believed to be the least detrimental option. Some have felt it important to publicise their views and describe their own practice in the hope that some consensus would emerge on an approach that would best protect the interests of the child and family. However, as pointed out in this study, knowledge about these life and death decisions in neonatal units was largely anecdotal, and it was impossible to know just how representative were the views of the minority of paediatricians who were willing to publish. Furthermore, as these decisions are as much moral as medical, it is important that we understand the views and relative roles in decision making of the other important participants, notably the nurses and junior doctors who are likely to be in the closest and most consistent contact with the infants and their parents.

This study goes a long way to filling this 'data vacuum'. Sensitively and meticulously, the views of key participants in a representative number of Scottish neonatal units were carefully collected, not by impersonal questionnaires, but by detailed personal interview. The results are important and make fascinating but in some ways uncomfortable reading. *Inter alia*, the study indicates the awesome responsibility assumed by those who make such decisions; it shows the need for discretion and tolerance while making sure that the interests of individual patients are protected, and it indicates the important elements of 'due process' that should precede such poignant and troublesome decision making. To many neonatologists it will be reassuring to have evidence that their practice is consistent with that of colleagues, and that difficult decisions generally are carefully considered and are being taken responsibly, sensitively and in the best interests of the infants concerned. Some of the findings are disturbing and merit close attention even by those complacent enough to think that they have little to learn.

Good communication is such an important element of team leadership that it is upsetting to learn that it can be so poor among doctors and between doctors and nurses; and that some members of staff can be so insensitive to the feelings of others. Perhaps the consultant who steps briefly into the unit to switch off a respirator without a word to the staff may be trying to protect them from responsibility (or guilt?) and sincerely believes this demonstrates leadership. Decision makers must not only be comfortable with their own values and beliefs but they must be receptive and understanding of those of the others involved. Leadership imposes an important responsibility on the consultant to take careful note, not only of the wishes of the family, but of the views of the nurses and other key members.

It is also most unfortunate if the welfare of babies and families becomes jeopardised by an inconsistent approach to management and abrasive arguments that can be so damaging to team morale. A consistent and cohesive approach to the care of the infant is essential. There will be occasions when a change of mind is appropriate, but deviations from an agreed plan must be discussed thoroughly with the parents and team members. The authors' recommendations are worthy of careful study and implementation not only in Scotland but in neonatal intensive care units everywhere. These fundamental decisions about a baby's future should depend on the facts and circumstances of each case and not on ideologies or hospital politics, nor indeed on the great variation in individual personalities reflected in these interviews.

A.G.M. Campbell
Emeritus Professor of Child Health, University of Aberdeen

CHAPTER ONE

Introduction

Hamish is a premature infant weighing only 536g. He lies in an incubator wired up to a battery of machines hissing and whirring, alarms occasionally disturbing the rhythmic background sounds. His skin is grey, stretched tightly over his bony frame. His abdomen is grossly distended and dark brown exudate seeps into a bag lying on the mattress. Eight adults, all except one wearing light blue trouser suits, stand looking at his laboured breathing, their expressions betraying their concern. The 12 days since his precipitate delivery have been full of invasive procedures and grave prognoses. Scans reveal that his brain is severely damaged. Lungs and intestine show serious problems. Hamish's parents sit silently on low chairs hedged into a corner, to one side of the circle of uniformed doctors and nurses. They do not look into the eyes of the consultant neonatologist when he addresses them. Everyone is thinking the same question: should we continue to treat him? Is it in Hamish's own best interests? And all over the country the question is repeated, though the babies are all unique, and the circumstances all slightly different.

Birth and death represent two of the most significant events in the human experience, and these two poignant happenings converge in the Neonatal Intensive Care Unit (NICU) in a unique way. With advances in knowledge and expertise more infants are surviving but the deaths of the sickest and smallest have assumed different proportions now that so much is possible.

Medical technology and skill tend to gather a momentum of their own and as more becomes possible, more is expected. In the fierce battle against disease and death in NICUs, it is all too easy to lose a sense of perspective. Death can be seen as an enemy to be repelled almost at all cost. But in terms of human experiences, death is not always a harm and life is not always a good. There is a dark side to all our successes. What is professionally appropriate is not necessarily morally right,[1] and the difference is something which must be periodically revisited. New techniques create new situations and circumstances which in turn require new deliberations about moral choices.

> 'When scientific projects race ahead of ethical reflection, we see decisions based on pragmatic grounds and immediate interests and concerns. Although technological accomplishments can give ethics the slip for a while, sooner or later they will meet up and settle accounts.'[2]

Powerful and moving books have been written by researchers who have entered NICUs and described what they found.[3-5] What goes on within the walls of these rarified environments is so compelling that in a sense the outside world ceases to exist.[4] But making decisions about which babies to treat is one of the most painful experiences which staff and parents face. Parents themselves have captured the pain and the agony of both the total experience and the decision making in ways which make disturbing reading.[6-8] Though in terms of the total number of births in the country, these cases are rare, such is the burden of the decision about withholding or withdrawing treatment* that it can assume overwhelming proportions for all concerned.

The changing face of neonatology

The issues and responsibilities are not unchanging either. For with increasing capability new burdens are created and new dilemmas present. Questions now are less about whether we *can* save these babies – the very premature, the congenitally malformed, the severely damaged – but about whether we *should*. The potentially adverse sequelae for these infants and for their families are well known and widely reported.[9-13] Clinicians have been forced to consider the long-term consequences of modern neonatal care, and the disproportionate expense of treating babies whose outcome is uncertain or bleak when resources are known to be limited. The incidence of many congenital anomalies has already been reduced by antenatal screening, and increasingly clinicians are looking to the prevention of premature delivery as the way forward[14] rather than an even more aggressive pressing back of the frontiers of neonatal care.

Costs

Perception of the justification for such large expenditure, however, varies according to where the assessor stands. An administrator responsible for a budget for the whole of a region's healthcare may well look askance at the high costs of saving these infants. But one well respected paediatrician, NCR Roberton, after a survey of the data on outcomes, declared that the case was conclusive: infants of a birthweight greater than 500g or a gestational age of 24 weeks or more should unquestionably have 'proper' treatment.[15] Furthermore, he concluded that those in a satisfactory condition a little below these levels should also be treated. In relation to cost he considered that the current cost of treatment for premature infants at about £10,000–£15,000 per survivor[16] is not prohibitive – it compares favourably with the price of a new Ford Escort or a triple coronary artery bypass, and is far cheaper than a year of haemodialysis.

Nevertheless, even within the paediatric world, questions are not infrequently raised which ask about the justification of intensive care for infants. It is not simply a matter of counting the costs of immediate neonatal care. The long-term sequelae which add to the costs and burdens borne by society as well as by the children and their families cannot be neglected in any such assessment.[12,13,17] The most recent estimates[18] put the mean cost of medical care for low birthweight children up to age 8/9 with no disability at £2,737; which represents a cost 4.7 times greater than the cost of normal controls. The mean costs for the children in the lowest birthweight group, however, were more than 16 times greater. Those children who survive with disabilities are clearly more

---

*Throughout this volume the term *withholding* and *withdrawing treatment* is used to denote stopping aggressive or invasive procedures but not to indicate the withholding of basic comfort measures or caring.

expensive again: the mean cost was estimated to reach £19,593,[19] and these are conservative estimates based on 1979 prices, the rate recommended by the Department of Health.

Although many writers have cautioned that doctors need to be aware of the immense costs for marginal benefit of many medical interventions, Roberton[15] has made an impassioned appeal to those representing paediatricians to recognize the reality of modern treatment: babies over 500g have an excellent chance of neurologically intact survival. It is well known that in specialized centres survival rates are high.[20] Paediatricians, therefore, Roberton contended, have a clinical, moral and legal responsibility to treat these infants and the money must be found to do so. Arguments about resources are political not medical. He is not alone in believing that society has an obligation to fund neonatal care:

> 'society has the ultimate responsibility for providing adequate economic and human resources for the immediate and long-term needs of imperilled newborns and their families. Without this commitment, the discussion of ethical dilemmas often becomes academic.'[21]

The moral dimension

However, the decisions about which infants to treat and which should be allowed to die require more than simply reference to hard medical facts, economic evaluations, and the applications of guidelines or principles.

> 'The question of over treatment of seriously compromised neonates with life-prolonging hardware is, in the end, a weighing of values – a moral judgement. The most pressing issues of our time, it has been said, are not matters of engineering, but of human values.'[22]

Moral judgement is not as easily captured nor its wisdom passed on. For it is not a monolithic concept;[22] a system of values is not the same everywhere and for everyone. Nor is it an unchanging construct over time. Silverman, himself an eminent neonatologist, described his own changing views over 47 years of working closely with neonates, concluding that, 'As my social experience grew, so did my moral ambiguity.' Uncertainties and exceptions confound the picture on all sides.[22]

Ethical conflicts and moral values are rooted in our culture, giving shape and meaning to our lives.[21] These dimensions cannot be overlooked in any consideration of decision making on behalf of neonates. But ethical reflection is more than simply thinking about what we ought to do in certain dilemmas. It must be equally concerned with how we perceive and understand the dilemma,[23] and here philosophers, ethicists and theologians as well as clinical colleagues can assist us in our search for understanding.

The responsibility of making decisions on behalf of vulnerable patients puts a heavy onus upon us to think clearly and logically – a difficult thing to do when we are caught up in the personal tragedy of a given family facing these momentous choices.

For high flown theoretical ideas are of little use to the babies in our nurseries, rather what children need is a medical ethic that

> 'is practical, involved and personal; centres on the moral concerns of patients and those caring for them; learns from the thinking-feeling knowledge of everyone concerned; clarifies the problems in everyday terms that ordinary people can use; helps people to work together towards solutions.'[24]

CHAPTER TWO

Withholding and Withdrawing Treatment: The Debate

Issues relating to the so-called 'right-to-die' have become matters for widespread debate in recent years. Just in the two years during which this present study was underway there was considerable public interest in the question of withholding treatment. For example, the House of Lords Select Committee on Medical Ethics published a report on euthanasia.[25] A landmark case was brought to the courts in Scotland where medical staff wished to comply with relatives' request that treatment be withdrawn from a patient, Mrs Janet Johnstone, who had been in a persistent vegetative state for four years. The father of a ten-year-old girl, Jaymee Bowen, rejected a decision not to offer further expensive treatment for leukaemia to his daughter and as a result of his public appeal, a benefactor paid for a controversial new therapy. Jaymee lived for a further 17 months. The parents of Thomas Creedon were campaigning to have treatment withdrawn because of the burden of continuing existence for the severely brain damaged two-year-old boy, but he died before their case was heard. Doctors caring for Baby C in the Humberside area were granted permission to switch off the ventilator keeping her alive. Widespread coverage of the heartbreak of these families poignantly illustrated the effect of modern technology, the scrutiny of the lives of older children bringing into sharp relief the need to have a long-term perspective. Early triumphs in the nursery can later become disasters for families. These events brought into the open many questions relating to withholding or withdrawing treatment – the status of feeding as a medical treatment, reasonable grounds for not treating, the doctrine of double effect, competence to decide, and the place of paternalism.

The legal dimension

The law as it stands prohibits the killing of human beings. But grey areas exist around withholding and withdrawing treatment which have exercised the minds of both health care professionals and lawyers.

Society has produced an anomalous situation. A woman can terminate a perfectly healthy pregnancy up to 24 weeks gestation for no very powerful reason, and that is legal. Furthermore a fetus can be aborted after 24 weeks if a major impairment is diagnosed, and that is legal. In some circumstances a life may be destroyed simply on the grounds that it *might* be affected by a non life-threatening disease. For example, the male child of a woman who is a carrier of haemophilia stands a 50–50 chance of having the condition. Once she knows she is carrying a boy, she can terminate the pregnancy, even though the child might well not be affected; and even if he is, the boy could enjoy an excellent quality of life. That too is legal. It seems odd, therefore, that a society which countenances the destruction of human life for quite debatable reasons, still holds such strong preferences for preserving the lives of infants who are either born with serious impairments or develop them in the neonatal period.

The Dutch Paediatric Association have addressed these delicate issues directly and produced a report entitled *Doen of Laten?* ('To Do or Not To Do?'). They found a consensus among their members about the necessity to take quality of life into account when deciding whether to withdraw or withhold treatment, but there was a division of opinion when it came to euthanasia for this group of patients.[26] Even in a society where euthanasia is not always a criminal offence, clinicians vary in their thinking as well as their practice. However, while the current study was underway a test case was being examined through the courts. A doctor, Henk Prins, actively terminated the life of a severely malformed infant and by informing the Dutch legal authorities set in train his own trial for murder. To date he has twice been acquitted in the lower Dutch courts on the grounds that he faced two irreconcilable duties – to save life and to prevent suffering – and that he chose a justifiable course of action in the circumstances. But the case has been taken to the Dutch Supreme Court for constitutional clarification.

In this country the difficult position of doctors is well recognized. Recent cases such as *Bland*[27] and *Cox*[28] have exposed the tightrope which they sometimes walk. The lack of legal clarity has been variously applauded and condemned but a proposal has been put forward that at least for some well recognized circumstances, such as permanent vegetative state and progressive neurological disorders, suitable legislation could be framed which would simultaneously protect doctors and ease the trauma for relatives of patients for whom treatment is futile.[29] Something like a Medical Futility Bill, it is said, could eliminate many of the emotional responses surrounding euthanasia and obviate the necessity to take to court cases where treatment withdrawal is a clearly justifiable option. To date there has been no such firm proposal for infants.

An historical perspective

Most medical actions are carried out within some broader social, cultural and historical context. The withdrawal of treatment is no exception. As far as society in general is concerned, the majority of non-Western societies have at some stage accepted the practice of infanticide at least in some circumstances.[30] Nevertheless there is a widespread abhorrence of such practices in the Western world. The origin of the West's rejection of this practice appears to stem at least in part from a belief that unbaptised babies went to hell, or at best, into limbo,[30] and there are to this day concerns amongst Roman Catholics and some minority Christian sects, about the destiny of infants who have not had the necessary ceremony to place them within the sphere of God's protection.

In the professional medical world, paediatricians have for years been concerned about the tragic consequences which can follow an indiscriminate use of modern technology and expertise which does not take into account the effect of prolonged dying or of subsequent severe disability on babies or their families. When dilemmas about withdrawal of life-prolonging treatment for infants first came to wide public attention in the early 1970s, the issues mainly revolved around infants born with major congenital abnormalities.[31,32] Advances in prenatal diagnosis and in the management of babies in NICUs have changed the emphasis somewhat and dilemmas now hinge more frequently around infants compromised by extreme prematurity or neurological damage.

In all Units mortality rates have fallen. But although there is a fall in the absolute number of deaths, there is an increase in early deaths following withdrawal and withholding of treatment as more and more infants are born at the extreme edge of viability. However, although the practice of withdrawing treatment from infants appears to have gained momentum, it is conceivable that reporting has been tentative in view of potential public as well as professional reaction. In an American Unit in the early 1970s, 14 per cent of deaths followed withdrawal of treatment.[32] A decade later Whitelaw reported that 30 per cent of deaths in a London Unit occurred after such a decision,[33] and Aberdeen paediatricians reported that as many as 51 per cent of deaths in their Unit were directly related to the withholding or withdrawing of intensive care.[34]

In this latter part of the 20th century it is accepted that the unthinking and indiscriminate use of modern skills and technology can have tragic consequences and is insensitive to the harsh realities both for the children who are damaged and for their parents. The distinction is between 'having a life' as opposed to merely 'being alive'[35] or between the 'quality of life' as against the 'fact of life.'[34] Moreover it is understood in a clearer way than hitherto that resources devoted to this specialty of necessity are unavailable to meet needs elsewhere.

Although the issues around decision making in NICUs have fairly recently come into the public domain, it is argued that it is not the situation itself that is new but it is that these things have been newly exposed.

> 'There has been a sort of historic understanding, even a conspiracy, between medicine and the public. Doctors have not sought nor tolerated scrutiny of their decision making, and the public has not generally wanted to know how uncertain, idiosyncratic and capricious medical practice can be. Both medicine and its clients have collaborated in the mystification process.'[36]

The increasing involvement of the public in health related issues has brought about increasing interest in what goes on in NICUs and facilitated more searching investigation of the practice of treatment withdrawal.

Categories of babies concerned

There are basically three groups of babies for whom withholding or withdrawing of treatment may be an option.

1. The congenitally malformed – those infants with severe or multiple congenital anomalies whose imminent death is inevitable regardless of any medical intervention; for example, anencephalics or infants with no intestine.
2. The severely impaired who are receiving treatment – those who are dependent on life-sustaining treatment but whose prognosis for a future quality of life is so

poor that non-treatment is considered preferable to continued existence; for example, extremely premature infants or those with severe congenital abnormalities.

3.   The severely impaired who are not receiving treatment – those who are not directly dependent on intensive care but whose quality of life is expected to be extremely poor; for example, babies with severe birth asphyxia.

The Dutch Paediatric Association[37] has defined the groups more precisely.

1.   Those for whom it is inappropriate to initiate treatment;
a)   those who will die regardless of medical intervention;
b)   newborns with severe multiple congenital anomalies or extreme prematurity for whom the prognosis is so poor that non-treatment is morally preferable.
2.   Neonates who are dependent on life-sustaining treatment but who:
a)   will die regardless of any existing accepted medical treatment;
b)   might survive with intensive treatment but would have no chance of an acceptable quality of life; for example, very low birthweight (VLBW) infants with severe intracranial damage; severely asphyxiated infants; newborns with an extremely short bowel and severe complications.
3.   Those who are not directly dependent on intensive care but whose prognosis for an acceptable quality of life is extremely poor;
a)   neonates from Group 2 in whom withdrawing intensive care does not result in their death;
b)   neonates who were initially treated intensively but are no longer dependent on such support, but their future prognosis is poor; for example, severe birth asphyxia where the infant is breathing spontaneously but there is evidence of extensive hypoxic ischaemic encephalopathy;
c)   neonates for whom treatment was not started because of a poor outlook but who do not die; for example, severe spina bifida and hydrocephalus;
d)   newborns who survive but who are unable to communicate with their caregivers or those who face extreme suffering if they survive.

The conflicts

Excellent discussions of the issues around treatment withdrawal exist[30,38,39] and we do not propose to rehearse them all here. But in order to set a scene for the research which we undertook, it seems appropriate to outline some of the conflicts which complicate decision making in this sensitive area.

Background and perspective

Some philosophers and ethicists have little difficulty in making a logical case for helping infants to die.[30] Pro-life spokespeople argue persuasively in the opposite direction.[40] But for the clinician caught up in the human tragedy of these choices there is a very real difference between theoretical ethics and clinical ethics.[41] What may seem a perfectly logical argument in the lecture theatre or in an academic paper, assumes quite different proportions in the face of infant suffering or parental grief or actual medical responsibility.

Even within the nursery perspectives vary. Nurses' concerns about excessive treatment of patients have been well documented and conflicts do exist between medicine and nursing in this regard.[42] There is ample anecdotal evidence that nurses have long struggled with the problems of withdrawing treatment from neonates in a way not seen in medical circles. Tales of slipping fluids to babies whom doctors and parents had decided should starve to death, abound[41] and are testimony to staff's concerns. It has been called 'the nurse in the middle' problem[41] – caught between a responsibility to care and comfort while having few decision making powers, and yet vulnerable to criminal charges if they carry out the instructions of others.

The technological imperative

An inherent conflict already exists in the high powered environment of intensive care.[43] Highly specialized knowledge and expertise tend to encourage the pursuit of treatments, while a natural compassion for the individual may suggest that death is to be preferred to life. The medical instinct is to strive for recovery and it is easier to keep treating than to stop. Personal satisfaction comes from responding effectively to challenge. A sense of pride comes from averting an apparently inevitable death. Even if death occurs, if every possible therapeutic measure has been called upon, the doctor can feel free from guilt: he has discharged his responsibility in full, the patient has been given every chance.

The 'technologic imperative'[3] is a major factor in deciding to treat infants aggressively. It comes in various guises. One intervention leads to another producing an incremental process which creeps in small steps rather than in one recognizable and dramatic leap. Staff invest energy, time, money, effort and emotions into saving an infant and once embarked on a course of active treatment there is a reluctance to accept that the initial investment has not produced the hoped-for returns, or that the intervention has been over zealous. Furthermore a 'vicious cycle of commitment'[44,45] has begun. Having done so much already, why hesitate now? Reducing a baby to a set of pathologies makes it easier to continue aggressively treating symptoms; seeing the infant as a whole and within a family context raises doubts and ethical qualms. Doctors are uneasy about patients' dying because of a lack of technical treatment which they have the capacity to offer. Further pressure to pursue aggressive measures comes from fear. Fears are complex and multidimensional: fear of making an error of judgement which could cost a life; fear of criticism; fear of litigation; and fear of a burden of personal guilt which may have to be carried indefinitely for having 'failed' a patient. Personal pride can add pressure to try any new available treatment, even without previous personal experience, sometimes even at the cost of not transferring seriously ill patients to centres with expertise in the less frequently used procedures.

Within a short space of time staff can identify characteristics in infants which endow them with the status of unique and irreplaceable individuals. The acquisition of such a status makes justification of heroic measures easier. Many nurses and doctors speak of a baby 'making up his mind to die' or of an infant clinging to life against the odds or being a fighter resisting the onslaught of repeated medical catastrophes.[3] If an infant keeps battling it can sometimes create a moral obligation to continue aggressive measures even against the staff's better judgement.

Subjectivity

Treatment can be thought of in terms of the balance of benefits and burdens. If the benefits outweigh the burdens then the treatment is proportionate; but if the burdens outweigh the benefits it is said to be disproportionate. Inevitably judgements have to be made and it is not always clear on which side the balance falls. If we do think that in certain circumstances we ourselves would opt for death rather than a seriously impaired life, we are in effect saying that some lives are not worth prolonging. Competent adults and even older children can decide for themselves just when the burden of treatment becomes intolerable and a life not worth living; a neonate cannot. Nor can anyone else know what he would choose were he able to state a preference.

In making life-or-death decisions much hinges on the best interests of the child. Indeed it has been said that the 'only acceptable legal and ethical justification for deviating from the general obligation to provide life saving care is that doing so is in the patient's best interests.'[46] But this is a difficult assessment to make since a neonate has no history or established set of values to guide us. Trying to imagine oneself in the place of the baby is a common method adopted by those who encounter these problems firsthand. However Glover has argued that it is not a reliable guide to how that baby would feel were he able to understand his position.[47] Nevertheless it represents the least unsatisfactory alternative. He points out that,

> 'there is no adequate test for deciding the point at which someone's life is not worth living. Any general formula seems either too indeterminate or too contentious, or both. What is crucial is how much the person himself gets out of life. And where he is not in a position to express a view on this himself, the least unsatisfactory test is to ask what one would choose for oneself: would I choose death rather than have that sort of life?'

The problem arises from the fact that not everyone would choose the same thing. Each of us inevitably takes something of our own preferences with us. If music is something very precious to me, being unable to hear and appreciate sound might seem appalling. If my chief delight is in athletic pursuits the thought of being paraplegic might seem like a fate worse than death. Furthermore life with certain impairments may be impossible really to imagine. Can anyone truly appreciate the nightmare of being fully sentient and intelligent but trapped in an unresponsive body?

Moreover, there are even greater complications than these. There is a 'vast and ill defined gray zone'[48] into which many cases fall where uncertainties in diagnosis and prognosis make it impossible to predict with accuracy the outcome in terms of mortality, morbidity or pain. Thus any assessment is predicated on factual uncertainty as well as subjective bias.

Personal conviction and approach

There are widely divergent views on the morality of withholding or withdrawing treatment from infants and a massive literature exists on this subject. At one end of the spectrum are those who argue that severely impaired babies do not have the requisite characteristics of 'personhood' to qualify for the same rights as other babies; at the other end are those who believe that life is sacred and must be preserved irrespective of outside measures as to the quality of that life. In between are very many shades of opinion. Culture, upbringing, religious persuasion and life experience can all influence an individual's perceptions and beliefs and attitudes. What seems like a moral imperative to one might be a flimsy scruple to another.

Each person will draw his or her line at a different point along the continuum from death to life and this point may well change over time and with experience. To some extent it is only a matter of degree.

> 'staff too are likely to have mixed feelings – their instincts and training are transgressed by withholding or withdrawing support, and the dividing line between a 'passive' measure which allows death to occur naturally [withholding antibiotics] and an "active" measure which promotes earlier death [reducing the concentration of oxygen] is only one of degree when so much of the life at stake is already dependent on synthetic measures.'[43]

Rights and duties

Much is said about rights of individuals to decide whether they live or die. Neonates, of course, cannot voice their preferences. But that has not stopped others arguing for the rights of parents to decide on their behalf, or the duties of doctors and nurses to advocate for them. Nor has it inhibited people from appealing passionately for the rights of the infant to live or to die. Any such debate is constrained since there are few absolutes and many rights have corresponding duties which place burdens on the shoulders of others. It is one thing to accept martyrdom for oneself but another thing entirely to place oppressive burdens on others, be they babies or parents or health care professionals. Campbell has argued that,

> 'It is doubtful if absolute "rights", moral or legal, either to life or to death can exist in any modern society. "Rights" must be relative to responsibilities and obligations and will depend on circumstances.'[49]

The slippery slope

In any discussion about allowing people to die the spectre of a slippery slope tends to rear its head and the Nazi atrocities are cited as dire warning of the potential consequences of liberal attitudes. Indeed a notable exponent of the right to die with dignity, Dr Jack Kevorkian, (often styled 'Dr Death' because of his advocacy of the suicide machine) has written,

> 'One of the most powerful forces energizing the rule approach is fear of the so-called wedge or slippery slope [also known as the camel's nose under the tent, a foot in the door, and give an inch ...] argument. All of these catchwords imply eventual moral disaster through supposedly inevitable abuse of any "radical" innovation, no matter how small or innocuous its beginning. This dread of gray zones and of imaginative novelty ultimately rests on a lack of confidence in one's ability to control – and is, in effect, an admission of character weakness.'[50]

In medicine and particularly in areas such as neonatology, slopes can indeed be slippery. Whether the salient determinant is quite so simple as a matter of strength of character is debatable but the fact remains that these slopes can be slippery however far up them one sets a foot. Venturing nothing because of a fear of extremes can have equally problematic consequences.

Quality of life issues

Perhaps the widest and most prolific part of the literature on this topic relates to quality of life. Quality of life is seen to be,

> 'a polymorphous collage embracing a patient's level of productivity, the ability to function in daily life, the performance of social roles, intellectual capabilities, emotional stability, and life satisfaction.'[51]

It encompasses functional status, perception, and symptoms brought about by both the disease and the treatment.

Since so much hinges on individual meaning the decision is relatively straightforward if a competent adult is asked to choose. He has experience and understanding of the implications to guide him. If relatives have to make a decision on behalf of a patient who has already lived a life, they too have some foundation on which to base their thinking since the individual will have demonstrated in many ways his own philosophy, tolerances and preferences. But as we have already seen, newly born babies have no history or set of established values to guide us. It is clearly impossible to predict for infants what they would regard as an intolerable quality of life – these are very subjective measures. Things are further complicated by the fact that the child himself may be quite happy with his lot; it is those around him who are not and who mourn the loss of the potential he might have had if circumstances had been otherwise.

Yet some sort of evaluation has to be made. When assessing the projected quality of life of an infant, there are important matters to consider:

- the physical and mental burden of that infant's life and the extent to which that burden can be lightened by caretakers;
- the infant's capacity to interact meaningfully with his environment;
- his capacity for self-sufficiency and independence from caretakers;
- his future dependence on the medical system;
- his expected life span.[37]

Since every case has unique aspects, it is not possible to set fixed parameters or design any kind of scoring system which provides an unequivocal answer to the question of whether to treat or not.

A major impediment to clear statements on these matters is the existence of people who are already living with severe impairments. It is difficult to say that some lives are not worth living without seeming to devalue the lives of human beings with such deficits. But it is perfectly possible to value them whilst at the same time not wishing to impose such a burden on others. As Kuhse and Singer observe, 'it is one thing to say, before a life has properly begun, that such a life should not be lived; it is quite different to say that, once a life is being lived, we need not do our best to improve it.'[30]

The opinions of different individuals on these issues vary greatly. It seems doubtful whether anybody really believes that all human life has equal worth. The Baby Doe regulations in the USA were introduced by the US government in an attempt to prevent discrimination against impaired infants. But it became apparent that clinicians, even the most ardent advocates of the sanctity of human life, have to differentiate between babies. A treatment that will extend the life of a normal child is not necessarily appropriate management for a severely compromised infant. Distinctions have to be made between ordinary and extraordinary means of treatment; extraordinary treatment being taken to mean 'all medicines, treatments and operations which cannot be obtained without excessive expense, pain or inconvenience or which, if used, would not offer a reasonable hope of benefit.'[30] Even followers of the religious organizations which are staunchly pro-life, may draw the line at prolonging or preserving life which is totally dependent on the application of extraordinary measures.

Most clinicians appear nevertheless to subscribe to the idea that human life is inviolate irrespective of whether or not they hold particular religious convictions. Life is not something to be destroyed at will. To kill a baby or an adult in pain is not seen as morally equivalent to destroying unwanted kittens, or putting an aged or ailing pet to sleep. Yet in spite of this native respect for life, paediatricians in general do not support a 'life at all costs' policy.

'Most doctors reject an absolute adherence to the sanctity of life as inhumane vitalism that takes no account of tragic errors in development or the realities of disease and human suffering. On the other hand they are wary of suggestions that the swift, painless putting-to-death of deformed or brain-damaged infants would be more humane and should be sanctioned by law. Paediatricians generally prefer an intermediate position which recognizes that there are occasions when withholding or withdrawing life preserving treatments and allowing an infant to die is best for the child and the family and is probably best for society. There may be no *moral* distinction between "killing" and "allowing to die" but I believe that there is a powerful *psychological* distinction which is important particularly to parents and to the staff of intensive care nurseries.'[52]

Quality of life judgements are ubiquitous, then, and it is widely accepted that the indiscriminate application of treatment is inhumane in some circumstances.

Whilst clinicians speak from the vantage point of experience in real-life situations, philosophers explore more theoretical realms which can sometimes shed light on clinical dilemmas. Kuhse and Singer[30] have gone to considerable lengths to demonstrate that the 'sanctity of life' principle is 'impossible to defend in rational, non-religious terms.' Rather it is, in their view, 'the outcome of some seventeen centuries of Christian domination of western thought.' Glover[47] has taken the matter further. He has argued persuasively that a viable alternative to the doctrine of the sanctity of life is to consider the autonomy of the person whose life is at stake, the extent to which his life is worth living and the effects of any decision on other people.

Life may indeed be in the best interests of the baby. But it may not. Much depends on the quality of the expected life. Mere biological life is not sufficient. Opinions differ as to what constitutes a minimum level of life which is preferable to death but there is a general sense that awareness of pleasurable states of consciousness, ability to perform some rational and purposeful action, or to achieve some human goals are appropriate values to consider.

Decision making

The manner of decision making and responsibility for its conduct are further areas of debate and hinge on a number of issues. One part of the debate centres on the question of *futility* : Is this treatment futile and if so, under which circumstances should it be withdrawn or withheld? It is important to note that the value of the concept of futility has been called into question since imposed value judgements, imprecise definitions and lack of certainty cloud the judgement of what is futile.[53,54] As we have just seen a second hinges on the *quality of the infant's life*: What is a minimum standard for an acceptable quality of life? Whose interests take precedence in the event of a conflict of interests? Yet another part of the debate relates to just *who should make the decision*: Can the parents, caught up so intensely in the emotion of such a circumstance, make an informed choice? When do social circumstances come into the equation? Where parents and doctors disagree who should decide? A fourth aspect of the discussion deals with the matter of *costs*: What are the costs in terms of pain, handicap, guilt, distress, grief and finances? Is the cost too burdensome for the commensurate benefit? Is a life expectancy of two years with constant suffering and medical dependence, a good or a bad outcome?

There are decisions which rest in the domain of the doctors. The responsibility to assess whether a treatment is physiologically futile is one such. Here the parents do not have responsibility,[37] although they may well be involved in decisions about whether continuing treatment is desirable for other reasons, even though it will not effect a cure, such as in the case of a child with cystic fibrosis. When it comes to other factors, such as the potential impact on the family of a severely damaged child, parents may be the only ones who can come near to making the assessment. Whatever the extent of the responsibility each will assume for the decision, it is vital that communication and negotiation are good.[25]

Problems in prediction

Part of good decision making involves accurately predicting probable outcome and 'good ethical decisions begin with good facts.'[48] But the field of neonatology is littered with uncertainty.

Even the context for neonatal decisions is hazy. Viability itself is a movable concept and it is only relatively recently that fetuses which once were legally classed as abortions, have become viable infants. Indeed many countries have been struggling to define a proper cut-off point between abortion and the birth of a potentially viable infant. Following a series of international consultations the World Health Assembly[55] recommended a consistent form of gathering perinatal statistics which included all fetuses/infants weighing 500g or more, 22 weeks gestation or more; or 25cm crown–heel length. The choice of these criteria helped to overcome some of the problems of differentiation but there are arguments for criteria other than these.[56] Even within the UK the term 'capable of being born alive' is open to various interpretations and some clarification of the Infant Life (Preservation) Act has been called for.[56]

It has been said that 'a modern clinician's main challenge is to make predictions',[57] but neonatologists are agreed that prediction is very difficult in their area of expertise since every baby is unique, exceptions to every rule cloud the issue, so-called objective data are often unavailable or unreliable, and reactions to therapy often only become apparent over time. In response to the statement that, 'A science does not truly become mature until it develops a predictive capacity',[58] it has to be said that the multiplicity of variables to be considered in medical science makes it unlikely that prediction will ever be applied with the precision possible in the pure sciences of physics or chemistry.[59] Nevertheless advances in neonatal neurology and modern investigative tests, combined with careful follow-up studies, are together resulting in a gradual sharpening of the predictive accuracy of neonatologists[33,34] and some people believe that scoring systems might potentially offer refinements in assessment.[43]

Scoring systems

In the struggle to make informed choices about which babies to treat, efforts have been made to develop predictive scoring systems[60–67] although some people have cautioned that there are inherent dangers in making such categorizations.[66]

Guidelines for practice have also been promoted as a way forward out of the uncertainty. Countries have tried to develop such frameworks. For example, Denmark has tried to combine a lower limit of gestation with maturity criteria and also take account of a consensual view between the health care team and the parents.[38] Certain organizational bodies and individuals too have tried to set parameters to guide practitioners,[21,46,69–81] with some of the later models trying to redress perceived deficiencies in earlier attempts. During 1995 the British Paediatric Association convened a Working Party expressly to debate these issues and draw up a document to address the difficulties. All the available models vary greatly in complexity and scope for practical application, but the essential components tend to revolve around combinations of some or all of the following factors: collection of facts; identification of the problem; identification of decision-makers, personal values and ethical positions; consideration of alternatives and their consequences; application of relevant ethical theories or principles; development of a plan of action and its implementation; and evaluation of outcomes. On first inspection these models appear to have a process of steps through which to progress, however the authors do not insist on a linear progression but offer these points as a process through which ideas are examined by means of questions and answers. Inevitably certain responses will take the decision maker back to an earlier point in the process and a different route will be followed.

There is no evidence in the literature or anecdotal reporting to suggest any of these frameworks is actually used in clinical practice, and indeed it seems highly improbable that ethical dilemmas will be amenable to a 'cookbook recipe' solution. Choices are too often framed in terms of the best solution under these circumstances rather than a definitive all embracing right or wrong course of action. Specific guidelines appear simultaneously too simplistic to satisfy ethicists, and too burdensome to be useful to clinicians in real life situations.

Practice in relation to withdrawal

However, even though there is a lack of definitive and authoritative guidelines, clinicians are having to make decisions. There appear to be a number of commonly accepted practices. Most paediatricians will offer a 'trial of life' to all infants born alive. This allows a period of assessment, consultation and reflection before a final decision is made. It is recognized that there are times when it is more humane to allow a baby to die rather than continuing to strive to keep him alive. Treatment is sometimes continued for a short period to allow parents to adjust to the inevitable outcome. When the outcome is unclear treatment is continued until a firmer prognosis is possible.

Rhoden[82] has identified and categorized certain strategies variously adopted.

*   The *wait until certainty strategy* adopts the principle that all infants are treated vigorously until there is virtual certainty that they are either not benefiting or are being harmed.
*   The *statistical prognostic strategy* withholds treatment from infants where the prognosis is uncertain or grim.
*   The *individualized prognostic strategy* involves starting treatment but then re-evaluating the situation regularly on the basis of clinical indicators of ultimate death or severe brain damage.

One study of international differences found that in general the USA adopts the first strategy; Sweden the second; and Britain the third.[83]

Euthanasia

When it comes to active measures to terminate a life the whole debate is clouded by emotion and strong feelings. Furthermore it is also complicated by a lack of clarity about the terms used.[29]

In various ways attention has been drawn to changes in the medical professions' view of assisted suicide and euthanasia. Such sources as the The Bulletin of Medical Ethics and television documentaries have exposed practices where doctors have actively procured deaths. Some have defended their practice as acting in the best traditions of medical ethics. It is difficult to gauge the strength of support for this point of view but an editorial comment in the *British Medical Journal* took the view that,

> 'most doctors – and most people – are gradualists. They accept that withholding treatment may be a compassionate decision when the infant's handicaps are largely irremediable; they are less sanguine about hastening death by heavy sedation and withholding food.'[84]

One area of less extreme contention but more widespread concern relates to what exactly constitutes euthanasia. Measures such as reducing the concentration of oxygen delivered to a ventilator, the chemical composition of fluids not being adjusted to match worsening body chemistry – are these euthanasia in disguise?[43]

Another thorny problem relates to a group of infants whose lives cause great anguish to all concerned. When babies' deaths are lingering and miserable the inadequacy of current legal provision raises profound questions. Staff are seriously disturbed by the effects of some non-interventionist courses of action, such as the practice of starving severely birth asphyxiated babies. Kuhse and Singer shared this disturbance. After a profound consideration of the issues they concluded that,

> 'Until we are willing to break with the past and use the most humane ways of ending the lives we have decided to end, the infants drifting slowly towards their pre-determined deaths in our hospital wards will cast a shadow on our claim to be a civilized, independently-minded society.'[30]

The parental role

As we have said there are matters relating to withdrawing treatment which might conceivably fall within the domain of parental responsibility. Involving them requires great sensitivity and tact. The death of a child is one of the most traumatic events a parent will ever have to face and yet the needs of parents have often been misinterpreted, underestimated or even overlooked by health care professionals.[85-87] Some publications have attempted to offer guidelines to professionals to help them to care sensitively[88-91] and a wealth of anecdotal literature written by parents offers clues about what they seek in the neonatal nursery.

It seems clear, however, that even where parental opinion is known, practice may be deficient. Parents have strongly pleaded for accurate and full information but even in those Units where staff advocate candour, researchers have found that euphemism and evasion tend to characterize communications between doctors and parents.[92] It has been amply demonstrated that parents are very vulnerable to persuasion after the birth of a defective child,[93] but there is little evidence that health care professionals recognize this in their handling of discussions.

Yet parents have 'a most private and precious responsibility'[22] vested in them for the care of their baby. Theirs is a unique and special place. They have much invested in this child. They will be the ones to bear the consequences of these crucial decisions on his behalf for the rest of their lives.

Transforming private agonies into public debates in the courtroom and the media has aroused powerful feelings of revulsion in many. For the eloquent lawyer or the articulate Pro-lifer it is easy to demand prolongation of every life no matter how frail, or painful, or limited its capacity, if it requires none of his own or the community's resources to maintain that life throughout the years ahead. Parents, on the other hand, can resent the implied demands that they should sacrifice their lives because of the judgements of others. In defence, it has been argued that,

'No one is requiring parents to "sacrifice their lives" either physically or metaphysically, and it is a corruption of both language and truth to suggest they must.'[94]

Nevertheless to the parents it can appear that this *is* what is required of them.

Helping parents to grieve and participate in the decision making is fraught with difficulties. Each family is unique with their own history, expectations, values and beliefs, support networks and vulnerabilities. From a range of studies it has become clear that the duration of acute parental grieving varies and may be prolonged in some cases for years. Several researchers have identified the critical effect that interventions by health care professionals can have on these grief reactions.[86] Positive interventions have been seen to include parents being allowed to see and have opportunities to care for their child prior to, during and after death; being informed; being reassured that the child did not suffer; having opportunity to participate in decision making; having the infant's existence and death acknowledged; having their expressions of grief and anger treated sensitively; having caring and supportive people present. However the authors of one qualitative study of 14 parents whose nine children had died in hospital, concluded that the uniqueness of every parent's grieving experience precluded staff from identifying specific actions as helpful or unhelpful; responses needed to be individualized to meet the needs of each bereaved parent.[95] Their very uniqueness makes it imperative that doctors and nurses should be,

'careful not to impose unwelcome choices on families through feelings of moral superiority, worries about the views of colleagues, or excessive timidity about the law; yet they may have to guide parents towards what is acceptable not only medically but morally and socially, and what is within the law. Thus much latitude in decision is to be expected and should be tolerated.'[54]

From the literature, which in this area is largely anecdotal or based on personal opinion, clinicians appear reluctant to see State involvement either enforcing life or determining when death is preferable to continuing treatment. These are tragic and intensely private matters. Legalizing infanticide is seen to carry the threat of substantially eroding the trust between doctors and parents upon which much of British medicine is predicated. Even though deliberating together on such painful matters where they each have personal investment causes anguish and uncertainty, it is still thought to be a preferable option more likely to take account of individual factors in deciding the least detrimental solution for an infant. What parents and doctors are seen to need from society and from government are not new laws but more understanding of the reality of what impairment and disability can mean for a baby and his family, and sufficient latitude to work out the dilemmas in the best interests of all concerned.

Some have gone further than expressing a general antipathy for State or legal intervention. In their judgements, the imposition of regulations like the Baby Doe Rules and the activities of 'pro-life' activists could force paediatricians to go too far in keeping babies alive beyond all reasonable hope of healthy survival, thereby increasing the suffering of infants and the harm done to families. Such pressures might even lead to parents taking legal action against paediatricians similar to the 'wrongful life' suits directed against obstetricians. Such a cruel use of new technologies to keep infants alive for no justifiable purpose, beyond a personal conviction about the sanctity of life or a fear of legal sanction,

> 'is in itself one of the worst forms of child abuse and constitutes a victimizing abandonment of our responsibility to do no harm to patients'[54]

Need for research in this area

The research evidence related to the withholding and withdrawal of treatment from neonates is scant. Current understanding is largely predicated on the writings of senior figures in the paediatric world. Based as these usually are on a wealth of clinical experience they command respect. But arguably they do not adequately take account of the views of others involved in the decision making or in the implementation of the decision. Their opinions are seriously under-represented in the literature except for the occasional anecdotal article.

A sign in a dynamite factory reads, 'Sometimes it is better to curse the darkness than to light the wrong candle.' Sometimes a last-ditch unknown therapy can seem preferable to certain deterioration. But too many practices in NICUs have not been adequately researched before they have been widely implemented. The sequelae of vigorous oxygen therapy is a well-known example of the dangers of untested practices. This present study was an attempt to explore the darkness around ethical decision making.

A large number of surveys have been carried out on attitudes to prolonging life, the right to die, euthanasia and related issues, almost all of which involved sending questionnaires to large numbers of respondents, with some incorporating vignettes to focus thinking.[96–127] A number of the reports of these surveys refer to the advantages of anonymity offered by postal surveys. While it is tempting to obtain responses from large numbers of people, there are major methodological questions over the quality of information obtained by these means. A current EU study is being undertaken in a number of countries throughout Europe, including the UK, under the title of EURONIC, which is exploring staff views about withdrawing treatment in relation to neonates (HMcH is involved in this research). Such large scale questionnaire studies provide a certain kind of broad brush picture. There is a need additionally for more in-depth enquiries to supply detailed information about the multiplicity of factors involved in these complex decisions, and this was the avenue chosen for this enquiry. The wisdom of choosing an in-depth interview method appeared to be borne out by the respondents' comments: many spontaneously commenting that they would not have supplied such detailed and personal information or shared such profound emotion through a written document.

The aims of the research

This enquiry had as its main aim:

- to explore thinking and practices amongst doctors and nurses in relation to decision making in Neonatal Intensive Care Units in cases where withdrawal or withholding of treatment are possible options; to do this with special reference to ethical reasoning, perceived dilemmas, sources of conflict and productive working practices.

Its overall objective was:

- to identify practices which facilitate appropriate decision making relating to the care of neonates, minimising tension and conflict amongst the caregivers and family members involved.

CHAPTER THREE

The Study Method

A descriptive survey design was chosen as the appropriate method for this investigation. In-depth interviews appeared to offer the best way to explore individual experience and perceptions in an area hedged about with sensitivities and taboos. In any investigation of such a delicate nature, it is vital that great care is taken in the early negotiations, during fieldwork and in later presentation of the findings, to protect individuals and organizations from identification or adverse sequelae to participation. Throughout our enquiry this remained a primary concern.

During the planning phase of the enquiry, the principal researcher (HMcH) discussed many of the issues with clinical colleagues in various settings. One result of these deliberations was an invitation to attend a meeting of the Scottish Neonatal Consultants Group to present the proposal and provide an opportunity for the most senior medical staff involved, the consultants, to ask questions relating to the study. A useful discussion helped to clarify clinical perspectives and identify potential anxieties. Following this event, the Chairman of the group sent a letter to the researcher, to the effect that the consultants welcomed this enquiry and would cooperate in any way they could. This letter accompanied the application for funding, in order to reassure the grant-giving body that the project had sound clinical support.

Selection of units

At the time of this investigation there were 23 Units offering special care for neonates in Scotland, five of which provided special care but not intensive care.[128] The official size of the Units varied from 8 to 40 cots, with between 1 and 12 of these designated as intensive care cots.

Regionalization of services has resulted in a concentration of expertise and equipment in a limited number of specialized centres. Decisions about withdrawing and withholding treatment are likely to be addressed mostly in those specialized Units caring for the sickest and smallest infants. It was decided therefore, to draw the sample from the larger NICUs. Size was assessed on the capacity, the number of intensive care cots, and the number of admissions to the Unit each year. Eight of the Units were selected and approached sequentially.

Initially letters were sent to the clinical directors (where such an individual could be identified) or to all of the consultants, explaining the nature of the investigation and inviting them to participate. Telephone calls and letters to administrative heads, both medical and nursing, followed up these negotiations. In two Units the researcher was asked to pay a preliminary visit to discuss the study with medical staff.

It had originally been intended to concentrate the fieldwork in five centres. However, it became apparent that there were essential differences between university based hospital NICUs and District General Hospitals (DGHs). The senior medical staff in the DGHs seemed less likely to be dedicated neonatologists or to work full-time in the Unit. Variations also appeared to exist in certain characteristics of doctors employed and in the responsibilities assumed by the nursing staff. It was therefore decided to select Units in four university-based hospitals and two DGHs.

Of the eight eligible Units, six agreed to take part. In one of the remaining two centres, no response could be elicited to either letters or telephone calls. The reason given for the other Unit not participating was that they were currently undergoing major organizational changes and it was not a good time to ask staff to take part in something so sensitive. Additionally in this second Unit the consultant in charge believed that staff would have reservations about such an enquiry.

Ethics committee approval

In only one Unit was it considered necessary (by the most senior consultant) to obtain ethical clearance for this project. There it took nine months from the initial approach to the final letter of approval from the ethics committee. During that time, however, data were collected from the other five Units.

Tools

A semi-structured interview schedule was designed specifically for this project based on the known relevant topics identified in the literature and from discussion with clinical colleagues. There were minor differences in the questions asked of doctors and nurses*, but the formats were kept compatible to enable swifter and comparable analysis. The schedule was scrutinized by other researchers and minor modifications made before the tool was tested with colleagues from NICUs other than those selected for this study.

Procedure

A period of about two weeks was allocated for data collection in each Unit. The principal researcher (HMcH) independently arranged accommodation close by each hospital so that she could visit the Unit at all hours, through the night, over weekends and holidays, as well as during normal daytime shifts. We considered it important to elicit the views of a range of staff across the spectrum and to include in the sample part-time nurses who work only at weekends, evenings or nights. By being around at all hours too the researcher was seen to appreciate the round the clock nature of neonatal intensive care. At the commencement of fieldwork, she negotiated with the appropriate staff an agreed procedure for recruiting respondents, and the setting and timing of interviews.

---

*The term *nurses* has been used to include midwives since they are known generally as *neonatal nurses*.

Initially time was set aside during which the researcher could familiarize herself with the layout, organization and procedures in the NICU, make herself known to staff and allow people to ask questions about her investigation. This initial period varied from a matter of hours to five days. In the latter case she was asked to hold a series of team meetings to alert all staff to the study before recruitment began. Efforts were made to build up trust and professional credibility, not only by evening, night and weekend working, but by meeting as many staff as possible informally.

Face to face interviews were then carried out with individual staff. It had been the intention to select respondents randomly from a total list of team members. This proved impossible given the fluctuating needs of the Unit, shortage of staff and the requirements of shift work. Therefore, a different system was adopted for nursing and medical staff.

For the nurses, the researcher asked the team leader to free up a respondent of a certain grade or position for interview. The period of time spent in each Unit was long enough for her to ensure that an appropriate balance of grades was achieved, including representatives from among part-time and night staff. All respondents were interviewed during their work time although two sessions were lengthy and consequently encroached into personal time. Only qualified nursing staff were eligible for inclusion. Those nurses currently undertaking a neonatal nursing course were excluded since they were sometimes studying in a Unit other than their usual place of employment and the issues could have become muddied by their inclusion of practices, policies and attitudes from elsewhere.

The doctors were more difficult to access since their workload was unpredictable and it was not always possible for colleagues to cover for them. The Neonatal Consultants Group had specifically requested that all consultants be invited to be interviewed since they felt they carried the ultimate responsibility for the decision. Accordingly all consultants were given this opportunity. For the remaining grades – senior registrars, registrars and Senior House Officers (SHOs) – as many doctors as could be recruited in the time period to give a representative sample of each stratum, were included.

The interviews were held in a room away from the nursery areas with a notice outside the door asking for no disturbances. However, it was made clear that the needs of the babies took precedence over those of the research; staff were free to interrupt for legitimate business. In five of the six Units a quiet room was made available for the researcher except for those times when it was needed for delicate discussions with parents. All interviews were tape recorded and every effort was made to ensure the exchange was relaxed and unthreatening. The interview schedule, specifically designed for this project, set the pattern for questions but the researcher intuitively tailored the extent of probing for each respondent.

A gift was left in the Unit for the staff at the conclusion of each period of data collection, and formal letters of thanks were sent to both nursing and medical staff.

Response rate and sample size

The size of sample required for this study could not be calculated in anticipation since with such an enquiry there is a theoretical necessity to continue until conceptual categories are saturated. However, it was planned to recruit a minimum of 50 doctors and 50 nurses. Given the fact that there are far more nurses than doctors working in these Units it seemed likely that it would be harder to obtain a large sample of medical staff.

The actual sample size reached 119 nurses and 57 doctors. Nursing staff themselves were keen to contribute and opportunity arose to investigate the perceptions of more of them in the time it took to recruit sufficient numbers of doctors. It was possible to tease out finer differences between the nurses as a result of the increase in sample size. The final sample represented approximately 1 in 3 (36%) of the total population of nurses and approximately 4 in 5 (79%) of doctors. By selecting a stratified sample the researcher was able to ensure that the different grades were represented.

Since requests to participate were often relayed through the senior nursing staff it was not possible to know how many if any declined to be interviewed amongst the nurses. Requests to the doctors were direct, however. Two expressed reservations about being interviewed. One consultant said he would participate if the whole procedure could be completed in 15 minutes; but as interviews with the other consultants had taken from one to three and a half hours, it was decided not to attempt to gain information in such a limited time. One house officer declined on the grounds that her spoken English was too poor. Two other junior doctors initially agreed but later said they were unable to participate at scheduled times because the pressure of work had increased since the arrangement was made. These 'official' reasons could have been a cover for an unwillingness to participate, although there were independent indications that their workloads were heavy at that time, and their original consent and later regret appeared genuine.

Coding and analysis

A coding frame was designed to enable the data from the tapes to be recorded in numerical form using Microsoft Excel Version 5.0. The principal researcher undertook this primary task herself. Given the confidential nature of this enquiry it was important to build in checks for scientific rigour. Accordingly a clerical assistant checked 10% of the tapes for reliability of coding – the conversion of descriptive data into numbers. A total of four errors in a total of 2,048 values was considered acceptable. Additional slight differences in interpretation enabled the researchers to discuss the issues concerned and develop a consistent policy for coding.

In addition to the coding checks, there were content checks. The co-researcher (PWF), himself a senior registrar in neonatology, listened to a random sample of the tapes (10%), excluding those recorded from interviews with colleagues whom he knew well, concentrating on themes and content. In his analysis, blind to the principal researcher's coding, the co-researcher did not identify any unreported themes, suggesting reliable content analysis. The two researchers then agreed the level of analysis which would be necessary for the reporting. When data were to be reported in quantitative terms, reliability was again assessed by both the researchers analysing the data separately. In the allocation of qualitative information into themes there is inevitably some margin for slight differences of categorisation, but no differences were found which might have affected the interpretation of the findings.

As the principal researcher listened to each tape she marked on a card those direct quotes which either substantially captured the essence of an idea or which illustrated a point well. The clerical assistant then transcribed those sections of the tape on to the computer, assembling a collection of illustrative material for each section of the report.

Analysis of the data was carried out using SPSS for the Apple Mac Version 6.1. There was a danger that the researcher who was also the interviewer, would have gained certain impressions from her fieldwork in the Units which could potentially bias her thinking. In order to minimize this risk, analysis was carried out initially using the numerical values assigned to responses as far as possible rather than the words which captured the essence of what respondents said. In this way it was less likely that responses could be forced into categories to substantiate hunches.

Confidentiality and anonymity

Great care was taken to ensure confidences were preserved. During her stays in each of the Units, the researcher limited her activities to the immediate environs of the hospital and her nearby hotel, thereby reducing to a minimum the chances of other people seeing her and making the connection with a specific centre. The responsibility of each respondent to keep their involvement quiet was pointed out at interviews although, of course, the researcher could exercise no control over what clinicians might divulge in a private capacity.

It seemed important to protect the identity of the Units themselves as well as of individuals. To this end only basic information about them has been reported in order to set a context for the findings and to enable the reader to assess the quality of the research and its findings.

Tapes holding each respondent's data were numbered to minimize the possibility of identification and kept securely locked away. In any reporting, only essential denominators have been added to direct quotes to protect each respondent. One respondent asked to have a copy of his tape so that he could listen to his responses and reflect on the issues raised. He was given a copy.

For three participants additional safeguards were necessary: these three all requested that no one else in the research team except the principal researcher should listen to their tapes. Quotes from these respondents were typed up by the principal researcher and their tapes were not entered into the pool for random selection by the second researcher to check the analysis and coding. Two of the three also asked that, following the coding of their information, their tapes should be destroyed. Accordingly their tapes were shredded immediately after coding and transcription of quotes, and a letter sent to each to say the process was complete.

In the small world of neonatal care in Scotland, it would be all too easy to divulge identifying information inadvertently. To try to prevent such a slip, unusual cases which might identify a Unit have not been included in the reporting. In addition, all written results have been scrutinized by both researchers and the project's scientific advisor who is a retired Professor of Child Health familiar with the Scottish neonatal scene. It was felt that if all three considered that the information was untraceable, the checks could be considered as stringent as it was within their power to make them.

Limitations

Ideally it would have been good to investigate staff thinking and practice in all the 23 Units in Scotland caring for sick and premature infants. It is conceivable that opinion would be very different in those nurseries which rarely encounter these difficult cases. Time constraints as well as limited resources made it necessary to select only six which deal with these situations most frequently.

Clearly single encounters with individuals do not take account of the changing nature of opinions and attitudes.[129] As Powell has pointed out:

> 'My person is not ... permanent and fixed; person implies a dynamic process. In other words, if you knew me yesterday, please do not think that it is the same person that you are meeting today.'[130]

The one-off nature of each interview is inevitably a limitation of this investigation, but it reflects the constraints which exist in the real world where research is of necessity bounded by time.

People play games both consciously and subconsciously.

> 'scars and ... defenses, which we use to protect ourselves from further vulnerability, tend to form patterns of action and reaction. These patterns eventually become so self-deceptive that we forfeit all sense of identity and integrity. We act "roles", wear "masks", and play "games."'[130]

It is possible that respondents in this present enquiry were not always in tune with their own thinking, or that individuals wished to create a particular impression of themselves. There is no way of knowing. But the method chosen which built in opportunities for them to come to know and trust the researcher over a period of time, went some way towards minimizing this possibility. The genuine distress so many showed in relating stories and feelings, and the generous and often self-critical way they unpacked their insights, make it more probable that they were as frank and honest as it is possible to be in these circumstances.

A recent nationwide study has shown that NICUs are operating below recommended establishment figures.[131] It was not desirable to add further to the load of staff in the study Units and when they said they were too busy to free anyone up for interview this was unquestioningly accepted. Although recruitment at haphazard times could potentially have skewed the characteristics of the respondents, it could also have added to the random nature of their selection, thereby reducing the risk of introducing bias.

Readers, particularly those with an inclination towards quantitative and rigorously controlled research, might well have reservations about the part played by the researcher in this qualitative exploration of a most sensitive topic. Certainly it was not possible to adopt a rigid technique: a degree of intuition and response to cues guided the questioning of each interviewee. But to ignore the human factor would be to deny the bases of interaction one with another. Some respondents needed more encouragement than others. Some appeared robust enough to have their views challenged and feelings probed, others were not. When individuals presented a response which triggered new ideas in the researcher's thinking, opportunities for deeper investigation were offered which might well have been absent in earlier encounters. Being receptive to such cues formed part of the tools the interviewer used to gain understanding of the subject. It was necessary in some measure to enter into the respondents' world of pain and distress in order to make sense of the dilemmas they face.

> 'Subjectivity is not the same as bias. The subjective scientist who is aware of personal perceptions and takes them into account is in closer touch with reality than the scientist who imagines that ignoring feeling and values is the same as excluding them. All data are perceived through the senses and are inevitably filtered through the grid of former experience.'[24]

By entering this specialized and intensely emotional world the researcher gained insights into thinking and feelings which would have been inaccessible by any other method. The results of this understanding are presented in the following chapters and will allow the reader to assess whether the inevitable limitations have detracted substantially from the value of the findings.

CHAPTER FOUR

The Respondents

As reported, 57 doctors and 119 nurses participated in this research. In order to protect the identity of the senior staff who were numerically few, those with additional administrative responsibility have been placed in wider categories. A breakdown by grade is given in Figure 4.1.

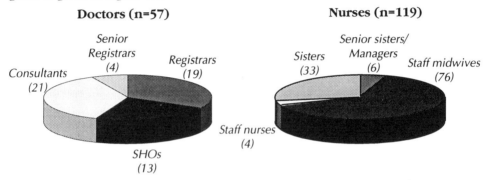

Fig. 4.1: Grades of doctors and nurses who participated

The doctors

Some staff held research posts but, to protect their identity, they have been classified according to their level on the clinical scales. A small number of the SHOs had had exceptional backgrounds in terms of experience either in paediatrics abroad or other specialties such as General Practice but again these factors have not been linked to respondents since they would identify the individual too closely. Three of the 57 medical respondents were employed on a part-time basis in the study Unit.

Communication is an important factor when it comes to dealing with families where treatment is being withdrawn. It is noteworthy, therefore, that three doctors had foreign accents which were quite difficult to understand. A further seven had fairly pronounced foreign accents but they were easily understood by the interviewer.

The nurses

There was much greater diversity amongst the nursing staff. Of the 119 respondents, 25 (21%) were part-time; 13 (11%) rotated into different areas of the hospital so were not permanently in the Neonatal Unit; 8 (7%) worked exclusively on night duty. Administrators, clinical specialists, liaison nurses, in-service education sisters, and research staff, were also represented in the sample albeit in small numbers so they have been subsumed into wider categories to protect their identity. A greater proportion of nurses than doctors had local accents, but only one nurse had a foreign accent which was difficult to understand.

Gender

Thirty-four of the doctors (60%) were male and 23 female (40%). Very few male nurses worked in the study Units and only two (2%) of the nurses interviewed were men.

Experience

The medical staff's experience of working in this specialty ranged from less than a week to 30 years (mean 10.5 years, mode 2 years). Three of the doctors interviewed had been working in this field of practice for less than one month.

Only six of the 57 (11%) had never worked in another Unit. For the remaining 51 (89%), their experience had been obtained in a range of other centres – up to 15 different ones (mean 6, mode 3). In addition to their experience in the study hospital, they had worked in other Intensive Care Units (50), in Special Care Units (19), in District General Hospitals (9), and/or small nurseries with limited intensive care facilities (7). A quarter of the doctors (15, 26%) had also worked with neonates abroad.

The nurses' experience ranged from a few months to 24 years in this specialty (mean 8.5, mode 5). Ten had worked with neonates for less than a year, and only a quarter of the total sample had more than 10 years experience (28, 24%). Half of the 119 nurses had worked in other units (60, 50%). Those who had worked elsewhere had gained their experience in from 1 to 7 other centres (mean 2.5, mode 2). Sixty-six of them had experience in other Intensive Care Units; 12 in small Units with limited intensive care facilities; 14 in Special Care Units; and 2 in Hospitals for Sick Children. Two had worked abroad with neonates.

It was interesting to note the differing perceptions of the doctors and nurses in relation to time and experience. Doctors considered themselves quite experienced after 18 months working with neonates. However, many nurses with years of experience still regarded themselves as junior colleagues, especially where they had remained at the level of staff midwife/nurse.

Involvement in decisions to withdraw or withhold treatment

All except five of the 57 doctors had been involved in a decision to withdraw treatment from a neonate at some point in their professional careers. Only four of the nurses (3%) had never been involved in a decision of this nature. One person found it impossible to quantify since these experiences tended to come in spates. But for the remainder, the frequency was assessed and the results are presented in Figure 4.2.

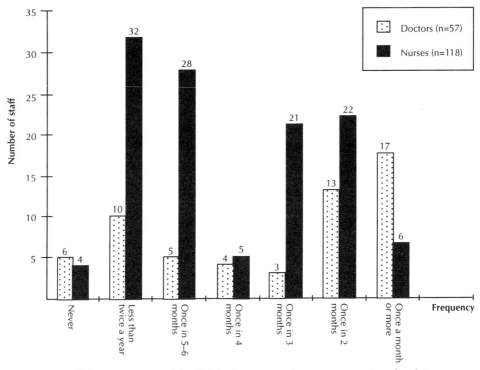

Fig. 4.2: Frequency with which doctors and nurses were involved in decisions to stop treatment

In addition 49 of the 57 doctors (86%) had been involved in such decisions in relation to patients other than neonates. In the majority of cases (40, 70%) these were on behalf of paediatric patients. Experience had also been obtained in adult wards or units and spanned general medicine and surgery, A & E, coronary care, oncology, haematology, vascular medicine, neurosurgery and geriatrics. A few staff additionally reported participation in antenatal decision making.

Fourteen of the nursing staff (12%) who had rarely or never been involved in these cases, nevertheless said they were sometimes aware of the discussion going on, while two nurses (2%) had never been conscious of the team deliberating about withdrawing or withholding treatment from a baby. As onlookers nurses sometimes formed their own opinion, however, and a minority (3, 3%) had in the past been uneasy about the decision reached on the grounds that it was not, in their judgement, in the best interests of the baby. It is noteworthy that a small number of nurses who professed themselves very religious and voiced very decided pro-life opinions, appeared to have had little exposure to these difficult cases. Other staff implied that the exclusion of these individuals was deliberate because of their extreme views.

Less than half of the nurses had ever been involved in decision-making in any other specialty. For the 50 (42%) who had, a much smaller percentage of nurses (10%) compared to doctors (70%) had obtained such experience in paediatric settings. Most had been working in adult nursing with specialties including terminal care, oncology, intensive care, geriatrics, neurosurgery, theatre, gynaecology, A & E, or haematology, as well as general medicine and surgery.

Experience of decisions about withdrawal or withholding of treatment

Early on in each interview respondents were asked to relate a case with a neonate where the option to withdraw or withhold treatment had been discussed. They were requested to choose one which had particularly stuck in their minds. The accounts were graphic and moving, and many people became quite emotional recalling the events. Listening to these stories it would have been easy to assume why the teller had not forgotten this particular case. But in order to be true to them, the interviewer asked them to specify why that case had made such an impression. In total 111 factors were cited. Proximity to a case made it come quickly to mind in some instances (10 doctors; 16 nurses).

The nurses' impressions

A number of categories emerged: personal factors for the health care professional herself; factors relating to the baby, the family, or to the management of the case; and the decision itself.

a) Personal

For the nurses a powerful factor was their own close involvement with that particular family. Where they became close and had shared significant moments with the parents, the detail and the emotion stayed with them.

> 'It was quite a traumatic time but it was also the first I experienced and it always stays in my mind. People say you can forget as a nurse, but you don't, because I can even recall the baby's name and I have wee sort of gifts that her Mum gave me, like the baby's teddy bear – the wee girl's teddy bear. I've still got that teddy bear. I was like her mother there – I didn't want to hear that decision. But it was the right decision.' (Staff midwife, less than 5 years experience*)

A considerable number indeed reported continuing involvement with those families long after the death of the infant.

---

*The years of experience denotes the total length of time spent working with sick and premature neonates, and not their time in this position.

'I think some parents don't like to let go. I got a letter from a Mum the other day, whose baby died here 7 years ago, last weekend. She still relates to me.' (Sister, more than 10 years experience)

Nurses spoke eloquently of their distress when these things happened to such 'nice' parents. In a few cases a sense of personal inadequacy was conveyed; they had felt powerless to give the parents real support because of their own emotion, inexperience or fears.

'He was such a beautiful baby and it was quite sad. It was very hard to cope. And I felt that I had let the parents down, because I was so emotional myself that I felt I couldn't help them as well.' (Staff midwife, more than 5 years experience)

Having personal doubts made it difficult to support parents and some staff suspected that certain cases were managed in a particular way because of the feelings of the professionals as well as those of the parents.

'The baby had been paralysed. He'd been on morphine. So we had to take away the [effects of these before the neurologist made his assessment]. He did it and then came back two days later and did another assessment and ... even though the baby did not react, one of our concerns was maybe the baby was in pain. We just weren't very sure. It's hard to reassure the parents when you maybe have, at the back of your mind, these doubts ... That's one of the main things they are concerned with, that he's not suffering in any way ... we did give him sedation – I don't know if the sedation was for the comfort of us, you know, or the comfort of the baby or the parents. And then we just did it slowly – over a period of 24 hours which was what they wanted. They wanted to see the equipment gradually being taken away. Such a sad situation but the baby did go very quickly. He died within about 5 or 10 minutes.' (Senior sister, more than 20 years experience)

A sense was occasionally conveyed that nurses did not like babies to die on their shift even though the death was expected. Although they realized it was a rather irrational belief, they felt it in some way reflected badly on them.

'It was a very small baby – 26 weeks or 28 weeks, I can't exactly remember. Christmas Day. He'd been very stable all morning. Came on to do a late shift and the baby had been fine. Sort of 2–3 hours into the shift, he wasn't so well. Sucked him out and were sucking him out [when] he wouldn't start breathing. We had to breathe for him. He had a cardiac arrest ... you felt like you'd done it. You'd sucked him out and started the whole [crisis], and he'd been so stable all morning ... The Mum came in obviously extremely shocked and upset. She knew her baby was poor, that he was unstable. But that morning she'd gone home and they said to her, what a good Christmas. What I remember is that [the parents] didn't stay in very long – she barely had him out of my arms and into her arms, and she gave him back to me. And they actually left quite quickly.' (Staff nurse, less than 5 years experience)

Being themselves pregnant or recently bereaved or grappling with personal problems at the time, made the nurses themselves particularly vulnerable. Some poignantly related incidents to their own circumstances.

Standing up for a principle or behaving out of line could create tensions which stayed with staff. One sister with 20 years experience reflected back many years to a case when she was on night duty and refused to give a dose of morphine to a baby. There had been a degree of unpleasantness with one of her nursing colleagues who felt she was passing the buck. But the respondent reported that she remained adamant in her stance and simply told her colleague that she too could refuse to do this thing if it troubled her. She had not, however, forgotten the incident or the feelings it had engendered.

b) The baby

Details relating to the dying could etch indelible memories. Graphic accounts were given of babies whose appearance, or the nature of their actual death, caused great distress. A considerable number of staff made reference to the difference between an extremely premature infant dying and a full-term infant's death. Where the baby was a beautiful, full-term child whose life was lost because of damage in the perinatal period, there was a more profound sense of grief.

> 'It sticks in your mind more, really. You don't expect a term baby to die as much as a preterm baby, I suppose. He was here for a long time as well, and you got to know his Mum, and his parents and family – that as well. It doesn't seem right when it's any baby. But if it's a bigger baby it's maybe harder to take.' (Staff midwife, less than 5 years experience)

> 'I think because the baby was so old and we obviously knew him very well. I mean, we bounced him on our knee numerous times. And obviously by that time we got to know the parents very, very well, so we were all on first name terms and were quite friendly with them. More of a bond there, I think. And with the baby ... all the staff felt a bond with the baby himself ... even after two or three months they have little personalities and some of them are so bad tempered!' (Staff midwife, more than 5 years experience)

Where the dying was prolonged there were especial traumas.

> 'The talking was over a period of about 5 weeks. And the reason for that was that they agreed that he wasn't progressing but it was coming up to Christmas and New Year, and they couldn't cope with taking the baby off over [that] period for the [other] children. But it was very hard to look after him ... we all knew what we were waiting for, and the staff in the Unit knew that after New Year we were going to switch him off and take him off, and it was terrible, absolutely terrible.' (Senior sister, more than 5 years experience)

c) The family

The family's response to events made a big impression on the staff – if they handled things well or badly. The nurses particularly had their own expectations of what constituted a 'good death' and if the parents rushed things or were not sufficiently involved, the detail remained in their memory.

One nurse described an incident at a funeral of twins one of whom was a still birth and the other survived only two days. The event left an indelible impression:

> 'I went to the funeral service. The father stood up and said, "The two days this baby was alive were the happiest days of my life." I thought, even if these babies don't make it, what we do while they're alive, dying, can be tremendously significant and I think that's what affects the way we think about bereavement care now.' (Staff nurse, more than 5 years experience)

Particularly tragic circumstances also made some families unforgettable. Examples included the death of the mother, subsequent infertility, and a series of additional traumas for the parents to deal with. Multiple births where one baby after another subsequently died had a profound effect on nurses who were trying to help the parents simultaneously to grieve and to hope, and then to go through repeated bereavement processes.

If parents did not visit the baby, or become involved in the dying process, the nurses felt especially protective of the child.

> 'So the baby was taken off the ventilator and he survived for about an hour, an hour and a half. But there were lots of problems with the Mum, and the Mum didn't want to come and see the baby. We eventually persuaded her to come along and see the baby, but she didn't want to stay with the baby once it was taken off the ventilator. There was no one there when the baby was [dying]. It was horrible. I could understand why the baby was taken off the ventilator. But we were very, very busy at the time. There was no one to sit with this baby. And it was the end of my shift, so I felt I had to go – it was the traditional thing to do, go off shift ... Then I *had* to come back and just sit with this baby – I thought, I can't leave this baby. It was just lying in the middle of the incubator ... And it was horrible ... took it out and ... cuddled it [until it died].' (Staff midwife, less than 1 year experience)

Other staff also reported spending time cuddling these infants to ensure they were surrounded by human warmth and love in the last hours of their short lives. An additional distress accrued from parents declining to attend the funeral. In some instances nurses intellectually recognized that religious beliefs and practices dictated procedure, but their overwhelming feeling was that important elements of grieving were being shelved by these practices. Knowing the theory of bereavement, it was hard to run counter to what they sincerely believed was in the best interests of the family members.

In some cases fathers or relatives or even the mother wanted to be involved, but were delayed in arriving at the incubator side. This sometimes meant that the baby died before they could see him, or that strenuous efforts had to be made to keep him alive until they got to the hospital. Both these scenarios made cases memorable for the nurses, who went to considerable effort in orchestrating the dying to meet parental and infant needs.

d) The management of the case

In singling out specific cases for mention, respondents recounted details which in their judgement indicated that the events were either well handled or badly managed. Where everyone had worked well together and the dying had been as sensitively handled as possible, a favourable impression was left. But many nurses' most abiding memories related to cases where things had not been so managed. The most common lament was about procrastination which protracted treatment until long after the nurses or junior doctors themselves had come to the conclusion that the best interests of the baby were not being served by prolonging his life.

> 'The week before Baby N died obviously things were going really badly. She'd had to be re-ventilated and was very poorly – absolutely no chance of survival whatsoever. Her lungs were just appalling, and the consultants brought the parents in and said she was probably going to die within the next few days ... I came back at the end of the week and she was still here. And I was absolutely irate because she was still here, because in the back of my mind is – she's supposed to be going to be a respiratory cripple and at the same time she'd been having fits as well. Her temperature control was all over the shop. And I just thought, what kind of a life has this child got? She's suffered this [for five months]. I mean, it's gone on long enough. I just felt nobody was making a decision.' (Sister, more than 5 years experience)

This sister went on to describe graphically the potential consequences of this delaying. Baby N's parents lived a long way from the hospital and there was a real possibility that if the baby collapsed in the night they might not get there in time before she died. The alternative was to have a controlled end which the respondent felt would be 'so much more bearable for them.'

It was not just the baby and family who suffered when decisions were protracted. Nurses were obviously distressed themselves recalling such circumstances.

> 'That baby, he had a very swollen abdomen and they literally started drawing blood. I think in the end his liver had been punctured. That had quite a grave effect on a lot of people, and you were literally standing there saying, "Baby R, just die. Please God, just take him." The baby was just grotesque and I don't know what he was to the parents.' (Sister, more than 10 years experience)

> 'She was grossly oedematous ... I remember going and somebody saying, "I can't suck this baby out." Her oesophagus was so oedematous you couldn't even get a catheter down ... it was like looking after a living corpse – they were stiff, woody, you just lifted them in one piece.' (Sister, more than 10 years experience)

Whatever the cause of the delays – medical indecision, bad management, or conflict between staff, or between parents and staff, or between parents – the consequences for the baby could be grave and this upset nurses. On the other hand they found it stressful when doctors unilaterally decided to withdraw treatment, or when they did so for social, or resource, or idiosyncratic reasons when in the nurse's own judgement the baby was not sick enough for death to be preferable to life. A small number of nurses related in minute detail cases where a doctor had withdrawn treatment in such a manner, vividly recalling their own feelings of bewilderment, anger and uncertainty. However, they specifically requested that this information should remain confidential so these accounts cannot be reproduced in this report.

Respecting a baby's dignity was clearly important. Cases where this right was infringed remained with the respondents.

> 'You felt that the baby lost its dignity, that's what sticks in your mind. I do feel that [the doctors] just forget that this is somebody's baby. And well, they did forget this was somebody's baby, because they were putting a needle in two or three times into the baby's heart, and that was terrible. I wouldn't want them doing that to my baby.' (Staff midwife, less than 5 years experience)

Inherent conflict made cases remain with the staff. Examples were given of doctor-doctor, nurse-doctor, parent-doctor, and parent-parent conflict. These situations were stressful enough without an additional layer of tension.

Another different but peculiarly stressful circumstance for the staff was where feeding was withheld from babies who had suffered severe birth asphyxia. Some Units routinely tube-feed such infants and their deaths are brought about by untreated infections or sudden collapses. But in Units where nourishment was on occasions withheld, and babies were perceived as starving to death, the nurses experienced profound emotions.

e) The decision itself

It was only rarely that the nurses cited cases where the decision itself had really troubled them, but such experiences were particularly worrying. Long after the event they agonised over the consequences.

> 'She was very preterm and had quite bad intraventricular haemorrhages and her head scans weren't particularly good ... That's probably the only time that I haven't necessarily [agreed with the decision] ... It was decided to discontinue care in view of the poor prognosis. It was an unwanted pregnancy in the first place, the mother was from very poor social circumstances, and I think she had booked too late for a termination, and I just felt this was all involved [in the decision] as well. The Mum was distraught at the baptism, probably one of the most distraught parents I've seen ... it wasn't that she didn't agree or anything. She was going along with the decision. But [that baby] appeared too well. Compared to other ones that I'd been involved with, really ill babies, I felt she just appeared too well. And she responded.' (Staff midwife, more than 5 years experience)

Where resources appeared to limit treatment the nurses felt very angry.

> 'There were three admissions coming in and all needing intensive care, one set of twins and one singleton. And the singleton wasn't treated ... It was very difficult. It was very stressful for me for a good few days afterwards, because people didn't understand why the baby hadn't been treated. There was no discussion or anything. Just that was it – the twins were treated, the singleton wasn't ... I was to take that baby away.' (Staff midwife, more than 5 years experience)

The doctors' impressions

Not all the doctors described a specific case which stuck in their minds. As has been pointed out five had not yet been involved in a case of treatment withdrawal from a neonate, but one of these doctors did outline a paediatric case. A few very senior clinicians were able to list those factors which made a case memorable without reference to an individual case. But 44 respondents described a particular baby or babies. Similar categories emerged as those cited for the nurses but the detail differed.

a) Personal

Getting to know the baby and family well was a powerful factor for a small number of doctors but they were more inclined to reference their sadness at being unable to save these babies. Some even used the term 'failure' to describe their feelings when such infants died. In other instances where they were intimately involved, they cited the consequences of their involvement as the reason why these babies stayed in their minds: for example, personality clashes with certain 'difficult', demanding or confrontational parents.

A few cited cases where they had doubted their own judgement, or that of senior colleagues, or where they were left with a troubled conscience.

> 'I don't feel happy with every decision I've taken. There are some that have left me feeling that factors that I thought were important at the time, these were not the important ones. From a moral point of view, I've been left feeling guilty about it because I know it influenced my decision whether to resuscitate the baby or not. It's on my conscience that I let that baby down. I didn't give that baby the chance it should have had.' (Consultant, less than 10 years experience)

Junior staff could feel particularly vulnerable. They did not have the experience to decide readily but there could be qualms of conscience in carrying out the general instruction to resuscitate until senior help arrived, if the child was clearly badly impaired. Going against the opinion of senior nursing colleagues carried its own burden.

> 'The baby was a normal pregnancy. Nothing was expected and this baby came out with multiple abnormalities. Obviously I was concerned as to how much I should be doing, how much I shouldn't be doing. So the baby was brought

along and given some oxygen. I really wasn't doing much, so I phoned the senior registrar and phoned the consultant as well. This was usual. The problem then was that the baby went very blue and because the others hadn't arrived at that point, I was going to have to give a decision as to whether I was going to resuscitate this abnormal baby. And what made it extra difficult was the nursing staff were really not happy for me to resuscitate the baby and asked me to take the decision not to do anything. And at the time I just thought, "Well, I can't, because I don't know what I'm doing. I need a senior registrar or consultant coming in." So I just started resuscitating the baby, but there was some indecision around, because they were older, more experienced nurses. And I thought maybe I'm doing the wrong thing.' (SHO, more than 1 year experience)

Some looked deeply into their own feelings and acknowledged the danger of letting personal considerations influence them.

'You can't be justified in resuscitating this baby, you know, just for an hour or two days, just to make *me* feel better. I don't believe that we do no harm. I mean we *try* not to do harm, but I don't believe that we do no harm. I think we've always got to remember that the natural outcome for these deliveries in the past would have been death, and we are artificially prolonging [that life].' (Consultant, less than 10 years experience)

The first cases in which they were involved, or had themselves to decide, stayed with some doctors for a long time and clearly made a big impression on them. A few generously shared experiences where they had acted but had subsequently regretted aspects of their management of the case.

b) The baby

Where the deterioration in a baby's condition was very marked but the death protracted, junior doctors reacted very much like nurses did – it was like 'looking after a living corpse.' Doctors generally dwelt more on those cases where the infant was a full-term baby, or had suffered a suspected obstetric accident, rather than the extremely preterm infants. To lose 'a potentially good baby' raised serious questions which troubled them; losing preterm infants was to be expected.

'To be brutally frank, the older children make much more of an impression than the neonates, and I can remember some of these much more vividly in terms of what was done, and what was said, and so on. I'm not suggesting it's a terribly commonplace situation in a neonate but a lot of these babies have such a precarious hold [on life] that one tends not to bond quite so much with them, I suppose.' (Consultant, more than 25 years experience)

Additionally children who had lived for longer became real little people with identifiable characteristics and attachments grew stronger, making it harder to watch them die.

'He was here for one year. There was hope all the time he was here for his getting better. But his last few weeks were really horrendous. And it was a very, very difficult decision to make, because having held on to him for a year, and then to let him go was really difficult ... You get to know him, not as a patient but just as a baby. And it's more like he's *somebody*, rather than one of your patients. I missed him terribly when he wasn't there. [For] probably the next four weeks or so, you'd pass by and [think] "that's his corner".' (Registrar, less than 5 years experience)

One doctor differentiated between the deaths of these two types of babies in a spiritual sense. He described seeing a spirit leave the larger infants which was not seen with the preterm babies. Indeed he specifically looked for this phenomenon.

In making these difficult decisions, there is already much perplexity because of the uncertainty of prognosis. In reported cases where a baby had defied medical predictions, worrying questions were raised which further complicated the dilemmas attached to this type of decision making. These cases profoundly affected the medical staff involved. An example was where they had seriously considered stopping treatment, but the child had continued to live and grew up with only minor impairments. A subsequent baby in the Unit presenting a similar picture could resurrect these doubts and make the decision harder to take.

Certain types of death which were physically repellent and distressing to witness (for example, those from pulmonary haemorrhage) had a marked impact on some doctors. They instanced cases not only where the baby had actually died in this way, but the tension that built when they had to care for other infants and the potential presented for a repeat experience. Waiting and fearing over a period of time took its toll.

Withdrawing and withholding treatment is not undertaken lightly. There is a basic instinct to treat which several doctors acknowledged.

'It's actually quite hard not to treat babies. You have to actually put the brakes on. Everything makes you want to jump in and do everything you can do.' (Consultant, less than 10 years experience)

c) The family

Parents' reactions did affect the medical staff and dramatic accounts were given of those parents who had made the situation exceptionally difficult to handle. In one Unit several doctors described a single case where a baby appeared to endure months of suffering because of entrenched parental beliefs. Not being able to do what they considered to be the best for the baby produced its own enormous stress; having to deal with the ongoing distress of other team members compounded the tension. A few doctors betrayed a degree of irritation with such parents. They compared their own considerable knowledge and experience with that of the parents and felt it was unreasonable for such people to take inflexible positions when the victim of their stubbornness was a baby who relied on others to protect him.

d) The management of the case

'Good deaths' were remembered as well as those which doctors felt had been mismanaged. There was satisfaction in orchestrating things so that parents had the best experience they could in a difficult situation.

> '[These parents] expressed a worry about whether she would choke and go blue and thrash out her arms and have a very unpleasant time. I had a further meeting with them ... and it was a very easy and natural thing then to suggest that the baby had morphine as a – firstly as a feel-good drug for the baby, secondly as a sedative ... because she was a big baby, she didn't like the tube ... it was potentially unpleasant for her to thrash around despite the use of other drugs and we agreed then that we should give large doses of morphine even though – and they were very clear about this – even though this would really not be giving her a chance in a sense, it would almost necessarily suppress her breathing when she came off the ventilator. And so we started her on morphine as an infusion and she had a much more settled night ... All the staff remarked on how peaceful she looked whilst still alive on the ventilator ... We actually planned for the parents to come in the next day with the grandparents ... to go through this in the proper way. She didn't cough and struggle and throw out her limbs as she'd done in the previous accidental extubations – which was very nice. But she made a lot of noises with her breathing. She had this rather shallow expiratory effort and I was aware that noisy breathing is quite unpleasant for adults, because you think of drowning or choking and that's probably one of the most unpleasant sensations people experience. She was more or less snoring, but with rather sharp intakes of breath. But it was quite clear that her face looked very peaceful, she wasn't thrashing around and I talked them through this, rather than do anything else at this stage. I said, "This is quite normal for this to happen, with a big baby like this. It's that their drive to breathe is overwhelming." But this carried on for several minutes and I didn't give her a further dose of morphine. Her colour had continued to get worse but she'd continued very peaceful. The parents themselves were amazing in that they were both talking through this as well. The Mum was very tearful, they were both hugging the baby in turn ... From what they've said to me since, they had a very pleasant surprise about how peaceful this had been. They steeled themselves to a much more unpleasant situation. So we gave her several more doses of morphine intravenously.' (Consultant, less than 10 years experience)

Protracted decisions were cited by a fifth of the doctors as reasons why cases stayed with them. Graphic accounts were given by junior staff who were required to keep treating infants knowing that treatment was later likely to be withdrawn. Although they sometimes understood the reasons for the delays they vividly recalled their own painful emotions as the medical staff most intimately and frequently involved with the babies and parents. It was hard to keep repeating invasive procedures or to keep discussing matters with families when they felt so ambivalent about the management themselves. One registrar gave a detailed account of a case where junior staff had struggled all weekend to keep a sick premature baby alive, fully expecting to be given the go-ahead to withdraw on Monday when the consultant did his round. When, instead, he ordered further delaying tactics the junior staff were incensed and commented that in their view, he would have been more sympathetic if *he* had been up for two whole nights battling with this child. It appeared to them all too easy for such a senior colleague to pronounce a judgement and then walk away leaving other people to bear both the practical and emotional consequences. Senior staff however alluded to the difficulties they faced when either families or staff appeared to them unready to have treatment withdrawn. There was a peculiar poignancy in having to order continuing treatment which they too thought was not in the best interests of the baby, knowing that other staff were struggling with this decision.

Discussion

There was tremendous enthusiasm for this enquiry and staff cooperated willingly, not only in actively participating at interview, but in generously covering for their colleagues and attending sensitively to the comfort and convenience of the researcher. Respondents gave most generously of their time and experiences. The interviewer was enormously impressed by the generosity of respondents in sharing these intense emotions and traumatic experiences. But as has been said, 'It is impossible to overemphasize the immense need humans have to be really listened to, to be taken seriously, to be understood.'[129] Many respondents in this enquiry volunteered that it had been therapeutic to think through these issues in a structured way, and to share their doubts and pain with someone who had the time to listen and who understood the world of sick neonates.

Introducing the opportunity to share an intense personal experience at an early point in the interview was, however, a deliberate move, since recalling the events and relating personal feelings helped the teller personally to engage with the subject, and to take some sort of control of the situation. In addition it encouraged a more relaxed tone for the exchange. Each person could recognize that he or she had a unique contribution to make. When people became particularly distressed during the interview they were given the opportunity to take a break or move on to something less painful but no one took advantage of this offer. Some indeed commented that it was cathartic to share their feelings after sometimes many years of suppression.

A number of interesting issues emerged from this consideration of the real-life experience of these 176 practitioners. Four specific ones were identifiable.

The impact of different types of death

Staff become very involved with the babies and families who come into the NICU, particularly those who strike a chord with the doctor or nurse, or those who spend a long time in the Unit. The deaths of both full-term and long-stay babies tend to be more stressful to deal with than the very premature ones; grief at the loss of a loved person, an element of unexpectedness or unacceptability, and sometimes a sense of failure or a suspicion of medical inadequacy or negligence can compound the emotions in those situations where larger babies do not survive.

The timing of events

Protracted dying is a source of great distress and nurses frequently attribute this to medical procrastination and harbour resentment against those who have to make the final choice. Doctors, however, are more likely to experience a sense of failure when babies do not live whereas the nurse, though she may mourn the loss of a baby she has cared for with affection, has an opportunity to demonstrate a special skill in caring sensitively for the family at this uniquely precious time. The emotions they experience when an infant dies may well be different. Senior doctors too, are very conscious of the need to be sure that everyone is ready for this irrevocable step and that the prognosis is as certain as it can be. The final responsibility rests with them and they are all too aware of the consequences of precipitate action.

It appears to be rare that staff disagree about the final decision but the timing of the death causes much tension. However these feelings are often disguised or suppressed and doctors and nurses do not always share their concerns and misgivings. It was fairly common to hear both sides of situations and to see why these different perceptions were held. But if the nurse is unaware of the real reason for the delay in deciding and is left to spend 8–12 hour shifts with a baby and his family, unable to escape the burden of pain and suffering and sense of futility, she is understandably aggrieved when nothing appears to be being done to relieve this intolerable position. On the other hand if the consultant is still unsure whether the parents have totally grasped the full implications of continued survival, he is understandably cautious about proceeding. Or if he has a niggling doubt about the outcome he may well remember an earlier baby who defied predictions and be in no hurry to make an erroneous judgement. He may well detect an undercurrent of hostility in the nurse's approach but attribute it either to her sadness that the baby is not improving or to her preoccupation with the parents' distress.

Junior doctors are particularly vulnerable and sometimes get caught up in these tensions because of their inexperience. If they are instructed always to wait for senior opinion on the one hand, but on the other, nurses are pressing them to leave a severely abnormal baby alone or not to resuscitate a badly damaged long-stay premature infant, they are caught between two irreconcilable forces. Additionally if they are up day and night struggling to keep a baby alive over a weekend (as in one reported case) and the consultant, well rested and relaxed, appears on Monday and orders further delays they can feel very used and unsupported. It appears to the tired and anxious SHO so easy to breeze in for a few minutes and order demanding and agonising commitments from others. The other onerous responsibilities the consultant is also juggling with are invisible to the staff exclusively employed in the NICU. But unless each person shares their reservations there is ample margin for misinterpretation in all such situations, especially because they are already heavily overloaded with powerful emotion and stress.

The dying experience

Nurses attach great importance to 'a good death'. Considerable efforts are made to ensure that comfort and dignity are preserved and the actual dying is sometimes delayed just sufficiently to enable the significant people to be present or to be informed, or to prevent the death coinciding with other important anniversaries. Where families either do not or cannot provide the expected comfort and presence, the nurses will often substitute for them, exceeding their professional duties in the interests of making the experience of dying as acceptable as is within their power. The sensitivity of the nurses and their great caring is impressive. But there is satisfaction for both doctors and nurses if the death is seen to be well managed.

The family

The attitudes and behaviour of the family can substantially alter the staff's feelings about an experience of withdrawing treatment. Doctors find it particularly stressful if parents are aggressively questioning or seemingly hostile, while nurses additionally find withdrawal from the baby a difficult parental behaviour to accept. But such experiences are relatively rare and many close relationships develop between staff and parents which endure sometimes for many years; a living testament to the personal investment of those working in this specialized environment.

CHAPTER FIVE

The Law

The whole issue of selective treatment has engaged the minds of doctors and lawyers for years and considerable literature exists to demonstrate this. In the area of neonatal care it is clear that it remains a topical issue in the 1990s with many countries continuing to grapple with these complex problems.[132-136] Specific cases, such as Baby K, an anencephalic child being kept alive on mechanical ventilation on the basis of her mother's strong religious conviction,[133] or the baby being incubated in its dead mother's body reported widely in the German press during 1992, occasionally hit the headlines and resurrect old arguments in new forms.

In relation to withdrawing treatment from neonates, there are three issues to be considered: What is the law in these matters? Should the present law be annulled or new laws introduced to permit these complex situations to be dealt with more adequately? Given existing prohibitions, what should doctors do? This study attempted to address each of these aspects.

The current position in Great Britain

Selective non-treatment of infants with severe impairments and an unfavourable prognosis has the clear backing of both doctors and lawyers.[137] However, there are limits, some of which have been explored through legal proceedings.

Some cases appear relatively clear cut. For example, in 1981, surgery was authorised by a Court of Appeal to correct an intestinal obstruction in an infant with Down's Syndrome even though his parents objected. The judges considered that the child's life with Down's Syndrome would not be so 'demonstrably awful' that he should be allowed to die.[138]

Also in 1981, after lengthy deliberations, Dr Leonard Arthur was acquitted of the attempted murder of a baby with Down's Syndrome.[30] The trial hinged around two main points: a written instruction which said that the parents did not want the baby to survive and he was for nursing care only; and the administration of a lethal dose of DF118. The prosecution claimed that these two factors showed Dr Arthur had intended that the child should die. At post mortem one of the pathologists involved had discovered the baby had additional abnormalities of his lung, heart and brain. It could not, therefore, be conclusively proven that death from pneumonia was the result of the DF118 or from natural causes. Eminent medical practitioners testified at the trial that it was normal practice to give 'nursing care only' orders and the judge in his summing up, suggested that it was unlikely that standards had evolved amongst men of such standing which amounted to a crime. In polls taken at the time, there was huge public support for the sanctioning of doctors seeing to it that such infants died, although members of the anti-abortion group, Life, were naturally seriously alarmed by the verdict.

The sensitivities involved and the difficulty in choosing words precisely to capture meaning, has led in other cases to wrangling in the courts between opposing factions. In 1989, a High Court judge agreed with a decision that a four-month-old girl with severe cerebral palsy, who was microcephalic, and blind, should be allowed to die.[139] The Official Solicitor, however, was unhappy with the comments of the judge, which seemed to give authority for the doctors to take active steps to end the child's life. The Lords of Appeal accepted the misgivings of the Official Solicitor, but their judgement concurred with the earlier one: the goal of any treatment should be to ease the child's suffering not to prolong her life.

In 1990, the Official Solicitor appealed a further decision of the courts that doctors should not be required to intervene in an emergency to save the life of a gravely ill child who was born at 27 weeks gestation and had undergone weeks of intensive care.[140] Baby J was known to have suffered brain damage but was not at that time dying. The Official Solicitor claimed that courts were never justified in withholding consent to lifesaving treatment whatever the ensuing quality of life. However, the Court of Appeal did not in this case accept the submission. It took the view that there were some circumstances where the quality of life would be so intolerable as to make it acceptable to withhold treatment from a baby who was not otherwise dying. Lord Donaldson emphasized the point that severely handicapped people can find a quality of life rewarding which to the unimpaired might seem to be intolerable. But he concluded that exceptional cases do exist where the burden of pain and suffering resulting from treatment would outweigh any commensurate benefit.

It is not just legal experts who challenge court decisions. In a case brought in 1992,[141] a consultant had recommended that a 17-month-old male child who was profoundly handicapped following a fall at the age of one month, should not be given intensive treatment were he to suffer a further life-threatening incident. The little boy was in foster care and suffered from cerebral palsy, microcephaly, epilepsy and blindness. The courts, the Official Solicitor and the Health Authority all upheld this decision. However the local authority in charge of the child, and the mother, challenged it. The Court of Appeal ruled that the doctors should be left free to treat the child according to their best clinical judgement. In effect this meant that they were not dictating either way. The clinical situation should be the determining factor. Lord Donaldson stressed that although no one could dictate to doctors which treatments were appropriate to initiate, cooperation with parents was essential.

Scots law varies slightly from English law. In essence in Scotland there is more latitude for doctors to make decisions and to practise in the best interests of the child without recourse to the courts. Nevertheless, no landmark case has so far tested the support of the Scottish courts where withdrawing treatment from infants is concerned, so there are no legal precedents north of the border to guide clinicians.

Judicial decisions are clearly not foregone conclusions. Ambiguity persists about the defining criteria for quality of life measures. In effect, legal support remains at a fairly general level and there is considerable uncertainty in the minds of clinicians about their true position in various circumstances. It appears to require further cases to go through the courts to establish whether legal support would be sustained in reality given different conditions and different mitigating circumstances. The adoption of specific and authoritative non-treatment guidelines have not so far been accepted by either discipline although, as has already been mentioned, efforts are being made to draw up some kind of statement which might provide a measure of accepted practice.

It is interesting to reflect that a number of the cases which have made legal history in Britain and in the USA have revolved around children with Down's Syndrome. No respondent in this present enquiry cited Down's Syndrome as a circumstance for selective non-treatment, and indeed a considerable number specifically singled out this condition as one in which they most certainly would not consider withholding or withdrawing treatment.

In the last few years much of the legal debate has hinged around issues such as whether feeding is a medical treatment. The case of Thomas Creedon mentioned in Chapter 2 brought this matter to the fore but also focused on the point at which death was preferable to a demonstrably poor quality of life, since Thomas was severely physically, as well as mentally impaired and was believed to be suffering unrelieved pain. But he died before the case came to court. At the time of writing, a case before Sir Stephen Brown, president of the High Court's family division, is being considered in which doctors caring for a severely brain damaged baby girl are requesting permission to switch off the ventilator keeping her alive. It is clear that efforts are still being made to address legal and medical uncertainties in this area.

The position in the United States of America

Criminal prosecution of a doctor in the US is almost impossible in cases of withdrawing or withholding treatment. Doctors are protected if they act on good faith judgements that are not 'grievously unreasonable' by medical standards.[142] In spite of this fact there is evidence that doctors are very concerned about this area of the law. These anxieties have been attributed to a number of factors: different states have different laws and this causes confusion; doctors perceive there to be a medical malpractice crisis; numerous court actions are brought in this area; and conservative legal advice may have unnecessarily exaggerated the perception of risk.[142]

It is difficult for those outside the clinical setting to appreciate the subtle nuances of any given situation. When, in the early 1980s, the Reagan administration attempted to formulate policies on the treatment of severely handicapped newborn infants, issuing guidelines which were to be posted in every delivery ward, maternity and paediatric ward, and intensive care nursery, there was enormous unrest amongst paediatricians. One is reported to have commented:

> 'Because of the fear I had in being "reported", I recently spent an agonising hour trying to resuscitate a newborn who had no larynx, and many other anomalies. The sad part was that both the parents in the delivery room watched this most difficult ordeal. It was obvious to me that this was in no way a viable

child but I felt compelled to carry on this way out of fear someone in the hospital would "turn me in". I am sure that you who sit in Washington are not faced with such difficult decisions at two o'clock a.m.'[30]

In fact, many American paediatricians misunderstood the regulations believing that they were being required to treat all infants intensively until death was certain.[127] Terminally ill infants were consequently given overly aggressive and futile treatment at great emotional and financial cost to those concerned. The regulations were actually intended to protect children from 'medical neglect'. However, such a distinction could well seem like a technicality to clinicians whose careful considerations were held up to the scrutiny and subsequent criticism of people not versed in the nuances of neonatal care.

Deciding within the current legal constraints

In principle it is understood and agreed that medical decisions should be based on the best interests of the patient. Where babies are concerned there are particular difficulties in establishing not only what those interests are, but also who is best able to represent the child's interests. It is well recognized that the stakes are high for all concerned. Obviously the infant has the most to gain or lose. But he cannot speak for himself. Typically, parents speak on his behalf, and most often, they choose from a vantage point of parental love. But other concerns inevitably enter into the equation: considerations of family stability; the impact of impairment and subsequent disability; emotional, social and financial costs. And parents can have difficulty understanding or accepting the medical circumstances.

From a consideration of the few cases which have come to court in Britain it might be thought that the law favours medical opinion over parental choice. Indeed it has been clearly stated that 'the principle of the professional standard is deeply entrenched in British law.'[143] British and American legal experts, looking at the law on both sides of the Atlantic, summed up something of the complexity of the situation when they concluded that,

> 'The parents, who have conceived the infant and who have the responsibility to raise it, should be given the right, within closely and carefully drawn confines, to elect non-treatment when their child is born severely deformed. Additionally, society should not, without strong reason, dictate standards to physicians, which compel treatment in circumstances in which ethically minded doctors would feel it was medically inappropriate.'[143]

Clearly there are potential conflicts from a legal point of view.

The courts have lingered over issues such as competing interests, the probability of a 'demonstrably awful existence', and the quality of life the child or the family could expect. In the USA there has been opposition to quality of life judgements on behalf of neonates. The *best interests* standard is seen to be forcing professionals to make impossible comparisons. It is one thing to compare better life with worse life; such comparisons can and should be made. But it is not possible to compare the advantages of life – even a life with severe disability – with death.[144] However, some renowned legal experts have stated firmly that,

> 'Quality of life – not in the sense of social utility or worth but solely as judged by a physiological existence without intolerable pain or suffering – may properly enter such treatment decisions.'[143]

From the literature this is clearly the position taken by clinicians dealing with these babies in the UK.

Matters are further complicated by the liberality of current abortion legislation in this country. Making arbitrary cut off points may seem questionable, but lines do have to be drawn for legal and practical purposes. Traditionally the law has found it convenient to draw a line at the time of birth to distinguish between abortion and infanticide.[145] Abortion up to 24 weeks is legal yet it is recognized that infants born at 22 or 23 weeks can survive with apparently little impairment or subsequent disability.

Results of the present enquiry
Knowledge
Knowledge of the law was found to be hazy amongst both doctors and nurses in the present enquiry. Considerable numbers of staff at all levels openly confessed to being unsure what the legal limits were. This awareness of ignorance could have been inhibiting, so in order to encourage further participation, the researcher was circumspect in her probing for deeper insights in this area.

For some the law offered fairly crude limits.

> 'I view laws as saying I'm not allowed to take a phial of potassium chloride and inject it into a baby to cause the baby's heart to stop beating.' (Registrar, less than 5 years experience)

Many more suggested that the law set broad boundaries, but areas of greyness existed which were potentially troubling. Some indeed added that only a certain kind of doctor would go into intensive care of neonates because it was necessary to tolerate such uncertainties and run the risk of litigation. The absence of clear precedents left doctors unclear about legal support in a number of scenarios. Situations were identified as areas of difficulty or legal uncertainty: circumstances where parents do not agree with medical opinion; pain relief; sedation; the use of paralysing agents; and the withdrawal of certain forms of treatment such as feeding.

> 'Here we certainly make certain that babies are not in pain when they die, and that can involve giving them large amounts of opiate analgesia. It may make a difference [to] when a baby actually stops breathing but I don't think legally that would count as us actively causing the death of the baby. I mean the baby is going to stop breathing because of the pathological process that's caused us to make that decision in the first place but we don't actually cause the babies to

stop breathing by pharmacological means. We maybe make the baby comfortable and maybe make that time for the baby to stop breathing a bit earlier than it would otherwise have been. That's certainly a sort of grey area from the legal point of view.' (Registrar, less than 5 years experience)

Constraints

The majority of the doctors (36, 63%) felt the law offered little constraint with a few suggesting that things like media misunderstanding and shortage of resources were the actual causes of difficulty. Problems accruing from legal boundaries were perceived to be largely theoretical: in reality there was rarely a conflict between legal requirement and clinical practice. Because the law was not framed too precisely and areas of uncertainty existed, it allowed them for the most part to practise in the ways they thought appropriate, although awareness of legal limits remained in the back of their minds.

There were two main influences which the law exerted. On one level it offered some form of protection and guidance (for example, it prohibited the active ending of life), but on the other hand the threat of legal repercussions made it imperative that, in exercising their clinical judgement, doctors had to be able to justify their actions to outside agencies. This latter influence resulted in a tendency for clinicians to treat more aggressively than they otherwise might. As part of the decision making process they paid great attention to objective measures, consulted colleagues, involved the parents, and erred on the side of preserving life. One very senior paediatrician said he always welcomed independent scrutiny of deaths by the procurator fiscal because it relieved him of the responsibility for having to try to explain his assessment of the cause of death to parents, removed any question of inappropriate conduct, and gave the parents the benefit of an impartial view.

It was interesting to note that some junior doctors suspected that it was not actually the law which was constraining consultants. They might well be hiding behind a seemingly respectable veneer.

'I suspect that it isn't so much the law that is stopping people ... it's their own fears, their reluctance to face up to the necessary but difficult decisions.' (SHO, less than 1 year experience)

The nurses' perceptions were rather different. Only about a quarter (32, 27%) considered that the law had little influence on practice. For a small number there was a difficulty in knowing how far it was the law which was actually making the doctors manage cases in a particular way. Like the junior doctors they suspected that personal views, inclinations and fears were the things that motivated the consultants. However, the majority felt that the law had the effect of making medical staff behave defensively: treat aggressively, and involve other people in the decision making. It also prevented them from actively ending lives. They were, moreover, conscious that individual doctors interpreted the law differently. To some extent individuals could manipulate the law to suit their purposes. In two Units, for example, nurses reported that only one of their consultants was prepared to make the decision to allow a baby to die. He appeared able to justify doing so. The other consultants used the law as part of their excuse for holding back.

Need for changes in the law

Approximately equal proportions of doctors (30%) and nurses (33%) would like to see changes in the law, although some highlighted the difficulty of couching laws in terms sufficiently flexible to accommodate the enormous advances occurring in neonatal care. It was not so many years ago that 32 week gestation babies were regarded as at the lower limits for intact survival: at that time it was inconceivable that the limit of viability would drop to 24 weeks. Although there is a prevailing sense that the limit of human achievement must be close to current skills, some respondents did make reference to the possibility that today's impossibility might become tomorrow's expectation. Laws tended to be too inflexible to allow for such changes.

Essential differences were noted between the emphases of the doctors and nurses. The doctors looked for greater protection while the nurses felt the law should recognize the value of clinical judgement.

Being vulnerable had the effect of making paediatricians careful in their practice, but a fifth of the doctors (12, 21%) would welcome more protection in the form of clearer guidelines, or specific avenues by which advice could be sought such as a consultative body or a type of neonatal ombudsman or legal/ethical expert. Some, however, were ambivalent on these matters.

> 'I would like to have more protection because I worry about perhaps one year spending a very, very large amount of my time in a law court ... On the other hand I think there are advantages in being vulnerable – it makes you extra careful about what you do, so that you document everything very carefully, you make sure that everything is done in a very open way and that there are other people as members of your team who are giving either nodded or verbal or written agreement that this is the right way to go forward.' (Consultant, more than 15 years experience)

Understandably consultants did not want to be the one to make legal history.

> 'I certainly have heard it indirectly said that that is what they predict is going to happen, particularly in Scottish law, where somebody is going to be prosecuted so that it can be a test case that will clearly come down in favour of the medical profession because of the common sense of Scots law ... but I don't want to be that person!' (Consultant, more than 25 years experience)

Some indeed volunteered that they always erred on the side of caution. Only ever adopting a line that was generally acceptable, always applying to eminent paediatricians for a second opinion, and obtaining the signed agreement of their peers, were just some of the ways in which consultants who were fearful of legal repercussions tried to protect themselves. It only needed one experience of an apparently innocent action ending in trouble for an individual to feel decidedly vulnerable.

It was generally recognized that formulating and interpreting laws is a difficult and skilled occupation. Even some of those who broadly accepted that current legislation was adequate in principle, felt that changes in wording might give better protection and guidance to clinicians. Just over a quarter of the doctors (15, 26%) considered that the law should more obviously recognize the importance of clinical judgement and the limits of medicine. At the present time it failed properly to take account of quality of life issues and the difference between killing and compassionate ending of a life.

Clearly the majority did not wish the law to be changed. A few even considered that tightening up the law would imply lack of confidence in the clinical wisdom of doctors. Many believed strongly that legislative change was not the way forward, but that the current system allowed for the necessary flexibility.

> 'If you are open, really you've been judged already by a jury before the actual withdrawal of treatment ...We could then go as a body and argue a case quite easily, knowing in full confidence that a jury made up of randomly selected people from the same population would come up with the same answer. So in fact *we* are determining the law in some sorts of ways, and I think that's a very powerful place to be because it means you can then make subtle changes in it without having to go through these nignogs in parliament and convince them that these things should be changed.' (Consultant, more than 15 years experience)

A few respondents had actually participated in a formal discussion of these issues between the Royal College of Physicians and the Faculty of Advocates. They reported that the conclusion from both sides had been that it was better that the law did not intervene in these delicate matters. Everyone recognized that it was extremely difficult for laws to take account of all the fine nuances attending these real life tragedies.

> 'The law has to be black and white and medicine never is.' (Senior Registrar, more than 5 years experience)

Some comfort could be drawn from a knowledge that their predicament had the sympathy of the advocates. If a civil action was taken to court in Scotland, it would appear unlikely that it would go against a paediatrician if he had done all he could to ensure that the best interests of the baby were respected.

The process of decision making was cited as one way in which the law was unlikely to be flouted. Involving a range of people offered some protection. Internal scrutiny kept the issues alive.

> 'I remember writing up a dose of morphine and the nurse saying she thought it was a bit too much. So I scaled it down so that we both felt comfortable... you're sensitive to how they feel – you don't ask them outright.' (Consultant, more than 15 years experience)

A far greater proportion of the nurses looked for better recognition of clinical judgement and the limits of medicine (42, 36%), while only 13 (11%) considered that the law should offer better protection to the staff involved in these decisions. Since many nurses considered treatment was overly aggressive but that doctors interpreted the law in their own way, their more marked concentration on change which better protects the interests of the baby is understandable.

The unique position of the paediatricians themselves was seen as a major factor in any consideration of what was legal.

> 'I don't think you could frame a law in such a way that you could change things. No, I couldn't envisage it because the main people whose advice would be sought would be doctors anyway so you'd really simply be putting into law what they do.' (Staff nurse, more than 5 years experience)

Some broadened the issue further to include others in the team in NICUs. For them, it had to be the staff who worked with these situations who decided what was legal. Without experience of the complexity of these real-life traumas, other people could have no accurate conception of what was involved, so they could not realistically formulate laws.

> 'I think the people that say it's against the law [to help a baby to go to sleep peacefully] have never had to deal with anything like this. I think [with] a lot of things that go on, if you said to a lay person, they would be absolutely aghast at what happens.' (Sister, more than 10 years experience)

Potential changes in practice following changes in laws

Half of the staff (54% of doctors; 50% of nurses) considered that changes in the law probably would not materially change practice in their Units. A further 10 doctors (18%) and 22 nurses (18%) were unsure or said that it depended in what way the law changed. For those who felt that behaviour would be different if the law were changed, the results indicated that much hinged on the kind of change the respondent was considering.

Six doctors feared that changes might add to the burden on medical staff and result in less sensitive care of infants and families. The existing ambiguity allowed them to act in the best interests of individuals: conformity to set rules might preclude this. Five, however, believed that change would be for the better in that it would enable them to make appropriate judgements about treatment or assisting death without fear of legal reprisals, and without undue influence from inexperienced parents.

A number of nurses expressed a feeling that the law could be changed to good effect if it allowed doctors to withdraw treatment earlier. In the present climate, fear of legal repercussions sometimes made doctors continue treatment long after everyone in the Unit had concluded that it was futile. But the need to wait for parental acceptance of a poor prognosis went against the baby's interests at times.

'We would obviously be able to let babies like Baby S go a lot earlier. We know that he's going to die. Really we've got to sit here and wait until he takes it into his own hands. He has periods where he gets worse and worse and you think, right, this is it. And then he just picks up – but picks up to just a borderline level. He's had very large brain haemorrhages. His heart is dreadful as well because of all the strain, and his kidneys. Everything's knackered. His whole body is knackered. You just think, it's not just his lungs now, it's his total system. So I feel really strongly babes like that – What are we doing? It's just wrong.' (Sister, more than 5 years experience)

'That baby went on – maybe another ten to twelve days, and just got to a stage she was just like a blob lying in the incubator, discoloured, totally unrecognisable to those parents as a baby.' (Sister, more than 20 years experience)

On the other hand, a sense was conveyed by some staff that there were fundamental dangers in bringing these issues more into the open.

'My fear would be that it would change behaviour, not because of the law itself, but because of the *process* to a change in that law. Because you would increase public awareness of the fact that doctors are switching off ventilators, taking away life support machines. And it would also increase political awareness and the agenda of the public in general. If we're actually keeping the public in the dark about this, as I think we are, public opinion and political opinion shouldn't necessarily influence how this is done. My fear would be that heightened awareness in the public about the law would lead to a lot more cases being brought to court, hence a sort of American system – litigation consciousness. There's a danger we're moving in that direction now but I resist it very hard.' (Consultant, less than 10 years experience)

Positive suggestions for change

Two main suggestions were offered as specific changes which might help the present difficulties. One was to introduce guidelines. The other was to legalise euthanasia in certain circumstances.

Since the law was too unyielding adequately to allow for the flexibility of real life circumstances, a few clinicians felt that specific guidelines could offer some help to doctors grappling with these difficult decisions. They could be designed by people who really understood the issues, be written in terms understood by the profession, and provide a recognised authoritative description of 'accepted practice'.

'I think if guidelines could be produced by the BPA and given some support in law, that would be appropriate. I don't think it's something really which lawyers or politicians could make decisions about. At the moment you have just got to take a chance on what you do. If there was a complaint about it and you'd gone about things well, you probably would be supported, but you could never be sure. So it's a risk we take.' (Registrar, less than 5 years experience)

There was widespread recognition that certain babies presented grave moral dilemmas. Continuing to treat infants when in the perception of most people, every indication existed that death was the preferable option, was distressing for all concerned. But sometimes the law precluded intervention to end that life and medicine provided no acceptable alternative. A considerable number of respondents would welcome a law which permitted them actively to assist a baby to die when treatment was futile and all other options would either prolong the dying unnecessarily or involve an unacceptable degree of distress.

But respondents were realistic about the difficulty in effecting this particular change. The process which would necessarily precede a change in the law would involve a sacrifice which few would willingly accept: it would require a paediatrician going on trial for actively killing a child.

> 'I think we're sometimes very cowardly in not being more positive. For me that's because I don't think I would have the nerve to stand up in court and say I've actually taken some positive step to end this life because I felt it would have no quality. But in myself, I feel much worse about say withdrawing treatment if you've got to a stage of withdrawing feeding and fluids, or even just carrying on doing nothing. I actually think that's worse than it would be to do something more positive – morally I think that's wrong.' (Consultant, more than 25 years experience)

It was clear that both doctors and nurses were troubled by their inability to treat babies in the most compassionate way in certain circumstances. When it was impossible to match what seemed morally indicated with what was legally allowed, compromises had to be made. By no means all doctors reported having such dilemmas however. Some were much bolder in their practice and appeared to engineer events so as to minimize the time it took from the decision being made to the actual death. It was not uncommon to hear phrases like: 'We break the law all the time'; 'Technically we are mass murderers'; from those clinicians who were prepared to withdraw treatment earlier, and use opiates, with or without paralysing agents on board, in sufficient doses to possibly hasten the dying process. For these practitioners there was less pressure to change the law although they too would welcome more security.

Discussion

Court cases have brought into the open issues such as the constitutional rights of babies, the rights of infants to receive life sustaining treatments, the rights of parents to make decisions on behalf of their infants, the rights and duties of heath care professionals to decide and to initiate or withdraw treatments, and the rights of the courts to interfere in treatment decisions.

It is very clear that there is a wide range of opinion about what is legally permissible. Tolerances of risk also vary from consultant to consultant. At the time of data collecting for this study a much publicised case was going through the Dutch courts. Euthanasia, although illegal, is permitted in the Netherlands under certain conditions, but until this point it was always when patients had explicitly requested this course. This case was the first to be brought which involved a person unable to express a wish in this matter. Dr Henk Prins, with the consent of the parents and the agreement of other medical colleagues, gave a fatal injection to a child who was born with microcephaly and spina bifida. He was found guilty of murder but was not punished for the offence because the court ruled that his action was justifiable under the circumstances. Indeed the lawyers praised his integrity and courage.

Current practices

In the Units studied for the present enquiry, practice varies enormously. Some consultants only ever withdraw treatment when death is imminent and inevitable. Others stop treating infants when they are not dying but have conditions which make their future quality of life poor. It is uncertain how much these differences relate to varying perceptions of the law and how much to the personality and inclination of the doctor concerned.

Although there is considerable support for the theoretical possibility of active measures to end life, no one appears keen to establish a new precedent in the UK by going through the courts themselves. Some, however, are 'sailing close to the legal wind' in their practice. For the most part these clinicians who were prepared to take greater risks are confident of the backing of their teams and they make great efforts to air the issues openly. In this way there is opportunity for opponents to voice their objections, but also for other staff to keep an eye open for dissension in the ranks which can be followed up. In this way legal repercussions are minimized.

There is wide recognition that much thought and agonising goes into these difficult decisions. Some consultants actually imagine themselves in court having to defend their decisions. Even junior staff who are not always in agreement with the way things are done, respect the fact that consultants deliberate long and hard, and often consult widely before acting. On the other hand they are sometimes perplexed when different consultants appear to have very different perceptions of what is permissible. In all of the Units studied where such differences exist, there are communication problems and it is difficult for junior staff fully to appreciate how final decisions have been reached.

Omissions and commissions

A huge literature exists on relevant issues such as the point at which a baby acquires personhood, the difference between active and passive acts, and the quality of life, and clearly all these issues are relevant to a legal defence. Philosophers, theologians, lawyers and health care professionals have all entered into the debate. But the question of whether a baby is a person from the moment of birth was not raised by our respondents. Nevertheless doubts do exist in the clinicians' minds about the borderline between an abortion and a very premature infant, and between withdrawing treatment and actively procuring a death. These distinctions present real management dilemmas to those at the cutting edge of practice. It is one thing to argue a theoretical possibility and quite another to implement the consequences of such discriminations. Whilst philosophers might argue persuasively that a distinction between not treating and actively assisting a death cannot be logically sustained, emotionally these acts are poles apart to the people caring for infants. That is not to say that all clinicians reject the idea of euthanasia. As has been stated, it has its supporters.

Recent official deliberations on the issue of euthanasia have shown that at least certain segments of British society are not yet ready for such a change. Both the House of Lords Select Committee on Medical Ethics[25] and the Government Response to its report[146] reinforced the view of medical and legal practitioners who were consulted, that euthanasia or the deliberate taking of a life should remain illegal. Neither Scottish nor English law accepts a defence of an unselfish motive as an answer to a charge of murder, and both legal and political authorities are agreed that there should be no new offence of 'mercy killing' created.[25,146]

In almost all cases where these treatment decisions are being considered, judgements about the quality of life are involved. As we have seen, the courts have established that such considerations are legitimate. Some impairments result in a life which is worse than death. When it comes to deciding just how to implement a decision not to treat, however, there are varying shades of opinion. The position reported in 1981[84] appears to hold true today: most doctors – and most people – accept that withholding treatment may be a compassionate decision when an infant is severely impaired, but are less sanguine about the wisdom of hastening death by heavy sedation and withholding nourishment. Nevertheless, there is weighty support for clinicians exercising prudent discretion in these matters from the House of Lords.[25] In their judgement the risk of double effect is not perceived as a reason for withholding medication, provided a doctor acts in accordance with responsible medical practice with the intention of relieving pain or distress, not of killing the patient. Much hinges on intention. But from long discussion in this research with those whose intentions are in question, it appears that it is difficult to separate out the sure knowledge that a certain course of action will hasten death from the actual intention to relieve suffering and distress.

For some infants with a poor prognosis there is no obvious way to assist them in dying. They are not being mechanically ventilated and they have no need of pain relief. Some doctors withhold food, others abhor this practice and wait for infection or some other medical emergency to provide a window of opportunity for non-treatment. The point is well made that doctors have a duty to consider each new treatment carefully to determine whether it is in the patient's best interests.[25,146] When it comes to the withdrawal of nutrition and hydration, taking the line of considering the efficacy of the treatment seems a more appropriate way of looking at the issues than to come from a perspective of what is and is not euthanasia. If feeding is evidently burdensome to a person then it may be withheld on the grounds of this general principle. There are problems, however, in applying this principle to infants and doubts remain about the answer to this difficult area of decision making.

Changes in legislation

After the high profile Dr Arthur trial, eminent doctors concluded that changes in legislation were not the answer but would probably create more difficulties than they would resolve.[147] Paediatricians could well be forced to practise defensive medicine.

Furthermore the indications for certain treatments would become legal rather than medical, making the patient and the parents the prime victims of such changes. This was also the conclusion drawn from the responses to this present study, although others continue to argue for changes in statute which might help to clarify the terms used in the debate and also offer some protection to doctors without the need for recourse to the courts.[29]

Whether or not rewording and amendment would help, an inability to be certain about prognoses, and the range of circumstances which can influence decisions make it necessary to be fluid about these matters, clinicians believe. Hard edges do not fit soft contours. The flexibility which current laws allow, enables clinicians to practise in the way they feel is right for their patients and the infants' relatives. Once things are enshrined in law they can lose this capacity to take account of individual factors. Nevertheless in the minds of many consultants doubts remain about whether the law would actually back them in the event of a legal action, and they would welcome some more concrete indication or assurance of protection.

Common misperceptions
It is not unusual for decisions to revolve around a mistaken view of what the law demands. Staff not infrequently believe that if parents want heroic measures for their baby, doctors must conform to their request or run the risk of litigation. But one thing is clear: if a treatment is medically futile there is no moral obligation to provide it, even where a family insist on everything in the medical repertoire being done. Withholding physiologically futile treatment does not constitute medical neglect. Indeed to administer futile treatment may itself be morally indefensible. However, there may be other compelling reasons for at least initially complying to enable the parents to come to terms with a hopeless prognosis: the important thing is not to mistake compassionate compromise for legal imperative.

Conclusions
Clinicians' knowledge of the legal limits relating to non-treatment of infants is vague. Practice varies widely between Units and between practitioners but some at least could be reassured by a clearer understanding that what they are doing is both legally and medically accepted practice. Doctors who appear to risk more tend to operate within a context of team discussion and the involvement of a group of people holding a range of views tends to ensure that practice remains within acceptable bounds. This wide consultation, they believe, also minimizes the risk of court action.

Few people at the cutting edge of neonatology feel that changes in law would answer present uncertainties. Variations between cases, and the uncertainties of prognosis and of outcomes, make it essential to retain a degree of flexibility. Indeed a considerable number feel the element of risk ensures that everyone remains constantly vigilant, and thereby the interests of babies and their parents are best protected. The introduction of new laws could well result in a less sensitive approach to each individual case. Nevertheless some paediatricians would welcome more concrete evidence of legal protection.

CHAPTER SIX

Current Policies and Practices

As well as the law, hospital policies can potentially influence behaviour. Recent television programmes have drawn attention to the fact that policies vary in different Units, and that such policies can dictate which babies are treated and which are not. If, for example, senior paediatricians in a given Unit believe that below a certain level of gestation it is inappropriate to attempt resuscitation, some infants are screened in Labour ward: the extremely premature are not given a chance of survival, and do not therefore present dilemmas in the NICU.

If the policy is to treat all live births, however, difficult decisions have to be made further down the line, and events can gain a momentum of their own. Once treatment has begun it appears to be more difficult to stop it.

> 'The more we give care to see if we should give care at all, the more we find ourselves committed to giving more and more care.'[23]

Unit policy

The majority of the staff questioned (46, 81% of doctors; 100, 84% of nurses) reported that, in their Units, there was no policy which dictated whether infants were treated or not. Decisions were made on a case by case basis. Furthermore there was a strong feeling that policies could not take account of all the fine variations in circumstances which are germane to any decision making.

> 'I wouldn't go along with any policy simply because then you lose thought. I could find you an exception to every policy. I wouldn't go along with the hospital telling me *anyway* what its policy is – as an independent practitioner. But I think that [a policy would be] unhealthy because it's a dynamic situation. The situation that we're dealing with now is different from that five years ago, or in the seventies – in terms of the criteria that we're using; in terms of expectations – people's expectations, parents' expectations have changed radically in that time. Maybe *our* expectations have changed radically in that time – maybe not.' (Consultant, more than 10 years experience)

Having a set policy was perceived as like having a set law. If it existed staff would have to stick to it.

'The trouble with policies is that they blind everybody. People tend to look at them as written in tablets of stone.' (Senior Registrar, more than 10 years experience)

A small minority however, did have a sense that there were certain understood guidelines which did not necessarily amount to policies. For those who gave concrete facts for their perception of the guidelines, these were as set out below.

Treat all babies who show active signs of life	6 nurses	1 doctor
There are cut off points re gestation		
(range 22–24 wks)	11 nurses	3 doctors
Time limits exist re.		
• onset of spontaneous respiration (range 15–30 mins)		
• cardiac output (range 8–20 mins)	2 doctors	2 nurses
Once started must continue	1 nurse	
Policies vary according to consultant	1 doctor	1 nurse

The small numbers of staff who reported these policies indicated that there was no well known or documented policy in any of the study Units. Four doctors however, did specifically mention that there was a rule that a senior person was consulted in any case which was on the borderline of viability or where heartbeat and spontaneous respirations were not established after a reasonable attempt at resuscitation had been made. Although only four volunteered this as a sort of policy, the practice of referring any questionable cases to senior staff emerged in conversation elsewhere with many other doctors as accepted practice in all the Units.

For junior staff there was sometimes a difficulty in understanding the dividing line between a policy and a practice.

'As far as I can see, a lot of it depends on which consultant's in charge. Different consultants appear to have different views on how far we should go, and unfortunately that can vary sometimes from night to night, depending on who's on call. Certainly from week to week, depending on which consultant covers the Unit that week. And I think that's not acceptable. While obviously consultants are individuals and do have a right to practise as they see fit, I think when you're talking about babies who are here for long periods of time there has to be greater consistency. I don't think that's very good care of the patients. It puts horrendous pressure on junior and nursing staff – they're totally bamboozled. And having spoken to parents here, one of the complaints that comes again and again is the inconsistency, that they get different stories each time. And the policy appears to be changing.' (SHO, less than 1 year experience)

Unit practice

Given that clear policies did not exist in the study Units, respondents were asked about what was actually practised in relation to treatment. From the literature[82,83] and from discussion with a wide range of staff involved in the care of infants, it appeared that there are basically three main approaches to treatment decisions:

a)   to wait until the prognosis is virtually certain before withdrawing treatment;

b)   to withhold treatment from the outset if the prognosis looks bleak;

c)   to start to treat, evaluate and re-evaluate over time, before withdrawing treatment.

Respondents were presented with the three alternatives to help focus their thinking.

Here again there were important differences in the perceptions of doctors and nurses. Proportionately more doctors (34, 60%) compared to nurses (49, 41%) considered that the choice was tailored to individual circumstances.

> 'If it's a 23 week gestation, unmarried mother of 16 who's on Labour ward, then you will go down and talk to the mother and you will more or less say, "Look, this baby is non-viable at 23 weeks" – even though we know we've saved a number of babies of 23 weeks. But all the other pressures are so great and the likely disruption to her future life, even with the best baby in the world, is so significant that one would opt out of care early. More usually it's a less extreme scenario, where you've got a 26 weeker, where if you do nothing, yes, it will surely die on the Labour ward. On the other hand, if it's 27 weeks maybe they'll survive, even without you on Labour ward, but be damaged in the survival process. So in the majority of cases you're instituting full care until you know that there's irreparable damage, and then you're withdrawing, because what you don't want is irreparable damage which was avoidable. And finally there's the scene when they are up on the wards and [you've been through all the treatments] and then you make a conclusion that the time has come that you can't do any more. So I think [our practice is to go for all three options] depending on the individual case.' (Consultant, more than 25 years experience)

In the perception of the majority of the nurses, treatment was usually started and only withdrawn after a period of evaluation and assessment (65, 55%) whereas only 20 (35%) of doctors perceived this to be the case. A number of the nurses also volunteered that they personally believed that treatment should always be started.

> 'I think that everyone should be given a chance, a good chance, and I think the best possible treatment should be given. I would treat. There are babies – say a very tiny baby – even though a lot of people might say, "It's too wee, it can't survive, not at this stage". I think it should still be given the best possible chance of survival and I think it should still be resuscitated.' (Staff midwife, less than 5 years experience)

Problems and conflicts

One source of problems for paediatricians was when uncertain or conflicting messages came from Labour ward.

> 'I know sometimes obstetricians here [are rather half-hearted]. We had one last week – [they] didn't monitor [the Mum] in labour, but they wanted us to do things. If you've got a heart rate of 60 in your fetus, then it's going to be worse

and worse and worse for us [the paediatricians] ... If *we're* going to be aggressive, then *they* have to be aggressive. And there has to be discussion.' (Registrar, more than 5 years experience)

It sometimes happened that obstetricians had decided that a baby should not be treated after delivery, but when the doctor left the delivery area, the midwives rang for a paediatrician. Elsewhere obstetricians did not communicate with paediatricians sufficiently well and decision making was fragmented to the detriment of the infant's welfare and the confusion of all concerned. However, it did appear possible to institute a system where there was consistency. Some senior doctors reported developing a practice where they had detailed antenatal discussion with the obstetrician and agreed a course of action in conjunction with parents.

The nurses could see things differently on occasion, however. A decision might well be made in anticipation of an event. But there were certain imponderables and circumstances could alter.

'I think why I always call a paediatrician is in case Mum has made a mistake and maybe – you think you're delivering a 24 weeker, then this baby pops out and it's quickly assessed as a 28 weeker.' (Sister, more than 20 years experience)

Another potential difficulty arose when different consultants adhered to different practices. One very senior consultant described a case where he had had lengthy discussion with parents about their extremely premature infant. He explained that even though their child had done well for the first five weeks, his longer term outlook was not good and he might suddenly collapse. They had agreed together that heroics would not be appropriate. Only two days after this discussion, the baby did collapse, but another consultant was on call who decided to transfer the infant to a hospital far away for surgery for a perforated bowel. The respondent worried about the impact on the parents of such inconsistency and suggested that perhaps a policy of some kind might have avoided this situation. Having spoken to both consultants concerned, the interviewer suspected that this was a question of communication rather than of policy.

Elsewhere there were consultants who reported that they always handed over the care of 'their' babies to colleagues with a detailed discussion of the management and decisions involved. One senior doctor ranked this practice as a personal policy.

Personal preferences

It seemed possible that Unit practice might not reflect the preferences of each individual and the possible discrepancies were explored. Staff did indeed reveal that their own inclinations were sometimes at variance with practice in their Unit. Such discrepancies were uncomfortable for junior doctors and for nurses, but for a consultant himself to be at odds with the prevailing practice, there was a heavy burden to be carried. One very senior consultant divulged information which showed that for a large number of years he had been practising defensively, only withdrawing treatment when death was inevitable and imminent. His own private philosophy was that the quality of life of numerous impaired children was sufficiently appalling, and the burden of care on the families so weighty, that life was not to be preferred to death in many cases which presented in the NICU. But he was so fearful of being sued that he never took chances. As a result he was constantly grappling with his conscience as babies lingered and suffered longer than he felt was right but he could not bring himself to take an earlier decision.

When it came to their own preferences, there was considerably more uniformity between the two disciplines. The majority of the doctors (32, 56%) and of the nurses (67, 56%) would prefer that the choice was tailored to individual babies. Twenty four of the doctors (42%) and 47 of the nurses (40%), however, felt that treatment should always be started, giving time for proper assessment and adequate time to be taken over the decision making.

A considerable number commented that the real test was, 'What would I want done if this were my baby?' But the answer was often not simple.

> 'I always try and think, if it was my baby, what would I want, and then weigh that up against what I know as a professional. For instance, if I delivered a 23 week gestation baby, my *heart* would want them to do as much as they can to save that baby. But my *head* says, "No, it's not meant to be." And I wouldn't like that child to suffer. And the outcome is quite poor. So I wouldn't want them to pursue any active treatment. But it's *not* my baby. These babies are never my babies. And how do we know what the prognosis is going to be? Nobody can play God, so you have to assess and evaluate all the time that you're going along. We have to give them a chance.' (Staff midwife, more than 5 years experience)

Personal policy

Medical staff who had to undertake resuscitation or take responsibility for the decision might be expected to have some kind of guidelines or policies for themselves. When questioned on this, however, over half (32, 56%) had not. A further three volunteered that policies could vary with circumstances: working in different countries and with different cultures changed one's priorities. Where there is a dearth of resources (for example, in third world countries) premature infants are not allocated the same share of the budget, technology or expertise, which they enjoy in Scotland. Some foreign doctors were aware that returning to their own countries might be difficult now they knew what could be achieved. Earlier yardsticks would now be harder to apply.

Policies could be formulated within different parameters. Some people directly looked at the medical facts. Thus, nine reported personal policies related to the combination of factors which that doctor took into account: for example,

- gross system failure + prematurity + neurological damage
- gestation + medical condition + cerebral damage
- loss of haemostatic control + ischaemic anoxic insult to the brain.

Four other policies were couched in more general terms and hinged on the idea of withdrawing treatment where survival was not possible or the quality of life too awful to make life worthwhile.

Two consultants had a policy which referred to leadership: one never delegated the decision or the tasks around it to junior staff and the other accepted full responsibility for the decision but involved everyone else in the preceding discussion.

Junior staff recognized that they were in no position to take major decisions, so their policy was to resuscitate until a senior colleague appeared to take over the responsibility. As has been stated this was commonly accepted as a wise practice by junior staff and expected by senior doctors.

Discussion

It is well known that practice in different NICUs varies. What appears to be less well appreciated is that to some extent the place of delivery also influences the way these births are classified.[148] In reality the overall figures for perinatal morbidity may well be influenced by a lack of a standard recording system.

None of the study Units has clearly set out policies for treatment withdrawal although junior doctors are given some basic guidelines to help them to operate without always calling for a senior opinion. Decisions are made on a case by case basis. Given the dynamic nature of the circumstances, there is widespread agreement that it is neither desirable nor possible to set rigid parameters around decision making.

Actual practice varies considerably between Units. In the perceptions of the majority of the doctors, decisions are made on an individual basis, but most of the nurses perceive the practice to be one of treating in a fairly routine kind of way to buy time to carry out assessments and tests before withdrawal is considered. It seems likely that in Labour ward, the paediatricians are actually screening the babies who are sent to the Neonatal Unit. In some instances the consultant has already agreed with obstetric colleagues and with parents, that certain infants are not for resuscitation. In other cases, paediatricians are attending deliveries, making assessments on the spot and the outcome results in some instances in the death of the child in Labour ward. Those babies which do survive go to the NICU and the nurses there participate in their treatment. This could well explain the differing perceptions of the two disciplines, since the neonatal nurses do not always see the decision making which goes on in Labour ward.

Discrepancies are not limited to those which occur between the two disciplines of medicine and nursing. Different consultants involved in a given case may follow very different approaches, and then extremely complex and troubling situations can arise. The inconsistency is sometimes between obstetricians and paediatricians; at other times, between paediatricians themselves. Conflicting advice can cause major problems for other team members who are caught in no-win situations. Imagine that today Consultant A says Baby X is for aggressive new treatment and orders a battery of investigations as well as ongoing invasive procedures. But tomorrow Consultant B takes over in the Unit and he rules that treatment is futile and the child should be allowed to die in peace. The SHO is put in an unenviable position. Does he or does he not run the tests? He cannot please both consultants. These sorts of conflicts can also be extremely distressing for the nursing staff and seriously undermine the confidence and trust of parents. Such examples were cited.

Given that the majority feel that choices should be tailored to individual circumstances, it is not possible to lay down rigid parameters for practice, and therefore some individual latitude is necessary. It is almost inevitable that there will be differences of opinion in some instances. It was also to be expected that nurses' preferences would be less likely to be accommodated since the doctors are the ones principally deciding on the medical management of infants in their care. If the actual practice and personal preferences of the staff selecting the two main options are compared, it can be clearly seen that proportionately more nurses than doctors feel that things should be managed differently (Figure 6.1).

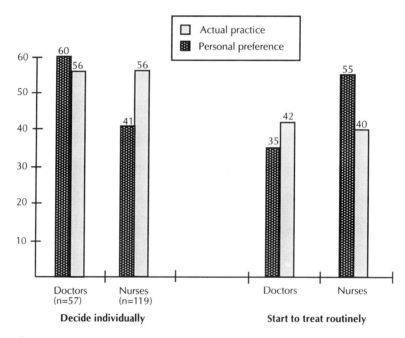

Fig. 6.1: Comparison of actual practice and personal preference in relation to decision making approach

Where discrepancies are inevitable, the management of them becomes critical if Units are to function harmoniously and to foster a sensitive approach to families. The issues which appear to keep the differences within workable bounds relate to communication and awareness of other people's points of view. Where communication is open and honest, where team members feel free to participate in decision making, and where senior people who make the final decision are sensitive to others' feelings, are good communicators, and are held in high regard by the rest of the team, there is a greater chance that those who have reservations about the decision will nevertheless feel that an appropriate course of action has been chosen. This issue will be developed further in a later chapter.

Given the potential for conflict where there are no set policies, it might be tempting to draw up guidelines for practice. However, in the USA where attempts were made to impose standards on clinicians, a survey of neonatologists found that application of the Baby Doe regulations resulted in over-treatment, restricted parental and medical discretion, poor use of resources and insufficient attention to suffering.[127] The end result did not show more uniformity and harmony.

It seems almost inevitable that clinicians must accept some degree of vulnerability. Applying the best interests standard, taking account of individual circumstances, would seem to be a healthier and more compassionate approach than applying externally devised policies which may offer protection to the doctor but lack the necessary sensitivity to the important subjective elements in the decision making. But asking paediatricians to carry such a burden is asking a lot. Their reputation and peace of mind are wrapped up in the consequences of these decisions. As Campbell concluded,

> 'it is sad but understandable, if paediatricians simply refrain from doing what they believe to be best for their patient because of concern about their own interests and those of their hospital.'[149]

However, the results of such defensive behaviour have been witnessed in the States where 'politically and publicly exploited concern' about discrimination against a few impaired infants has created a situation where harm is being done to others by the extensive overuse of painful and extremely expensive treatments.[149] It is important to point out, however, that even in the States, where the threat of litigation forces clinicians to act defensively, there appears to be a change occurring from a 'wait until death is certain' policy to a more individualized approach based on the prognosis for a given baby.[150]

The success of decision making individually tailored to each case, as we have suggested, hinges on the quality of the staff's communication and sensitivity, but the organization behind healthcare can present barriers to an environment which encourages sound ethical reasoning. Thus for example, an ethos placing high value on efficiency and economic factors, may well run counter to a commitment to family autonomy. It takes time and resources to listen attentively to parents struggling with the arguments for withdrawing treatment from their baby. Each hour of delay means that expensive equipment and personnel are caught up in a situation the outcome of which will carry no benefit for the Unit or for the wider society. Allegiances and loyalties may be divided and strained. Compromises may be inevitable but will probably add to the tensions experienced by the staff. Some of the factors which might influence decision making are addressed in the following chapter.

Conclusions

Flexibility and individual case by case decisions are the best answer to the multiplicity of factors to be taken into account in deciding which babies should be treated. If tension and conflict are to be minimized and confidence fostered, great attention needs to be paid to good communication within the team and consistency of approach. If there are no rules or fixed procedures, the way these cases are managed is crucial to harmony and good practice.

CHAPTER SEVEN

Influencing Factors

There are many factors aside from the organizational and environmental constraints which can potentially influence decisions about withdrawing or withholding treatment from infants. These factors relate principally to two main issues: the interests of the different parties concerned, and the perceptions, beliefs, values and attitudes of the professional him or herself.

Interests of the people concerned in the decision

The baby and family

When respondents were asked whose interests they took into account when deciding whether or not to treat, the results as far as the baby and family were concerned were quite clear. Everyone took the baby's interests into account, and all except two doctors and one nurse thought that the parents' interests had to be considered. A few went further and said they would listen carefully to the views of other family members apart from the parents who might have a special role to play in relation to this baby. However, a small number commented that it was actually very difficult to know what a given baby's interests were.

> 'I suppose in pseudo-philosophical terms, I'm saying I really can't judge the baby's interests. What I *can* judge is the likely outcome, and whether or not there's going to be any pleasure in this family from having this baby. And if it's all going to be hell, then I really can't see that it's in the baby's interests.' (Consultant, more than 25 years experience)

Isolating a baby's interests from his familial context was easy to do in a NICU especially where extremely premature infants were concerned: staff said it was sometimes more difficult to relate to them as individuals. Being involved with the family helped to set a human context. It also provided a context for appraising competing interests.

> 'When you see a baby in isolation, it is very easy to be completely cold and clinical towards the baby, outside of the context of the baby's family. So I always think it is better to know the parents and that somehow protects the baby in some way. Because when you look at a 24, 25 week baby, you don't react with them in the same way as when you look at another adult who is able to speak and to communicate and is able, in a sense, to force you to consider them carefully and value them carefully. So I think it's really important to see the baby in the context of his family, of the parents. That's important for me.' (Registrar, less than 5 years experience)

Differences of opinion emerged in relation to the importance given to family factors. Some respondents were quite clear that, since the parents were the ones whose lives would be irrevocably changed by this baby, their interests should weigh heavily. Others, however, felt that it was unfair to penalise a baby just because he happened to be born to parents who could not cope with problems as well as other families might.

> 'I feel quite strongly about [this] – I think it's unfair for some poor baby to be born having its health care decided on because his mother's only 15.' (Consultant, more than 15 years experience)

Sometimes, however, the parents' interests took precedence over the baby's and then respondents could see the potential for disaster. For example, pursuing treatment for the sake of the parents when it was physiologically futile for the baby, on occasions resulted in prolonged suffering for the infant, and profound distress for the staff. For those closely involved in the care of the child this could feel intolerable. But sometimes there appeared to be no choice and the parents' immediate needs were compelling.

> 'I can think of 25 week twins, and one of them ... I'd say it was still born, its heart rate was nothing. I resuscitated that baby. Now, it was just – I walked into the room. This baby was flat, white, no heart rate, no resps, and her mother said, "Please can you do something with my baby?" And it suddenly struck me, I really want the baby to do something for her. I resuscitated the baby. The other twin died as well. They both had grade 4 intraventricular haemorrhages. I felt really we could have stopped treatment earlier ... I take account of the parents. And I felt in those circumstances at least it gave them some time to be aware that their babies weren't going to make it ... they knew that we tried.' (Registrar, less than 5 years experience)

> 'There was another baby, a hydropic baby, that really was incompatible with life. Now the mother had been spoken to by one of the consultants who wasn't going to actively manage the baby. But it was a different consultant that was on, and he wanted to do everything. So we did resuscitate this baby, from the point of view of draining its pleural effusions, its ascites, and we ventilated it as well. But its heart rate never would have picked up. It wasn't going to make it. But the mother said – we turned off the ventilator after a consultant discussed it with her again – she said afterwards, "I'm really glad that my baby was resuscitated, because at least I feel now everything had been done for it. If it hadn't been, I would never feel right." So I think for her case it was obviously a good thing. It's very much an individual thing.' (Registrar, less than 5 years experience)

A considerable number of staff had analysed such situations and could rationalize the switch in priorities. They saw that the balance changed over time. Initially while efforts were being made to save the baby, his interests took precedence over all others. But when treatment became medically futile, the parents' interests became of much greater importance. Getting the management and the timing right for them could make a huge difference to how they would remember this experience and deal with their loss.

The staff

Staff's interests came second to the family's. Indeed some went so far as to say that if staff couldn't deal with these issues appropriately, and felt that their interests were important, they were unsuited to this specialty. It was difficult to unravel exactly what professionals thought the staff's own interests were. Some doctors specifically qualified their answer by saying that if taking colleagues' interests into account meant listening to what they had to say, then they did take account of their interests.

There was a difference in the perceptions of the two groups of staff. Of the nurses, 81% (96) said that when they were trying to decide what was best to do, they certainly took account of the opinions of other staff intimately involved in this particular case. Furthermore as many as 60% (71) would also take on board the views of other staff who were peripheral to the management of that baby. By contrast, only 61% (35) of the doctors felt that they took account of the interests of other colleagues. Others admitted that they would listen to their views, but that these opinions would not influence their decision making. Still others felt that staff's interests were only passing ones and therefore not to be compared with the intense and lifelong interests of the family.

> 'The interests of the professional staff are by comparison ephemeral. They get very upset. They get very involved with these babies and that's a good thing. It's healthy that they get emotionally involved, very upset when these babies die. It isn't as if they don't care. And they need a bit of support for a day or two ... but eventually that will go away and they'll get on with their lives.' (Consultant, more than 25 years experience)

There were some consultants who hand-picked the staff to be involved with them in these sensitive cases. By such selection they dealt with these difficult cases by working only with those staff whose basic philosophy matched theirs, leaving no room for those with extreme or different attitudes.

> 'I know the ones in the nursery who can deal with anything, and in a difficult situation, they're the people that I'm comfortable with. They're the people who've had enough bad experiences, who can actually get [beyond the death experience itself]. I'd rather there were certain people there when we withdrew treatment than that there were others. It's experience of life we're talking about. The worn ones, those are the ones you want.' (Consultant, more than 15 years experience)

When respondents were challenged on this point, they explained their position by saying that very often new recruits to NICU held idealistic and unrealistic positions, which were simply a feature of their naiveté. Staff who had had experience of life themselves, and had been through treatment withdrawal many times, had a greater understanding and recognized the wisdom of such a decision. There was no merit in courting trouble when the situation was already heavily overlaid with emotion. There was enough distress from parents and the nurse looking after the child without adding anger or upset from those who were felt to have too little knowledge or experience to be useful contributors.

The doctors

The doctors were asked expressly if they took their own interests into account. A number asked what their interests were. Replies included things like having a clear conscience, and avoiding conflict or litigation. Just under a half (27, 47%) felt that this featured in their thinking. Fourteen of these were consultants who would be accepting the final responsibility for the decision, but nine were registrars or senior registrars, and four were SHOs. Some appeared to have an instinctive resistance to the idea of being concerned about themselves, but a further two of these doctors on reflection said that in some circumstances their own interests might come into the deliberations.

> 'I'd like to think, no. But I'm sure your own feelings have a part to play. I'm thinking of experiences I've had where there's been a particularly bad week, for example, when several babies have died ... and I think there's a limit to the emotional load that one can actually take but I'd like to think that that would never influence the decision. I wouldn't be surprised if sometimes it actually influences the *timing* of the approach. I'm sure that happens.' (Consultant, less than 10 years experience)

The point was made that to some extent doctors had to consider their interests in that they had to protect themselves. They could not cope with the heavy emotional toll if they allowed themselves to become too involved in all the cases it fell to their lot to decide.

> 'I did [consider my own interests] to start with, but you develop a professional thick skin. You have to. All SHOs and registrars go through periods of intense emotional involvement with all their families. But if they carried on doing that they would, a) either go mad; b) leave neonatology; or c) commit suicide. All three are known.' (Consultant, more than 10 years experience)

This degree of detachment could, however, be misunderstood. One SHO observed that because no one appeared to take any account of junior doctors' feelings and opinions, it was all too easy to fall into the same way of operating and ignore the feelings of one's colleagues; a phenomenon she called 'group-think'. It had come as something of a shock to this respondent to discover that there were people in the team who held strong views which were quite different from her own. Sometimes these only emerged when colleagues became upset about other incidents. Instances were reported where consultants appeared to completely overlook the long hours and nights a junior member of staff had been struggling to keep a baby alive against their better judgement. They had come in, after a good night's sleep, to do a round, and publicly criticised that doctor for not having performed other duties. Such perceived injustices could prompt peer groups to share their reservations along with their hurt. In this way doctors came to understand better the effect of these decisions on colleagues who had appeared unmoved hitherto.

Society

Though many were clearly alive to the implications for society in treating these infants, the majority of the staff (44, 77% of the doctors, and 75, 63% of the nurses) indicated that they would not take the interests of society into account at the point of decision making in individual cases. At that time, emotions are running high and concentration is on medical factors and family issues. However, a minority felt that they would consider society's interests (10, 18% of the doctors and 37, 31% of the nurses). Some outlined the reasons why society had a vested interest: the initial high cost of care; ongoing needs for health and social services; the long-term burden on society of caring for very dependent people.

'If you're saying, OK, it ends up blind, spastic quadriplegia, with palsy and a gastrostomy and blah, blah, blah – it's going to be a million pound child, then I suppose it crosses your mind. But I don't think it's a thing that looms large at that particular time. The particular situation where that thought process is more in the front of your mind is in situations where you've got big hulking term babies – normally formed term babies – who've had an ischaemic anoxic insult and so on, a cord prolapse or an abruption or something of this kind, who are very knocked up, but they will survive anyway, because they've got the resources to and they've often not bled into the head and they will survive. And certainly one thinks, "Gosh, this is bloody awful", because we've got a baby who we know in the next few days is going to get over this insult but you know full well that in many of those cases will go on to be a profoundly handicapped baby and child, and is going to, in society's terms, cost an arm and a leg. But in terms of the context that you're talking about, actually withdrawing treatment ... then it's seldom on my mind.' (Consultant, more than 20 years experience)

'The cost to the Health Service, the government, is phenomenal. It's fine if they go on to be normal healthy children but of course, nobody really knows what they're going to be like as adults. But you can only just hope that they are going to be normal and have a normal life expectancy, but nobody's ever going really to know until they're a lot older. But you do think of these things ... the cost of intensive care ... who's going to care if they're not able to be [looked after by their parents] ...' (Sister, more than 5 years experience)

It sometimes happened that resource issues crept in because of the lack of staff or equipment. But then in some senses it was more a matter of society limiting options rather than staff consciously taking society into the equation.

'If you say, do I take the interests [of society] the monetary side, [into account], no. I will concede, however, that if we are extremely busy and the Unit is chocablock and somebody comes in at 24 or 25 weeks, and we haven't got the facilities, I will not compromise other babies that we've been working on and I will not institute intensive care ... I would either effect the transfer of the mother with the baby in utero, or assess the situation when it arose. But if I'd delivered the baby, I would not compromise those babies we had. Society may have a different viewpoint, and I think that's why I think what we do with a family is a very personal thing.' (Consultant, more than 20 years experience)

One consultant believed that society had forfeited the right to have an interest in as much as it had placed the responsibility on the backs of medical staff, and failed to provide adequate support for the families caught up in these tragedies. Society could not have it both ways. Either it gave doctors the responsibility and they bore the consequent burdens; or it put in place a perfect system of caring for all babies irrespective of their impairments which made choice simpler. Other respondents took an even more fundamental stance. As long as society funded wars, and trips to the moon, and plastic surgery, they would not accept that it lacked the resources to fund neonatal intensive care.

Although decisions were not influenced at the point of service delivery by society's interests, that was not to say such considerations should not be debated. As one consultant with a wealth of experience in community paediatrics pointed out, sensible discussions about society's interests could and should take place away from the nursery. But in the 'heat of the moment' clinicians reverted to doing what they had always done: treating babies to the best of their ability. For him there was a particular satisfaction in following infants through for many years. Decisions were able to be taken calmly and consistently and the importance of society's interests assumed a more balanced perspective.

'I think it's sometimes easier to have been with the family right from the beginning, to talk these things through, because at that stage you usually know the parents quite well, in a professional way, but it's not a face that's unknown, or an attitude that's unclear. And you're not trying to get over in half an hour in a clinic, what may take months to establish by discussing everything.' (Consultant, more than 20 years experience)

Priorities

Given the potential for conflicting interests, respondents were asked if they could prioritize the interests of the different groups. Most felt they could (93% of the doctors and 97% of the nurses). A few, however, having tried out some prioritizing, concluded that it depended on the circumstances of the case and they were reluctant to give a blanket response.

'I don't think I could [prioritize] because what we're trying to do right from the start is to have guided consensus and that, in a sense, is taking in strands of feeling from all over. I might give you a glib answer that it's the baby's interest that comes first, and I suppose, in a funny way, I believe that that is the case. But in practice what actually happens is, talking to the parents, they influence you, you influence them. This very thing happened to me about 6 weeks ago. One of the senior obstetric consultants and I sat down to look at a very difficult antenatal case, where there was a baby who had been seen on ultrasound scan to have large ventricles. And the question had come up, should we be going ahead with this pregnancy or should we not. And the obstetrician and I thought this was a very difficult decision and couldn't come to any recommendation, and we went in to meet the parents with some trepidation, I suppose, because it wasn't clear what our recommendation would be. But our recommendation evolved over the 10, or 15, 20 minutes that we spent with the parents. And by the time we actually left, it had become clear all along that the correct decision had been taken, but it was only the interaction between the staff and the parents that allowed that clear picture to emerge. That was a very interesting insight for me as to how we actually take decisions.' (Consultant, more than 15 years experience)

However, the overall pattern which emerged was:
1. the baby and his family
2. the staff
3. society.

A considerable number talked of the difficulty of separating out the baby's interests from those of the parents since the two groups together made up the family unit and interests were interwoven, and, as has been described above, the relative importance of each varies over time and with changing prognoses. In addition, circumstances could sometimes exist where it was impossible to know what the baby's interests were, and then the parents' interests might take precedence.

Given all these qualifications, 51 of the doctors (96%) put the whole family's interests first, with 32 (56%) specifying the baby as number one, 7 (12%) the parents; and 12 (21%) the baby and rest of the family jointly. Similarly 117 of the nurses (98%) put the family first, with 52 (44%) singling out the baby as top priority; 21 (18%) the parents, and 44 (37%) the whole family unit.

Influencing factors for professionals
Factors such as age, likelihood of long-term survival and religious affiliation have been identified as factors which are important determinants in withdrawal of treatment decisions. But it has been demonstrated that there is wide variability amongst individuals in the ranking of such measures.[151]

In this present study respondents were specifically asked about five different factors which could potentially influence their thinking: religious conviction, limited resources, fear of recrimination, professional experience and personal experience. They were then offered the opportunity to cite anything else which they felt had been influential for them particularly.

Religious conviction
It should be noted that the question related to personal religious conviction not affiliation to a specific religious organization, and a number of respondents were at pains to

reinforce this thinking that it was a personal belief in something rather than membership of a particular church that generated the influence. Proportionately more doctors (25, 44%) than nurses (34, 29%) were influenced in some way by their religious conviction.

Only a minority stated which religion they followed, and among those who did, the statement tended to assume that holding a set of beliefs was synonymous with church membership. Indeed the few respondents whose church held inflexible views about life and death which they too espoused, appeared to have the least difficulty with these issues. For them the issues were black and white, and they were comfortable with the fixed parameters which removed doubt or guilt. Even so, some were at pains to point out that, while their convictions dominated their own thinking and behaviour, they would not impose their own strong views on other people's lives. Learning more and more about the individual circumstances behind human tragedies, had increased the limits of their tolerance and compassion. They had come to understand that blanket judgements just did not fit real life situations. At the other end of the spectrum were those who, far from living by such clear demarcations, had difficulty even separating out the religious from a more generally ethical way of thinking and behaving. All shades of opinion between these two extremes were represented.

For the majority the influence was a fairly general one which led to their being compassionate, differentiating between right and wrong, and respecting others. A belief that there was a divine plan created a sense that not only did babies sometimes defy human prediction but that staff should be wary of giving up on babies who appeared to be doing badly, or making arbitrary judgements about the worth of a life from a purely human perspective. There was, moreover, an open acknowledgment that it was something to do with the sacredness of life itself which made staff ponder these things so carefully. This was not necessarily a belief in the absolute sanctity of life: only four doctors and three nurses believed it was an absolute. But because human life was something special and sacred, the withholding of treatment was something which should only be contemplated in extreme circumstances.

There were, however, limits to what doctors could do, and it was sometimes appropriate to 'allow nature to take its course'. A number of the respondents made reference to 'playing God'. Where it seemed appropriate to challenge their comments, the underlying thinking behind such a expression was pursued. A sense was given that it was God's prerogative to give or take life and it was therefore not appropriate for doctors to make such a decision. In NICUs an enormous amount of medical intervention goes on. It seemed relevant to try to discover what differentiated this intervention from measures which usurped God's authority. Amongst the small number of those who had an answer, it appeared that as long as doctors and nurses were striving to save a viable life, they believed they were acting on God's behalf. Where it was obvious that death was imminent, it was perfectly acceptable not to prolong the process of dying, and this too was acting along with God. But when decisions were made on the basis that that life was not worth living, then doctors were straying into God's territory. One sister with a strong religious belief, summed it up by saying, 'It's about allowing the living to live and the dying to die.'

Although it was predominantly a general religious ethic which influenced the respondents, a few had superimposed specific dogma which also had an effect on their thinking. Some instanced absolute prohibitions which for them had religious origins, for example, church opposition to abortion or euthanasia. Groups as diverse as Roman Catholics and born again Christians were represented in this sample. In terms of the neonate these underlying prohibitions could set limits to behaviour. Active termination of a life, for example, was out of the question. Staff with a Roman Catholic background were divided in their views here. Some of the staff who said religious conviction did not influence them, added a rider to the effect that, though it did not, it should. When asked to expand, they said they had been raised as Catholics but now no longer practised any form of religion. They retained something of the feel of Catholic prohibitions but most said they felt no more than momentary qualms of conscience now. Only four doctors and four nurses said without qualification that they subscribed to Catholic teaching in this area when it came to babies. A further three doctors and five nurses confessed that they no longer subscribed to all of the teaching of the organization to which they either were or had been affiliated. Working in a NICU exposed them to profound questions about life and death. Arguments that held up against abortion, were shaken when they encountered certain complex neonatal scenarios. It was not only the Catholic staff, however, who volunteered that real life encounters had challenged received wisdom forcing them to evolve their own more personal ethic.

A very few respondents acknowledged their affiliation to organizations such as humanism, and Quakerism, observing that in subscribing to this set of beliefs they also embraced a philosophy which made them compassionate, caring and sensitive to others' needs and pain. In this way their religious convictions influenced their management of babies and families. Additionally one doctor felt that her own *lack* of organized religion had forced her to consider the issues more broadly since she had fewer moral tenets to form the framework for her thinking.

For a considerable number there was comfort in holding a belief in a God and an afterlife. It helped them to see death in perspective and made it seem less of a tragedy when a baby died.

> 'In some ways, having gone through bereavement yourself, makes you less afraid of [death]. You see death as something quite real and also – certainly with my religious belief – I don't think of it as the end. And certainly in the period after you've lost somebody, you still really feel that they are still around. That death isn't frightening any more.' (Consultant, less than 10 years experience)

One respondent, a devout Roman Catholic, after confirming that her rejection of abortion was absolute in all circumstances, went on to give a detailed account of a personal experience where a close relative had had to make a decision about terminating a pregnancy for a very severe malformation which was known to be incompatible with life. Being closely involved had forced this neonatal nurse to look at the issues again. Her own position on abortion did not waver, but she subsequently withdrew her membership of an active pro-life organization because she felt that the emotive slogans they adopted simply did not square with the human agony she had seen and experienced at first hand. This was just one of several moving and eloquent examples of an individual coming to a realization that, when it came to infants, the tragedies of real life sometimes challenged cherished and long held but previously unshakable views.

Limited resources

Only seven doctors (12%) and 20 nurses (17%) felt that the fact that resources were limited influenced their thinking about when treatment should be withdrawn or withheld, although a number commented that they feared the day might come when they had to consider such factors in making their decision. The majority were totally opposed to this notion. One consultant described an illustrative case he knew of where a baby had been treated with Extra Corporeal Membrane Oxygenation (ECMO) in a hospital outside the family's own health area. Their health authority had phoned literally every day, 'not because they were interested in the baby, but because the costs were rising; and they did say at one point, it was now at £70,000.' He questioned what the health authority had wanted or expected them to do. But the incident made him realize that, 'It's now impinging more and more and clinicians are talking about [costs] because it's been hammered down their throats.'

Four of the nurses qualified their answer by saying that it was only when inappropriate treatment was being given that they allowed cost to enter into the equation: if treatment was being prolonged when there appeared to be no possibility of a good outcome it seemed a futile waste of resources. Others commented that resource issues did not influence the decision itself about whether to treat or not, but a *lack* of resources definitely influenced the quality of the end of babies' lives on occasions: if there were not enough staff to care sensitively over a prolonged period for a dying baby and for the bereaved family then the care given was suboptimal.

For one doctor, resources impinged when expensive treatments were available theoretically but were unavailable in his own Unit because of the high cost. But others made reference to these same expensive measures (for example, heart and lung transplants) and felt it was difficult to dissect out the resource implications from the morbidity and mortality which attended these therapies. The affluence of society clearly varies around the world. Two doctors were alive to financial implications because in their own countries treatments were not freely available and they realized how much more could be done in countries like the UK.

Resource factors which were perceived as influential included a range of issues. There was a general feeling that more should be spent on prevention rather than treatment of conditions such as prematurity. This smacked of closing the gate after the horse had bolted. The literature reinforces the relative inefficiency in terms of monetary considerations of ignoring preventative measures: it has been estimated that the total cost of giving a woman antenatal care as a preventative strategy would be less than half of the daily cost of neonatal intensive care.[5]

'My own honest opinion of this would be that in neonates, we've got the cart before the horse. That it's easier in terms of hospital numbers to look at a book and say we had X amount of admissions in intensive care, and we've got X thousands of pounds worth of equipment ... But it's much more difficult to quantify care outside: good antenatal care, good housing, good nutrition, all those factors the absence [of which] lead to the birth of premature babies. I think the balance has got lost a bit ... It reminds me of something that a medical doctor who is a missionary once said. It's like being at a river and seeing these bodies floating downstream. And you jump in and rescue them and take them out. And there's more. So you get lots of people to help you and soon you're taking bodies out [by the score]. But nobody thinks to go upstream and find out where they're all coming from ... We know the sociological factors that can bring babies in here. And I find that incredibly frustrating.' (Staff midwife, less than 5 years experience)

But to some extent a number of the conflicts in neonatology are the product of success in other departments. With developments in infertility treatment has come an increase in multiple births, for example. This has brought its own dilemmas.

'I do have strong feelings about multiple births and how damaging they are on intensive care funds. I've worked in places where triplets can go to three different hospitals, all to die. Or one dies and Mum's in one hospital, which one will she choose? Mercifully that issue is now resolving itself – in the last eight years anyway – and I think that reproductive technology is now much better controlled. But the strain that producing triplet births puts on the Unit is huge, really huge. I don't have a problem with looking after the babies. I just have a problem with someone else creating that [situation]. It's controllable. It's not acceptable to be producing five babies. Because some of them'll end up handicapped. It's not fair on the parents.' (Consultant, less than 10 years experience)

Shortage of staff and equipment was the expressed concern of only four doctors and eight nurses in response to this specific enquiry about factors which influenced decision making, although many more mentioned this reality in a variety of other contexts. Inadequacies meant that babies and families were not as well cared for as they might be and, furthermore, sometimes choices had to be made putting the welfare of one baby above another.

A realization that community resources were very under-funded and that disabled people were underprivileged, brought resources into focus for a small number. One doctor who had worked extensively with severely impaired people in the community and lamented the poor quality of services available, was aware that this experience definitely influenced his judgement when he was contemplating whether to treat compromised neonates. Whilst he was strongly supportive of disabled children he had reservations about introducing more damaged babies into the community when he saw firsthand how inadequate the infrastructure was. Two nurses however, had sympathy for the budget holders. They felt that it was right to consider what society was being required to fund after some of these prolonged and heroic struggles to save a life. For them there was merit in limiting the initial treatment in order to prevent long term burdens on society. Two nurses and one doctor went further: for them questions needed to be asked about the wisdom of spending such vast sums of money on neonatal intensive care in general. They found it hard to justify such huge expenditure for so dubious a return.

Fear of recrimination

Respondents were asked whether the fear of recrimination influenced them. More than half of the doctors (35, 61%) and 81 (68%) of the nurses instantly responded that it did not. Many of these, however, in their comments revealed that in a sense they avoided unpleasant repercussions by taking preventive measures. One consultant pointed out that you could not really prevent parents doing an about-turn. All you could do was build in practices like careful documentation and having witnesses at important discussion sessions. As he concluded, if the parents, after a few weeks, were going to change their minds and criticise the doctors, it was to a large extent outside of one's control, but 'at least you [can] make the chances of a legal action less.'

However, a few admitted that they did experience some anxiety after the event even though at the time they believed that no fear of recrimination influenced their decision. Those who had had experience of parents doing an about-turn were particularly conscious of the risk that parents could take exception to events later on even though they appeared to concur at the time. Graphic descriptions were given of such situations. While it was understandable that parents, in their hurt and frustration, should lash out at someone, staff who had painstakingly taken parents through every step of the decision making, found it hard to take criticisms of lack of communication or poor guidance. It made them extra vigilant about documentation, but could also influence them to delay taking a subsequent decision longer than they felt was appropriate. As one experienced sister put it, the thought goes through one's head: 'You're saying this [ie keep treating] to me now, but will you be saying it to me six months from now when you know how badly damaged your child is?'

A number of the junior staff said that the responsibility did not lie with them so they had no need to fear reprisals, and in any case, one doctor observed, junior staff were too inexperienced to do anything other than treat even where their instinct told them it was futile. Other staff observed that as it was a team decision, there was sufficient protection for individuals in the process by which decisions were made.

Twenty-two doctors (39%) and 38 nurses (32%) were, however, influenced by a fear of recrimination. Two doctors and five nurses felt that it was partly this factor which made the team keep treating when they might otherwise decide it was right to stop. The actual sources of recrimination included society (2 doctors, 1 nurse), pro-life organizations (3 doctors, 3 nurses), parents (3 doctors, 6 nurses), the press (1 nurse), and those who held the purse strings (1 doctor). One SHO worried about the repercussions where consultants were divided in their opinions about management. Junior staff were caught in a catch 22 situation, unable to please them all but dependent on these senior people for future references.

The majority conveyed a sense that an overall fear of possible consequences made people examine their behaviour and motives as well as their actual management of a case. Awareness that one might have to justify a particular course of action made one more questioning of one's own values and beliefs and practices as an individual as well as part of a team. That in turn led to a cautious approach. There were those who concluded that this was a positive effect; there should always be much soul searching when these momentous decisions were being made. But others were concerned that such measures prolonged the process of dying, and could add substantially to the burden of pain and distress for those most intimately involved. One consultant felt, however, that university employees were less burdened than NHS consultants. They acted in an independent capacity, were not reliant on the NHS administration for their salary, and were not obliged to conform to that organisation's rules. They were free to make a clinical judgement and give an opinion based on the medical evidence.

A considerable number were aware that a general anxiety to avoid trouble also made them careful in the way they managed these cases. It was at least to some extent this fear which made them meticulous in documenting and reporting discussions and treatment, circumspect about what they disclosed and to whom they divulged information, careful to establish a consensus or at least take the team along with them, keen to seek second opinions, and adamant about taking things very slowly.

One very experienced consultant volunteered that there could be no harsher recrimination than that of one's own conscience. He was, he said, his own most severe judge.

Professional experience

This was a powerful influencing factor for almost all of the staff working in neonatal intensive care. Only two doctors (4%) and four nurses (3%) stated that it had not influenced them. Many indeed spoke movingly of the impact working with neonates had had on their thinking. Prior to entering this specialty they had had fairly strong ideas about what was right to do in terms of treatment but the experience had confused their certainty. They saw for themselves that babies could not readily be categorized and compartmentalized. They were brought face to face with the advances in technology and knowledge whilst at the same time confronting the limits of modern medicine. There were profound and diverse influences preventing the drawing of straight and hard lines. Not least among these influences was the fact that children defied predictions. It was very sobering to consider withdrawing treatment on a baby and perhaps years later to be brought face to face with that child enjoying a good quality of life. The very uncertainty of medical prognosis could powerfully influence the direction people went in.

> 'I think you have to give them a chance to a certain degree, because I don't think you could live with yourself if you [thought you'd destroyed a baby's chance of a reasonable life]. Well, the thing is, you're not going to know. But if you withdraw the care you're not going to know if that child's going to make it or not. But I think you have to give them a reasonable chance to prove that they

might be OK, because we've seen babies with horrendous haemorrhages in their head, and they've been all right.' (Staff midwife, more than 5 years experience)

One group for whom the experience was different were those staff who had in their earlier years worked closely with severely impaired children or adults. Many stories were recounted of impressive courage and devotion. Some had spent impressionable years as schoolchildren or young adults in this way. Others had grown up closely encountering people with disabilities because their parents had been involved in working with them. Still others had personal experiences with disabled people, factors in whose lives were a testament to human love or endurance. Whatever the source of their experience, these respondents came to neonatology with a real appreciation of the impact of profound disability on the individual, on families and on society. This experience influenced them in one of two ways: either they now appreciated that there was value in even a severely limited life; or they were so appalled by the reality of severe impairment that they felt that babies should be allowed to die to spare the whole family such agony and prolonged suffering and indignity. It was sometimes a single incident with a particular family which brought the reality into stark relief and profoundly moved a person.

'I trained in Sick Children's [Hospital] and when I came to the Outpatient Clinic specifically, I remember very vividly, this old lady coming along – she wasn't old by her years but she was old because she was careworn – carrying a 13 year old mentally and physically handicapped child who was menstruating. Her husband had walked out on her and she felt so responsible for this person, so guilty about having given birth to this person, that it had wrecked not only her life, but her husband's life, and affected the whole family. I was only 17 or 18 at the time.' (Staff midwife, more than 20 years experience)

There was an overall acceptance that advances in knowledge and technology had made the hitherto impossible possible. These changes in some instances made it difficult for very experienced respondents to separate out the impact of these advances from their own personal development. Half of all of the respondents (28, 49% of doctors and 59, 50% of nurses) expressed a general anxiety about what they were doing with babies. Seeing certain infants defy predictions was scarey and the staff were troubled by the effects of so much uncertainty in prognosis. When they saw survivors returning to visit the Unit, attending follow up clinics or casually in the supermarket or street, enjoying a good quality of life, and realised that they had seriously considered terminating that life, they experienced considerable misgivings and sometimes regret. Five nurses actually described cases in detail where such a sequence of events had occurred. However, some staff worked exclusively in intensive care and never saw the effects of their work further down the line. For them it was difficult to get much feedback but they worried about the outcome nonetheless.

For considerable numbers of staff there had been a definable shift in their thinking as the result of experience in NICU. This could be in either direction. The doctors were equally distributed in both directions, but the effect on nurses was to make them much more inclined to limit treatment than to extend it. Compared with their opinion when they first entered the specialty, 13 doctors (23%) and 49 nurses (41%) were now less keen to treat aggressively. However 14 doctors (25%) and 24 nurses (20%), realizing what could be achieved, felt that more babies should be given a sporting chance by being offered aggressive treatment. A further 16 doctors (28%) and 16 nurses (13%) were ambivalent, moving in neither of these directions. For them there was a sense of increasing uncertainty which moved them from black and white to grey: each case had to be assessed individually. Summarizing these figures highlights the differences (Figure 7.1).

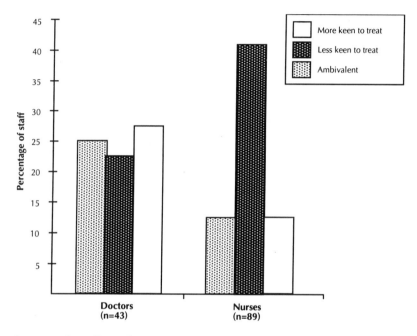

Fig. 7.1: The effect of experience in NICU on inclination to treat

Aside from the changes in their approach to the actual decision, staff were aware of changes in themselves. Fifteen doctors (26%) and 38 nurses (32%) said that with experience had come confidence in their own judgement. They could make the decision more rationally and less emotionally because it was based on medical evidence and their own knowledge of previous outcomes. More than one person specifically said that they looked back with regret at what they had been party to.

One problem which presented an acute dilemma for junior doctors was outlined by a senior house officer. Her own beliefs were quite different from those of the consultants in the Unit. As the most junior member of the team she was required to carry out instructions from her seniors and she was very aware of the potential consequences for her career if she raised objections. She was left wrestling with very troubling personal conflicts.

Specific opportunities for supporting families could also help staff to move on in their own thinking. Having the responsibility for follow-up bereavement work, or attending a funeral, or visiting parents some time after the death, rounded out the experience and helped respondents to see a broader picture than the rather narrow confines of the NICU permitted. Developing counselling skills and getting better at imparting bad news, took some of the horror out of dealing with distraught parents, and freed staff up to increase their sensitivity in managing these difficult cases. This in turn gave them more confidence in their own position.

Experience in Units also influenced the way staff managed cases. They felt they became more sensitive to the needs of different people at this traumatic time, instancing a variety of specific ways in which they had developed a greater awareness. These included the importance of ensuring babies died with dignity, taking sufficient time over the decision and the process of withdrawing treatment, and not leaving juniors to deal with the family or withdrawing the equipment.

Personal experiences

Staff's beliefs and attitudes and opinions could be influenced by things which happened in their personal lives, as well as by the experience gained working in a professional capacity. Over half of the doctors (30, 53%) were aware of these influences, with a further four unsure about the exact nature of these factors but believing that all of life's experience impinged on thinking in some way, so it was unlikely that nothing had influenced their thinking about life and death issues for neonates. They just could not pinpoint anything specific. A higher percentage of nurses (85, 71%) knew that personal events had influenced their thinking. The most commonly occurring events are presented in Figure 7.2.

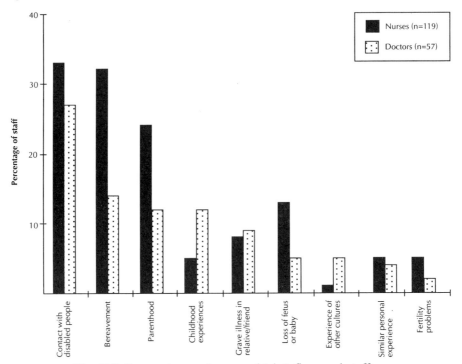

Fig. 7.2 Personal experiences which influenced staff's approach to decision making

EXPERIENCE WITH DISABLED PEOPLE

As has been mentioned in an earlier section, an impressive number of staff had been profoundly influenced by encounters with disabled people (16, 28% of doctors and 39, 33% of nurses). Experiences ranged from having more than one damaged child themselves to casual jobs taking people with disabilities on holiday. For the majority, the experience had given them a different perspective – a finer appreciation of the value of these lives and the joy of simple pleasures or extremely limited achievement. Even so, they sometimes commented that, whilst they could value existing lives and contribute to efforts to enhance them, they were uncomfortable with the idea that Units should continue to work so vigorously to save such damaged infants for a life of apparent deprivation and suffering. There was scope to limit the number of babies who endured these deprivations whilst at the same time enhancing the lives of the existing disabled.

PERSONAL LOSS

The pain of personal loss and bereavement is a profound one. It had influenced 8 doctors (14%) and 38 nurses (32%). But by their own assessment, this particular experience had helped staff to appreciate to some extent what parents were going through when decisions about their infant's non-treatment were being made. As one midwife commented, after the loss of a young relative in her 20s, she was more sensitive to parents waking up every morning to a feeling that 'something awful' had happened, and going through every day with a great cloud hanging over their lives. Having experienced these intense emotions, staff could understand why families sometimes wanted to delay the actual cessation of treatment. Such insight helped them to sympathise with a decision to wait until parents were more ready for this final step, even where the delays were painful for those nurses and doctors intimately involved with the baby.

More specifically, the deaths of close relatives or friends which had been difficult to tolerate, were instanced as leaving an indelible impression which was resurrected when decisions were being made in the nursery. Loss of dignity or intractable or untreated pain were two of the factors which left a strong resistance to allowing infants to die in such a manner. When nursing or medical care had been less than satisfactory it raised strong feelings in people which made them ask serious questions about their own caregiving as well as that of their colleagues. Some respondents had themselves been involved in making decisions on behalf of close relatives about withdrawal of treatment. Being on the receiving end of other people's communications and behaviours could make them see their own practices afresh. They understood the influence of powerful emotions on relatives' reception of information, and they saw for themselves the potential for misunderstanding.

As many as three doctors (5%) and 15 nurses (13%) had experienced the loss of a fetus or a baby. Three respondents had themselves had premature infants who had not survived, or had experienced cot death. Some of these respondents expressed a hope that such traumas had helped them to be more sensitive to the needs of other parents in similar situations.

PARENTHOOD

As in relation to professional experience, a considerable number confided that they would not want treatment for their own child in circumstances of extreme prematurity or impairment. Since a significant proportion of them had close experience of the impact of disablement and perinatal loss, their opinions were based on more than just intellectual argument. Many of the nurses (29, 24%) singled out parenthood as a profound influence since it gave them insight into the emotional investment of a parent for a child, and the strength of feeling when a child is ill or has an abnormality. A few doctors (7, 12%) also felt that being a parent had influenced them. They spoke of the effect of going home to normal able-bodied children and the rush of compassion they felt for parents faced with tragic choices. For those staff who had had problems with infertility or miscarriage (1 doctor and 6 nurses) there was also an acute understanding of the powerful desire for a child which helped them to understand why parents clung desperately to hope for their sick infant's survival.

EXPERIENCE OF GRAVE ILLNESS

A small number of the nurses had had personal experience of grave illness. They transposed to the baby their own emotions about having tubes thrust down their throats, enduring relentless invasive procedures with little rest, and the remembered feeling of powerlessness. It worried them that these infants might be feeling all the same horror and pain which they had gone through but without the capacity to protest or refuse consent. Empathising in this way tended to make them fiercely protective, warding off too many procedures, and facilitating periods of sleep rather than endless cleaning or taking recordings. It is noteworthy that some of the staff who appeared to have had the most gruelling experiences concluded that they would never say, 'I know how you feel', to someone else. They were acutely aware that experience is an individual thing. Their own had simply made them more aware of what suffering entailed, more ready to support others in their grief and pain.

Watching someone close to them fighting for life also affected people profoundly (5 doctors and 9 nurses). If they had been in a position of having to make a life or death decision on behalf of a parent or a child or a very dear friend themselves, (2 doctors and 6 nurses) they understood the pain of such a situation and agonised with parents in the NICU.

OBSTETRIC LOSS

A considerable number of staff had some experience of things going wrong for friends and relatives in their childbearing. Any kind of disaster could touch them deeply but mis-prognosis in relation to a baby they knew outside of work was singled out as having a profound effect. If a friend was told their child was irreparably damaged but he subsequently made a full recovery and survived physically and mentally intact, uncomfortable questions were raised. They could feel their own profession was being tried and found wanting. There was too, a particular poignancy in being asked to advise pregnant women about antenatal screening, or members of their family on the decision whether to withdraw treatment from a loved one. The nearness of the event and the uncertainties of which they were all too conscious, brought home to them the complexities and pain involved. But such experiences also helped to crystallise their own thinking.

MISCELLANEOUS PERSONAL EXPERIENCES

A few staff commented on their own long-standing love of children which made them feel protective. Occasionally a specific one-off event would impinge on an individual's thinking. One consultant described an experience of talking about neonatal care to a church group, and of being surprised to hear the strength of feeling against prolonging lives too aggressively. Getting married to someone who had very definite views about abortion and euthanasia had provoked one doctor into thinking afresh about these matters, and especially when the question of prenatal screening for their own child became an issue. The loss experienced from things as diverse as a broken relationship or the death of a much loved pet, could bring a new understanding which respondents felt could only be learned through being personally affected. Having experienced profound emotions they tried to empathise with the feelings which parents or babies might have.

Particular experiences could shape an individual's own approach to situations. For example, a doctor who had been excluded from family deaths as a child was now keen to involve more people in the process of dying. Another doctor whose own parents had become martyrs to a disabled relative felt his own thinking had been shaped by the repercussions he had experienced. One nurse was surprised by the strength of her own reaction to a fairly minor abnormality in her own child. Knowing these things firsthand could increase sensitivity but the point has also been well made that there is a potential for inappropriate bias. Each family is unique with its own strengths and weaknesses and to try to transfer values and reactions from one to another can be hazardous.

Less clearly defined was the influence of general childhood experience which was cited by seven doctors (12%) and six nurses (5%). Growing up in Ireland with its own approach to disability, abortion and family size, or in a third world country, or in a farming community, could inculcate a different view of death and disablement. Some staff clearly identified these influences as impinging on their whole attitude to selective non-treatment in the NICU.

Life experience could make individuals identify closely with certain families. This idea was borne out in the earlier description of babies and their families who had left an indelible impression on respondents.

Other influences

Eighteen doctors (32%) and 28 nurses (24%) identified other factors which had influenced their thinking. These fell broadly into three categories: the influence of other professionals (10 doctors; 4 nurses); new knowledge (5 doctors; 21 nurses); and personal philosophy (4 doctors; 7 nurses).

INFLUENCE OF SENIORS

More doctors than nurses were aware of the influence of their seniors. Indeed some doctors were eloquent in their praise of those people who had influenced their thinking by their wisdom and sound practice. A range of things were taught in this way almost 'by osmosis' as one person put it.

'Sometimes just a magical moment with somebody who is excellent at doing this, can influence you and change you. Sometimes you stumble across things ... a year ago I stumbled across the fact that when you take a baby from the ventilator and the child doesn't breathe, but the child's still alive, the parents may actually like to use the stethoscope to listen to their baby's heart beating ... I now use this on a regular basis with parents, and quite often they actually say, "You know, the most magical moment was having Judy in my arms and being able to listen to her precious little heartbeat". And that sort of thing is something you just kind of stumble across.' (Consultant, more than 15 years experience)

'I think I've matured a lot in terms of my ability to bring that decision to a conclusion. But also I've learned from my seniors not to make a hasty decision ... having seen how other people go through this decision making process and going the extra length for babies, going an extra day on ventilation, just to allow everybody to be happy about the decision ... and there have been times in the past where I've been surprised because I've given a baby time and it's survived, and one or two, I can remember, survived to be normal. So I'm very wary of hasty decisions ... I think I could have gone the other way had I had seniors who were very incisive, and [making] quick decisions. The colleagues I had were all very contemplative and very thoughtful about the decision they made and I kind of mirrored that.' (Consultant, more than 10 years experience)

NEW KNOWLEDGE

Increasing understanding of the medical facts, legal implications and the effects of treatment were mentioned by 26 staff. Nurses more than doctors tended to be influenced by what they read and what was reported by the media, but interestingly, only two doctors and one nurse mentioned the impact of legal cases.

PERSONAL PHILOSOPHY

Eleven staff cited their personal philosophy of life as an influence: for example, a belief in a right to die with dignity. It sometimes happened that a realization of their own stance on these matters gave staff a new courage to voice their opinions or to stand up for a certain form of management.

'[Another thing that influences me is] I think the knowledge of how small we are and how limited we are in what we actually know, especially when it comes to disabilities in children. We're still not really sure about what affects things. And I think that always comes home to me when you see all this equipment, but you still cannot save a life.' (Staff midwife, less than 5 years experience)

For some there was a profound challenge in what was done in the name of medical progress.

'We question nature too much. I just feel, how far are we going to go with medical science? How far are we going to go? Pregnancy was meant to be 40 weeks. How far into that will we go? Underneath I just have this feeling that sometimes we go too far against what our bodies are trying to tell us.' (Staff midwife, less than 1 year experience)

Nor was this feeling confined to the young and inexperienced. Even one very senior consultant said he was considering leaving neonatology because he was so troubled by its relentless erosion of accepted limits.

Discussion

Competing interests and a range of factors have to be taken into consideration when these difficult decisions are being made. With so much powerful emotion around, it is small wonder that feelings run deep. Such is the power of real-life experience that sometimes even the most entrenched of beliefs and values are threatened. This erosion of a baseline can in turn undermine the sense of security of the individual. It is impressive and to their credit that so many respondents had re-evaluated their own opinions and were prepared to share their doubts and errors of judgement so generously. Some had abandoned previously firmly held beliefs. Even if their own convictions were unmoved, others could sympathise with the pain people experienced and refrain from imposing their own inflexible stance on anyone else.

Interests

Whilst the interests of the baby and his family clearly take precedence over those of the staff themselves or of society, it is not easy to unravel where a baby's interests end and a parent's begin. Sometimes the interests compete. Keeping a baby alive for the parent's peace of mind may be at the expense of the baby's own comfort and wellbeing. Or withdrawing treatment may satisfy the parent's wish for an end to the baby's present suffering but not be in the long term interests of the child himself. Even knowing exactly what is in a baby's best interests is difficult since no one can know what he would choose. Furthermore, inevitably uncertainties in prognosis cloud knowledge of the probable outcomes.

Nor can the child be isolated in terms of the present family. As Kuhse and Singer have suggested, not only is it essential to take account of the interests of the parents and siblings, but in some instances also those of a potential 'next child'.[30] Having a severely impaired child can prevent a couple embarking on another pregnancy because they do not have the reserves or inclination to stretch their resources still further. The ramifications of any decision go in many directions.

Some people try to apply the acid test of 'if it were my child would I want this done?' and this does appear to be a fairly common approach to dilemmas of this sort.[24] But each individual is unique, and trying to transpose these beliefs is to some extent at least, an artificial exercise. The reality of this statement is underlined when we consider the wealth of factors which can influence what anyone thinks they would choose for their own baby. If a parent's own religious conviction is that all life is sacred and must be prolonged at all costs, have they the right to impose a lifetime of suffering on their child? As we saw in the chapter on legal matters, the courts do not support parents making martyrs of their children on a religious scruple. But is the lawyer in a stronger position than a parent to decide wisely and compassionately what is best for a child?

Some doctors see a conflict on occasions between their own interests and those of the baby and/or his family. If the parents are requesting that treatment is stopped because the burden of pain and suffering for the child and the family far outweighs any potential longer term benefit, the doctor might be tempted to concur. But if he does so and the parents learn later that a baby in a similar situation has survived with a good quality of life, they might well see things in quite a different light. Suing the neonatologist sometimes appears to be a knee-jerk reaction to a changed perspective and an understandable lashing out at someone when faced with a devastating loss and overwhelming grief with no adequate explanation of why things went wrong.

Only just over a half of the doctors in this study took account of the interests of other colleagues, many admitting that they would not allow the views of anyone else to influence their decision. Certainly the opinions of inexperienced junior staff are often dismissed since they are perceived as holding unrealistic and idealistic notions. But those same junior staff can encounter real conflicts of conscience if their firmly held beliefs run counter to what they are being asked to countenance or be involved in. The position of one SHO who held strong Catholic views about the sanctity of life, powerfully illustrates this point: the introduction to neonatology and the practice of selective non-treatment forced compromises which were not easy. Even those juniors whose unrealistic position is the result of inexperience rather than religious conviction, can still experience profound dismay if their perception of what is morally right or wrong is violated.

Although the interests of society are rarely in the forefront of the clinicians' minds when the actual decision is being made, the staff are nevertheless alive to the implications on the wider community of what they are doing. Although they do not for the most part at the moment have to consider money matters at the point of service delivery, many fear that there will soon be greater constraints put upon them, and some are now budget holders answerable to outside administrative agents for their decisions. In reality staffing levels are already perceived to be dangerously low in some places, which limits what can be achieved anyway.

But those who work in NICUs are not blinkered about what they do. They are not unmindful of the enormous costs of saving the life of an extremely premature baby; financial as well as psychological and emotional. They recognize that it would be difficult to defend the expensive measures sometimes needed when the outcome is uncertain and the concrete returns minimal. However, reluctant as they are to take on this financial component, they have serious reservations about having restrictions placed upon their activities by others who do not understand neonatology but are primarily concerned with balancing a budget sheet.

The danger of those outside the field of neonatology imposing standards on those inside has been demonstrated, albeit with a slightly different focus, by developments on the other side of the Atlantic. When the American Department of Health and Human Services issued the so-called Baby Doe regulations, not only were paediatricians being instructed to treat handicapped babies, but staff were being encouraged to report any violations of the rules. Clinicians strongly resented this ill-informed interference. One medical director of an Intensive Care Unit in Salt Lake City, wrote an open letter to the Surgeon General, C. Everett Koop, in which he declared that he would undertake to send him pictures of deformed infants they were being forced to keep alive, CT scans of destroyed brains or absent vital organs. He would also attach the monthly bills sent out to parents and insurance companies, and copies of the logbook documenting the new patients they were having to reject because of lack of space or staff.[30] The point was powerfully made that there are serious repercussions from such external dictats. Not only do such regulations force doctors to salvage babies against their better judgement, but other groups are also penalized. Resources are limited and more for one group inevitably means less for another. Furthermore, decisions which place certain groups outside the scope of treatment make a powerful statement about the value of those lives.

> 'If the political process refuses to provide a group such as the aged with hemodialysis, the clear assertion has been made that some lives are not worth saving. To the extent that our lives and institutions depend on the notion that life is beyond price, such a refusal to save lives is horribly costly.'[152]

British reserve about money matters and the existence of a National Health Service which, until recent years, was free at the point of delivery, have long made it unacceptable and unnecessary for clinicians to talk about the financial implications of treatment for infants. To a large extent they could ignore the problems, but while avoiding the issue avoids the cost of choosing, nevertheless, it does so at the cost of honesty and openness. But now that doctors and senior nurses are increasingly becoming answerable for the expenditure of the resources allocated to their areas, the focus has changed. It is widely recognized that the pool is not bottomless.

Calabresi and Bobbitt in *Tragic Choices* unpack the conflicts which society confronts in its allocation of scarce resources.[152] Ignoring some of the dilemmas might well help an individual to sustain a high level of care in a limited arena, since '[a]verting the eyes enables us to save some lives even when we will not save all.'[152] But although questions of logic and reason cannot be forever ignored, nevertheless when it comes to rational judgements there are problems: applying logical arguments to these sensitive matters can be less than helpful.

> 'Logic relentlessly and inappropriately pursued to its end can as readily lead to destructive results as can muddled emotions.'[152]

When one is dealing with so many unquantifiable matters as clinicians are in deciding whether or not to treat a baby, there are inevitably aspects of the situation which cannot readily be converted into money terms or mathematical expressions. Calabresi and Bobbitt concluded that, given even a limited number of such qualitative factors,

> 'It may be better to forgo market information, even as to those elements for which it is available and accurate, than to try to monetize the whole affair. A simple, muddled, collective determination may be preferable.'[152]

It becomes clear that there are no easy answers to simplify what is essentially an extremely complex and painful consideration. There are powerful arguments on all sides.

Influencing factors

To some extent staff working in NICUs control their feelings about what they are actually doing by perceiving their activities in certain ways. The language the respondents used and the interpretations put on various behaviours were testament to this.

> 'We can try to alleviate the dilemmas that we are facing in neonatal units by persuading ourselves that we are not really killing these children, but rather letting them die. We are "letting nature take its course". Part of the problem with this suggestion is that it is no longer clear what "nature" means in such contexts, as nature has become an extension of our technology's ability to keep us alive.'[23]

But beliefs about God's role in babies' survival or the idea that babies themselves decided whether they will live or die, only remove the responsibility to some extent. Staff have still to make certain decisions in the absence of divine revelation or the baby's verbally expressing his preferences, and inevitably a person's own perceptions, beliefs and values influence how he or she feels about these momentous matters, and constitute a major component in ethical decision making. Matters are further complicated because beliefs and attitudes are not immutable: past clinical and personal experience influence future evaluations.

PROFESSIONAL EXPERIENCE

Clinical experiences are profoundly moving and all respondents could relate stories which demonstrated that dealing closely with distressed families and being involved in decision making about forgoing treatment, leave indelible marks. The potential for getting it wrong is sobering. When the decision being made can result in the death of a much wanted and loved baby, the responsibility to get it right is weighty indeed. But many respondents could vividly recall circumstances where babies had defied predictions and prognoses had been very wrong. To see a child aged three running around enjoying a relatively normal life and realize that that life would have been ended had it not been for the parents' fierce clinging to hope against all the odds, gives staff much food for reflection. On the other hand, holding out for ongoing aggressive therapy, inflicting months of painful invasive treatment on a baby only to have him return to the follow-up clinic blind, deaf, with cerebral palsy, having severe fits and no prospect of an independent continent existence, seeing the parents crushed by the corrosive sorrow of an inescapable burden, can leave those who fought for his life feeling crushed too: crushed by a great weight of doubt and guilt. Yet in both cases intentions were only good. There are limits to knowledge and the limits of what can be predicted with certainty make this a decision fraught with problems. Where these errors of judgement happen to close relatives or friends of the doctors and neonatal nurses themselves, the issues are particularly acute and underline the serious nature of the consequences of decisions.

In any balance of burdens and benefits, much hinges on the perception of disability and it was interesting to find those who have worked closely with severely disabled people, are divided in their conclusions. Some see value in even the most severely limited life and go on to fight for each baby to be given a 'sporting chance'; others are appalled by the indignity and suffering involved and are persuaded that early death with dignity is preferable to a prolonged poor quality existence.

However, not all staff in NICUs have had close dealings with those who are seriously disabled. Working exclusively in a NICU can encourage a narrow and distorted view of life. Babies of 750g, babies dependent on ventilators, babies with rare congenital defects, become the norm. It can become habitual to strive to save any infant who draws breath; and the high powered technological environment can encourage a constant seeking for answers and a waging of war against death. If those so engaged do not see the long-term consequences of their activities, it is easy to measure success by the number of survivors. Those parents who return to the Unit to show off the baby subsequently are a self-selected group. It is salutary for staff to see the others too; the ones who have less or nothing to show off. But not all staff have this opportunity. Some, of course, do take a personal interest in certain families with whom they have established a special relationship. The lengths to which they go to support such parents are impressive, and to some extent following the families out into the community, attending the funerals, tracking their grief resolution, watching with them during a later pregnancy, are all activities which give a wider context for what has gone on in the NICU, although they are usually limited to one or two families. But consultants who see the infants repeatedly at follow-up clinics, community paediatricians or liaison sisters who continue to support families at home, can appreciate a longer term dimension which helps to give a more accurate framework for decision making. If the nurses and doctors in the Unit do not know that a family has disintegrated as a result of being burdened with a child who cannot even communicate with his parents, it is harder to appreciate the enormity of what was decided on their behalf by people who can go home after a stimulating day's work, enjoy a meal with their own children, take part in a game of squash, relax to Mozart, or take the dog for a long walk, their lives unruffled by the existence of someone else's profoundly damaged child.

The effect of experience in the nursery varies between individuals. In general nurses, seeing the results of their activities, tend to be concerned by the burden of pain and suffering often for limited gains, and move in the direction of feeling that treatment should be limited. But doctors are equally divided between this kind of concern and being excited by what can be done for these tiny patients, so wanting to give all babies the benefit of technological prowess. A number of explanations can be suggested for these differences. Being intimately involved with the babies' care the nurses are sensitive to their pain in the face of so many invasive measures. They spend long hours with the infants, dealing closely with the families and sharing their doubts and fears and tensions. Also when a decision is made to withdraw treatment, the nurse has a special role to play. It is often within her power to make the dying a meaningful experience for the parents, to ensure the baby lives out his last hours comfortably, surrounded by love and care. If she achieves 'a good death' experience for them, there is a resultant sense of satisfaction. She has done her job well. But the implications for the doctor are different. Neonatal care is dramatic and exciting work. Junior doctors, even though their work load is often immensely draining, can get 'a buzz' from the high powered experience. Seeing lives saved at the borderline of viability can initially impress them greatly. Not having known such results were possible they can be overtaken by a sense that anything is now feasible. Some very senior consultants confess that as time goes by they have lost some of their crusading fervour in the face of witnessing so much sorrow and suffering. They are then more cautious about inflicting a lifetime of unpleasant noxious stimuli on a baby, and sorrow and hardship on his family. Another factor relates to the perception of death by the two disciplines. If a baby dies, there can be a real sense of failure, and many doctors feel this even when death is clearly a preferable option to continued existence. Some do, of course, have a role in helping parents to adjust to a changed emphasis from aggressive hopeful treatment to comfort measures and the end of hope; others can prescribe analgesia and feel they are contributing to a sensitive management of a sad situation; but their involvement tends to be spasmodic. They do, however, unlike the nurses, have the advantage of having other happier work to help them maintain a healthy balance and keep the tragic cases in perspective. This difference in the role of the two disciplines, seems to explain their different viewpoints.

It is noteworthy that there appears to be a difference between withdrawing care which is simply prolonging dying and withdrawing care because one is afraid the child will live. In the former case once it is clear that treatment is futile the element of actively deciding that a child should die is absent. In the latter, it is apparent that one is considering and judging what constitutes a good enough quality of life and what is an unacceptable burden.

PERSONAL EXPERIENCE
Personal experience can also powerfully influence how people feel about these decisions to forego treatment. The range is wide and varied, but the commonest experiences staff can identify are having contact with disabled people, losing people close to them, and being a parent themselves. But whether their experience was of growing up on a farm where death was commonplace, or losing their own pregnancy or baby, or being involved in deciding whether to switch off the ventilator for their own mother, these events can have two effects. They can change the individual's personal response to the question of whether and when decisions should be made to stop treating infants. They can also affect their sensitivity to the needs of a baby's family. It was interesting to note the respondents' subjective assessment of the outworking of this increased awareness. There was some evidence that others did not always perceive that they had developed special skills.

Conclusions

Clearly there are many powerful factors at work – many unseen and often unrecognized – which are playing a part in the decision making process. Each individual concerned is bringing something of their own history, experience, values and beliefs to the situation. It is important not to underestimate these influences. But a degree of insight and critical analysis is required if the effects of these experiences are to be used positively. For there can be a danger that prejudice or ill-founded beliefs may have resulted which can subsequently sway their judgement. If senior figures too can gain understanding of their colleagues in the team, they will be better able to deal sensitively with potential tensions or conflicts. Not knowing about their background and beliefs can result in a denial of valuable contributions or violation of deeply held convictions.

These will always be agonising decisions and some unpacking of the components is desirable. But too much cannot be expected: tragic decisions need to be made 'which are not necessarily the easier for the understanding.'[152]

CHAPTER EIGHT

Impairments and Disabilities

It has long been recognized that, if a child is destined for a life of crippling disability which will prevent him from enjoying a meaningful life with a measure of independence, then for many people it seems perfectly proper to consider withholding or withdrawing extraordinary or aggressive treatment which would sustain or prolong that life. But clearly there are a number of questions which arise in relation to this practice.

Severe impairment as a reason for withdrawing or withholding treatment

Respondents were asked whether they felt that there should ever be an option to withdraw or withhold treatment because of severe impairment. (The term *impairment* was used rather than *disability* since for neonates the effect of many impairments on the individual's ability cannot be determined.) Some prefaced their response with a statement regretting the fact that society had produced a situation where parents had come to expect a perfect child.

> 'I think society's influenced us into thinking in a lot of ways that handicaps are terrible – they're abnormal ... the [kind of mentality] – if you don't have a perfect baby, then you don't really want second best. And I think, to some extent, that it maybe infiltrates our thinking too, that because we've got all this wonderful intensive care, we've got to be 100 per cent all the time. The babies have got to be 100 per cent. And they're not.' (Staff midwife, less than 5 years experience)

> 'I totally oppose a society who would just want very intelligent people walking around. And I think we could be all humbled by the child with a handicap, whether it is physical or mental ... Although I don't wish them on anybody, if they happen to be there, you don't differentiate.' (Consultant, more than 25 years experience)

Just over three-quarters of each group thought there should be an option not to treat on the grounds of a severe impairment (45, 79% of the doctors; 94, 79% of the nurses). A further two of the doctors, and one nurse, said that this was a very difficult question, and declined to give a definite answer. Two doctors and five nurses said they simply did not know. However, 8 of the doctors (14%) and 19 of the nurses (16%) felt that impairment should not be a criterion for withholding treatment. This last group included staff who were themselves the parents of impaired children and who spoke eloquently of the loss in their own lives if their children had been allowed to die.

Amongst those who considered that impairment was a reason to stop treating, all except a tiny minority (1 doctor and 6 nurses) said that the severity of the impairment influenced their decision. For the vast majority, the decision was based on a number of factors which included, alongside the severity of the baby's condition, the parents' wishes, beliefs and ability to cope.

A major factor in the respondents' choice to withhold or withdraw treatment in cases of severe impairment related to the futility of treating and the right to a dignified and pain free death. It seemed totally inappropriate to fill a short life with unnecessary invasive procedures and deprive a family of the opportunity to enjoy those precious hours in peace and privacy.

> 'I think in some conditions, if you say, "Well, we know that this condition is incompatible with life, so do we really need to have this baby on a saturation monitor, heart monitor, and this monitor and that monitor, and 5 drips in the baby? What does the baby actually need for it to be peaceful?" ... I think there are certain times when you have to take all these things away, and take the baby somewhere warm and quiet with the family and let them know a sense of – probably from a Christian point of view [the sacredness of this little life].' (Staff midwife, less than 5 years experience)

At other times it could seem appropriate to continue treatment for the family's sake even when the baby's condition was so severe that treatment would otherwise be futile. A number of graphic descriptions were provided. In one case a pregnant woman had died suddenly in a general hospital ward of a severe cardiac condition. The baby was delivered immediately by Caesarean Section. Though in poor condition and with a hopeless prognosis, the child was kept alive while the father and grandparents took in the enormity of the mother's death. In such cases the needs of the family were seen to take precedence over those of the baby.

Many people made reference to the problem of deciding what constitutes a good quality of life. To make decisions which end in a child's death based on a quality of life judgement is an awesome responsibility. It is also something that a considerable number were loth to do even though they subscribed to a general sense that some impairments were worse than death.

> 'It's very difficult because what one person's – [the] quality of life that they think is great, is not another person's ...If I couldn't run, if I couldn't think, if I couldn't feed – that would be dreadful for me. But obviously at the same time there are other people that as long as they can hear music or whatever, then that is quality of life for them. And I don't know how you resolve that ... So I don't know where you decide what disability is not worth it. I think pain has to be a big feature. If you think, or you know, that this child's going to go through years of agony at that hospital, lots of operations, I think that's a big factor, because I think, it destroys any quality of life if it's severe enough. That's a problem, but you just don't know how much awareness these kids have got. And if they're aware enough to know that somebody loves them, is that enough? I don't know how you answer that.' (SHO, more than 1 year experience)

Perceptions of mental and physical impairment

Proportionately more doctors (35, 61%) than nurses (53, 45%) differentiated in their own minds between mental and physical impairment. Almost all of these respondents considered physical impairment to be preferable to mental – this included all of the doctors who differentiated and all except three of the nurses.

> 'I don't think it's for us to decide what is a useful life someone can have or not, from the point of view of physical disability. I find it much more easy to feel that if someone is going to be a complete neurological and mental write-off, that they will not have a happy meaningful existence, and they won't be able to have a meaningful existence within the context of a family. And I don't have any problem with that. But there's lots and lots of very [physically] handicapped people who lead very fulfilling lives and physical disability wouldn't be an indication to not offer care, in my view.' (Senior Registrar, more than 5 years experience)

One nurse who was herself a mother of a child with severe learning difficulties, echoed the basic sentiment but from a very different perspective. She spoke eloquently of the problems accruing from having a child who looked normal behaving in socially unacceptable ways, volunteering that there was greater public tolerance of children with obvious conditions like Down's Syndrome. For her, physical impairments would have been infinitely preferable since the child 'would have a mind of their own.' Appearance was a factor mentioned by a few other staff too. Initially giving birth to a physically abnormal baby was seen to be a great shock to a mother because it was so visible, they could not escape the fact of the abnormality, whereas babies with mental damage could look perfectly normal. It was only later that the real enormity of a mental impairment impinged on parents. By that time many had become very attached to the child, there was no longer a readily available window of opportunity for stopping treatment, and in any case, withdrawal was emotionally a harder proposition.

The three who felt that mental impairment would be preferable, did so because in their judgement it would be extremely frustrating and damaging to be mentally alert but trapped in a severely disabled body, whereas a severely mentally damaged child could well be unaware of his handicaps. Much hinged on the degree of damage.

For a substantial number (18, 31% of doctors and 56, 46% of nurses) it was either difficult or impossible to differentiate. Eight nurses and three doctors observed that the two so often co-existed in babies that it was difficult to consider them separately. A few people volunteered that they would feel differently about this distinction if the child was their own, but they did not in practice differentiate for their infant patients.

Selecting babies for withholding or withdrawing treatment

It is clear from the literature that there is no absolute consensus about the circumstances in which it is appropriate to consider non-treatment. Attempts have been made to define 'customary medical care' without success.[30] There is, however, a general feeling that where there is no brain, or no intestine, treatment is futile.

For the present enquiry there were two reasons for asking respondents to outline those conditions in neonates which might prompt them to contemplate stopping or not initiating treatment: to understand the range of impairments or medical conditions; and to help them to concentrate on the scenarios which formed the basis for the subsequent quite deep probing for understanding. Early on in the research it was apparent that respondents frequently had difficulty identifying conditions, so unless they readily and spontaneously volunteered such information, a series of options were suggested for their consideration from anencephaly through to Down's Syndrome. Senior doctors readily understood the question and responded without prompting; very few nurses answered unprompted.

There is little to be learned from reporting absolute figures of the number of people who cited different conditions. Nevertheless a general picture emerged which sets a context for later analysis.

Even those staff who had a very high cut-off point which meant that they were extremely reluctant to withdraw or withhold treatment, all considered that it was futile to treat babies with conditions which were incompatible with even a short life, such as anencephaly. A few respondents expressed surprise that the question should even be asked.

There was more uncertainty where there was a possibility of a short life (for example Trisomy 13 or 18). A number of respondents felt that the emphasis should be on ensuring a 'good death'; only that length of life should be facilitated which was commensurate with dignity and freedom from suffering.

> 'I think with disorders that we know are likely to be fatal within the first days, weeks, months, even years, I would feel that we should be looking more at the quality of death. And if this child is going to die anyway, they can use death as peaceful for the child, and also as peaceful, and hopefully constructive, as possible for the family.' (SHO, less than 1 year experience)

Some staff mentioned the importance of giving parents the time to build up memories of their child. Furthermore a small number of consultants described cases where parents of such infants had requested that they be treated and the child had lived some considerable time against all expectations. If that was the parents' wish, these doctors were not averse to complying with it, provided the families were aware of the consequences of their choices. In a sense, since their prognosis was bleak anyway, there was nothing to lose from offering a little latitude.

> 'I would be confident that whatever I did for that baby, the baby would be dead in a year's time. So, you can make the wrong decision and nature will still help you out.' (Consultant, less than 10 years experience)

However, there were others who regarded this kind of compliance with parental wishes as inappropriate. Treatment in such cases was futile and should not be offered. This was especially so where the treatment itself was unpleasant for the child.

'Where the child's active life at the present is being made miserable by your treatment, that's the most important thing. If you have a child who has a strong chance of being retarded – you know that they might not be, but there's a good chance – and he's lying there in pain, has had days of misery and pain – not being able to have his IV sites out; infected; all sorts of things ... And you can imagine yourself in that situation and the pain and misery you must be in. And once the family then start to see, "What are we doing this for?", then I think the treatment should be withdrawn. It's a combination of things.' (Sister, more than15 years experience)

Extremely premature infants with multiple complications were a group where the majority of the staff working in these Neonatal Units felt it was appropriate sometimes not to treat. They should for the most part be given a chance initially but it was not a kindness to the child to pursue aggressive measures when it was clear the immaturity of the infant's systems precluded a good outcome. But where the child lived a long time developing complications and impairments sequentially it appeared harder to withdraw.

'Older babies, this is where I feel it's a difficult area. Babies who started off really small, and who have chronic lung disease and they're ventilated and their lungs are just really, really bad. They're really sick ... and they "go off", need to be resuscitated or re-ventilated. And it's like a scenario that goes on and on. And you get to the stage where you'll have had so many hypoxic episodes they obviously have some damage. That's a difficult decision to make.' (Sister, more than 5 years experience)

Birth asphyxia was a much more controversial area since the decision hinged on so many uncertainties. Many staff observed that the outcome was so unpredictable and babies not infrequently defied predictions. Seeing those infants for whom withdrawal of treatment had been seriously considered, recover relatively unscathed, added to their reluctance to commit themselves to a decision not to treat in future similar cases. There could too, be underlying worries about medical errors. As one SHO put it:

'A full-term baby – you feel extremely sorry. You feel shocked. It takes months to recover from that stressful, horrible situation. So you try your best to save them ... I'll feel guilty because probably there has been some lapse somewhere that led to this situation.'

When it came to congenital abnormalities, the clearest picture emerged for those babies with multiple anomalies. The odds were stacked against these babies and it was not a kindness to prolong their lives. One consultant described it as 'meddlesome' to intervene when all that was being done was to prolong the inevitable dying. Single problems, however, were generally more amenable to treatment, and children could be helped to maximize their potential. It was noteworthy that only relatively small numbers instanced severe neural tube defects as a reason not to treat. Kuhse and Singer singled out spina bifida with associated myelomeningocele as a form of severe abnormality which has occasioned much vigorous debate in relation to selective non-treatment.[30] However, nowadays this condition is rare thanks to a natural decline and the effects of prenatal diagnosis. A considerable number of respondents in this study reported that they had either never seen such a baby with spina bifida, or had seen too few to feel competent in assessing their outcome. The majority also commented that they could not give a blanket yes or no for this group of babies since it depended on a variety of other factors such as the site of the lesion, the extent of the damage to mobility and sensation, the expectation of pain and suffering, and the parents' ability to cope.

> '[Severe neural tube defects], that's more difficult, because I've seen spina bifida children – spina bifida adolescents – that are just magic people and they're so full of life, and love life, and are a joy to be around ... but then you see the other side of it, and you're restricted to what you do to a certain degree ... But it's very difficult unless you have some sort of crystal ball to be able to say, "This is how your child will be at 16 or 18" or whatever.' (Staff nurse, less than 5 years experience)

Where anomalies meant a future of repeated aggressive therapy, respondents had serious misgivings.

> 'The sort of heart things that I think are most tragic are the ones that are going to require several sets of surgery and not have a good long-term outcome ... complex congenital heart disease where you might rescue a child for a few years and then it'll die when it's in its teens, or be heading for a transplant. I think transplants and the traumas associated with that, and the anti-rejection treatments, and that – it's much under-estimated as well. Now, I wouldn't want a child of my own to have a transplant. And I think if I had an option to withdraw earlier, I would want to.' (Registrar, less than 5 years experience)

Some consultants had thought long and hard about the effect of traumatic treatments and had taken it upon themselves not to even mention certain options to parents. They were not unmindful of the ethical issues behind such actions.

> 'I personally do not believe that the outcome from the surgical attempts that are going on really warrant their use, and so I would recommend not treating – even to the extent of not necessarily discussing some of them with the parents. Now that becomes a difficult issue ... you're not actually giving them all the information that's necessarily around, but you are giving them – maybe – hopefully – what you think is a balanced opinion. I'm not sure what that is. Depends on the parents.' (Consultant, more than 10 years experience)

Nor was it only unusual treatments which produced reservations. A few respondents had their own reasons for viewing quite common invasive measures with misgivings. Such unease could materially affect their judgement about when the burden of treatment outweighed the benefits.

'I've actually been ventilated myself ... so I know from personal experience. Although we paralyse and sedate our babies, we didn't until quite recently. And I must admit, I kept saying to the nurses, "Look, you should try being on a ventilator." I was paralysed and sedated. Unfortunately, the paralysis was still working when the sedation was wearing off. So although I was paralysed, I could hear everything. And the worst thing I can ever remember was them coming to do ET toilet, because they are taking off your means of survival. And of course, if you're paralysed, you can't feel, you can't move. You're lying there and you are absolutely paralysed.' (Staff Midwife, more than 5 years experience)

Not a single respondent considered Down's Syndrome a reason to withdraw treatment. It was interesting to find that a considerable number knew people with Down's Syndrome and the idea of deciding those lives were not worth living was abhorrent to them. As one person commented, maybe if more staff knew survivors with other conditions, tolerance levels would change.

Defining the line

As was the plan, listing the conditions helped the doctors and nurses to focus on the specific groups who might be candidates for limited treatment. Once they had thought about these particular babies, respondents were then asked to try to define the criteria which helped them to draw their line. Since this question was completely open ended and no guidance was given regarding categories, descriptions varied widely. It would have been possible to subsume certain factors under broader headings, but in doing so something of the fineness of the distinctions people made would be lost. For example, many of the categories could reasonably have been categorized as quality of life factors but they actually captured something more precise. Therefore items have been reported separately better to reflect the subtlety of the differentiations made by staff working in clinical practice (Fig. 8.1). The exact numbers are not as important as the overall picture. It should be pointed out that staff were only too aware that a deal of uncertainty of prognosis attaches to many of the factors identified.

The predominant factor which weighed with doctors and nurses in their decision making was the quality of life the infant might expect to have. Where the pain and suffering were estimated to be extremely burdensome, with little compensating benefits the balance could be tipped in the direction of death. But where there was a commensurate benefit in terms of loving relationships and an ability to interact meaningfully with the environment and with other people, the balance might go the other way. Much appeared to hinge on the perceptions of the staff about what constituted a heavy burden and what was a rewarding level of attainment. Some freely admitted that what they would consider too burdensome for their own child was not the same thing as what they regarded as a burden too great to be borne by other people's children. This differential meant that they continued treating their patients longer than they felt intellectually they would choose to do for their own child.

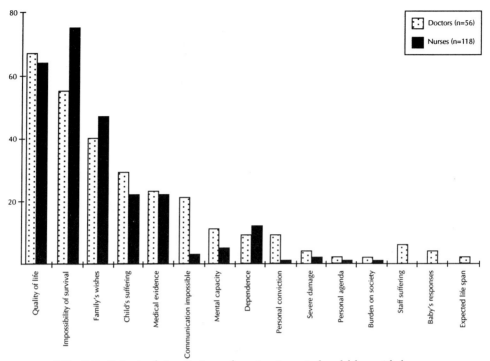

Fig. 8.1: Criteria determining when treatment should be withdrawn

In general, being unable to interact or communicate with others was seen to be a state of being worse than death. As one consultant put it:

> 'We're really nothing at all and we've got no potential if we're not thinking – communicating in some sort of way – humans. Because communicating is what separates us out from a collection of cells. We can keep all the other things going in terms of heart, lungs, kidneys and so on, but really what differentiates us is our capacity to communicate.'

For such infants, deciding to withdrawing treatment was relatively straightforward. The difficulty came in being certain of the prognosis.

Further along the continuum, where an infant was capable of some interaction, factors like mental capacity, level of disability, and extent of dependence on others or on medical intervention, all came into the evaluation. Again, however, the dilemma was in knowing the exact outcome for any given child. There was a marked difference between senior medical staff and the nurses in relation to this point. Whereas the nurses tended to cite 'poor quality of life' as a reason for withdrawing treatment, the doctors were more guarded in their categorization, qualifying their criteria with observations about the difficulty in actual practice of knowing how disabled a particular baby would be. This made it relatively easy to give broad statements about the factors which defined their line, but much more difficult to implement these distinctions in real life.

Another influencing factor which helped staff to draw their line related to the parents. Their reactions, wishes and values could materially affect the quality of life the infant might experience. However, there appeared to be a general reluctance to say that decisions about whether a baby lived were actually influenced by parents' wishes. Rather such information provided a context against which estimates could be made about how far the child might be expected to realise his full potential or be helped to enjoy the life he had.

Stories were recounted of families who had surprised the respondents by their reactions. For example, one consultant told of a family where a baby who was severely affected with cerebral palsy died following elective surgery. This baby had been largely looked after by her sister and the staff expected that she would feel relief at the lifting of this burden. They were surprised to find her utterly devastated by the loss and the consultant concluded:

> 'That's why I find life difficult now, because my perception of how families will cope is different from how families *do* cope.'

It also sometimes appeared that parents were setting things up to allow the child to die without having explicitly to request such a step.

> 'I think there comes a time when the parents come to the end of the line as well ... sometimes they get to the stage where they're relieved when somebody says that the next time [the baby needs resuscitating] we're not doing anything ... We had a situation the other night where a baby had a cardiac arrest. Now, I don't think any of us think that baby is ever going to get out of here – [she's] so badly damaged ... We couldn't raise the parents on the phone that night. They knew how ill the baby was. To me, if [someone] turns round and say, 'I can't hear the phone,' then I think they've reached the stage where they maybe don't answer the phone in the hope that someone's going to tell them that it's over, and they haven't had to make a decision. It's the way I look at it.' (Staff midwife, more than 5 years experience)

Overall the decision appeared to be based on a consideration of a combination of these factors rather than on any one alone.

Discussion

It has been suggested that quality of life judgements are based on discrimination:

> 'Stigma then is a socially created phenomenon ... Quality of life, too, is a socially (and politically) constructed phenomenon, forged in a crucible of discriminatory beliefs and practices.'[5]

Professionals working at the cutting edge of medical advances with infants regret society's prejudice against disabled people and emphasize the importance of valuing these individuals. They do not, however, wish to add to the number of people suffering from major disability and their acceptance of some discrimination between babies who should be treated is not seen to run counter to their wish to have the lives of disabled people enhanced.

Furthermore they are all too aware that life and death decisions are based on much agonising and discussion about what is in the best interests of the child, taking a wide range of factors into account. There is nothing cavalier about them. Their judgements reflect much more a compassionate understanding of the impact of severe impairment and disability on the lives of children and their families, rather than a prejudice against imperfection. Staff regret the influence of the media which appear to have promoted a belief in society that couples are entitled to a perfect child and that miracles are commonplace. They are themselves only too conscious of the limits of modern medicine and, working with an unusually high quota of babies for whom things have gone less than well, they are more alive to the potential for tragedy in childbearing than the majority of the population.

Actually making the decision is a complex and painful process. Many factors influence the final choice and it is this very variety which makes the use of a specific framework for decision making so difficult. But without such a yardstick there is great scope for individual pressures to bear on the decision with undue weight. Some have attempted to encapsulate the essence of what has to be decided, most notably clinicians in the Netherlands. Dutch paediatricians have addressed these issues squarely and produced a number of clear documents which spell out their consensus and differences. Although they recognize the uniquely personal aspect of each individual judgement they are also persuaded that prognostic assessments about the future quality of a child's life are part of the task of paediatricians faced with the momentous task of deciding whether or not to treat a baby. In essence when it comes to deciding the quality of an infant's life, they suggest there are five questions to be asked:

1.   What will the burden, both physical and mental, of the infant's life be compared to the joy of that life? The extent to which that burden can be lightened by caregivers is an important consideration.
2.   To what extent will this infant be capable of interacting meaningfully with his environment?
3.   Will the child ever become self-sufficient or will he always be dependent on others?
4.   Will the child remain dependent on medical services?
5.   What is the expected life span of this infant?[37]

In Britain there has been continuing debate about these issues taking up all these numbered points but so far no authoritative guidelines for clinicians facing these important decisions have emerged. The overall picture is one of general acceptance that some conditions are worse than death and that it is sometimes appropriate not to treat an infant if the burdens of doing so outweigh the corresponding benefits. Most such decisions hinge on what kind of quality of life that child can expect. Quality of life decisions are 'not only difficult and subjective but also common and necessary.'[153]

Quality of life

A good quality of life is thought to exist 'where there are good prospects for a child achieving a cognitive, sapient and interactive life free from the kind of crippling disability that would prevent normal relationships and independence.'[34] In 1988 three Aberdeen paediatricians wrote that they considered it entirely appropriate and ethical to draw lines limiting treatment at specific gestational ages and under certain circumstances.[34] They suggested 500g at 22–24 weeks was a logical point at which to set this demarcation. But this was no arbitrary limit: quality of life criteria justified the distinction. In 1996 there are very few people who appear prepared to set a specific limit on the lower edge of viability.

Differentiating between impairments

A general feeling prevails that physical impairments are to be preferred to mental deficits, although much depends on the severity of either deficit and the awareness of the individual. Certainly at the severe end of the spectrum where a child is incapable of making meaningful relationships, his life is considered worse than death. There is much written in the literature to support this belief since 'it is one's mental status that determines the essence of one's existence.'[50] But it becomes much harder to make judgements about the balance of burden and benefit when the level of awareness and capacity for communication and interaction is higher. There is then much uncertainty and difference of opinion amongst health care professionals. When this general insecurity is further confounded by the uncertainty of prognosis, there are major conceptual and emotional issues to be grappled with. Again and again this issue of the difficulty of being sure of the outcome was raised and it is clearly a dominant feature in any deliberations.

When it comes to the types of conditions which merit withholding or withdrawing treatment, a general pattern emerges. At one end of the scale, if the condition of the child is known to be incompatible with life, it is inappropriate to prolong it unnecessarily. At the other end, if a child has an abnormality which is not sufficiently severe to preclude the possibility of a reasonably good quality of life, then there appears to be universal agreement about the necessity to give that child every chance. In between are all types of conditions and all shades of opinion.

For children with the most severe intellectual impairment such as those with anencephaly, it has been argued that they can be seen not to have interests: interest in life only holds if that life holds some good for the child.[154] Where brain injury is so severe as to render the individual incapable of forming human relationships, human life is reduced to a level of mere biological survival.[155] Since the situation is irredeemable, treatment would be futile. The little girl with anencephaly kept alive in the United States of America mentioned earlier cannot be seen to have any kind of meaningful life from her own point of view: it is only her mother who gains pleasure from her continued existence not the child herself. Similarly for a child with no intestine there is no prospect of survival and the futility of treatment means that staff can accept with equanimity and what seems to be universal agreement the fact that prolonging dying is not indicated.

But there appear to be few conditions which come into the category where it can be said with certainty, from the infant's point of view, that continued existence is a fate worse than death. It is not appropriate to take the perspective of the normal healthy adult. The infant has no other experience and a disabled life would appear in most circumstances to be preferable to no life at all. Incessant unrelievable pain, or inability to even minimally recognize one's surroundings, or imminent and unavoidable death are the sorts of circumstances which might make death preferable to life.

Where the condition is not immediately fatal but carries a poor prognosis other factors impinge. The parents' wishes or the way the infant responds are additional criteria which help to decide the length of life and the extent of intervention. Infants in this category include the extremely premature and compromised, and those with multiple anomalies. Congenital abnormalities which are not necessarily fatal but imply a life of disability require decisions to be made about the cost to the child of treatment against the benefits of continued survival. It was pointed out time and time again that many treatments carry their own burdens. The effects of invasive procedures should not be underestimated just because they are commonly practised. More than one respondent had themselves been ventilated; some had had serious illnesses involving painful and debilitating or undignified treatments. They are all too aware of the horror of some of the things done to babies who can register no verbal protest and who cannot withhold consent. Since many of the germane factors are very difficult to assess, these decisions are often protracted and based on much soul searching for all those involved. But in general staff find it easier to accept the death of an extremely premature infant since their initial survival is a relatively recent triumph of medical intervention and against the normal laws of nature. The deaths of full-term babies or those who have survived for long periods in the nursery are emotionally harder to accept and are perhaps resisted more vigorously at times.

Full-term infants who are severely birth asphyxiated are one of the most problematic groups encountered. So many staff refer to them as 'beautiful babies' who look so normal. The stark contrast with what 'should have been' makes their case the more poignant. But their prognosis is difficult to be sure of and the window of opportunity for the withdrawal of treatment remains open for only a limited period of time. Practice as far as these infants are concerned varies widely. While some consultants withdraw after just 15 minutes of resuscitative effort, others continue to treat for protracted periods and may eventually send the children home to await an infection or a medical emergency which is then not treated.

At the far end of the continuum from the anencephalic children, are those with abnormalities which are compatible with a life of reasonable quality. Children with uncomplicated Down's Syndrome come into this category. But as Geddes and colleagues pointed out,

> 'A diagnosis of Down's Syndrome has very little prognostic value in itself; one must know about the particular combination of abnormalities from which the child suffers.'[156]

Some have accompanying defects which may or may not be readily correctable, and it is here that differences of opinion creep in. As we have already seen, much of the legal literature and a number of the landmark court cases have centred on children with Down's Syndrome, although there has been doubt expressed about the wisdom of certain court rulings.[154] In general the attitude in relation to Down's Syndrome has changed over the years. Now it is accepted that such children 'should not be denied a chance of happiness for want of a simple operation.'[157]

It is apparent then, that in drawing their lines beyond which treatment is discontinued, staff rely heavily on their perception of the quality of life that child may expect to have. The influence of parental capacity and expectations is clearly secondary to those factors which directly affect the prospects for the child himself.

As we have already discussed, the long-term consequences of severe impairments are not always appreciated by staff whose work is physically limited to the NICU. But as one respondent said whose job entailed trying to improve the potential of such babies after their discharge from hospital and after the diagnosis of devastating damage:

> '[Doctors in NICUs] look at a child and see this child needs oxygen, needs an IV. They are looking at an organism and trying to keep it alive. Maybe if they had more exposure to what these kids do as they get older, what we have to offer, what's required of them, maybe they would see that some heroic measures are only briefly heroic and may actually open the gate to a lot of suffering. I do think that a lot of people are going by the technological and legal imperative rather than according to an intuitive ethical sense or personal knowledge of what happens to children like these on a day-to-day basis.'

Actually knowing individuals with certain conditions sometimes opens people's eyes to the joys of that life in a surprising way. Many respondents have known people with Down's Syndrome or spina bifida who enjoyed a good quality of life. The point was well made that perhaps if more staff knew people with other conditions and saw for themselves their potential and achievements, they might be better able to appreciate the perspectives of a person who has known no other kind of life. When able-bodied mentally normal people are sitting in judgement their personal standards will inevitably reflect their own expectations and experiences.

It was sobering to hear so many people admit that the decision they think they would make for their own child is not the same as that they would make for someone else's child. Here again personal histories, expectations and hopes will influence attitudes. Of course, it has to be borne in mind that few can say with certainty what they would do in this hypothetical situation unless past experience has tested their resolve, and several nurses acknowledged the power of a maternal love which desires the life of the child almost at all costs. This very uncertainty about how any family will respond when faced with a severely impaired child adds to the other factors which make it so difficult to make this grave decision about whether or not a child should live.

Conclusions

A great deal of uncertainty bedevils decision making on behalf of neonates. It is impossible to lay down hard and fast rules or even firm yardsticks for practice. Only in those cases where the condition is incompatible with life are the issues clear cut. In every other case benefits must be carefully weighed against burdens, keeping the interests of the baby to the fore although recognizing that these decisions have wider implications for others too. Tolerances of families vary enormously. But deciding on behalf of another human being, especially one who has only just embarked on life, what constitutes an acceptable quality of life, is an awesome responsibility. It is right that much agonising goes into every such decision.

CHAPTER NINE

Current Procedures

In order to understand staff attitudes and opinions it seemed important to obtain a picture of the general context for what currently happens in the different Units. Respondents were invited to describe the procedures involved when treatment was being withdrawn. A number of factors should be borne in mind in the interpretation of these findings. This was an open question and staff were not always comprehensive in their responses. Some clearly assumed basic understanding of what was done and simply supplied detail about areas where there might be variations, while others recounted every step of the process.

Individual experiences varied and did not necessarily reflect a standard way of dealing with these cases. A small number, for example, volunteered that they had only watched one consultant in operation so could not say how the practice of the others compared with what they had seen. Certain circumstances – particularly well managed ones or those which were badly handled – tended to stay in the memory and were sometimes described in detail. It was not possible therefore to compare in any rigorous way the perceptions of the different members of staff in each Unit. Rather the data have been used to provide an overall context for practice in each centre. Strenuous efforts have been made to protect the identity of Units.

As well as information gained at interview, there was opportunity for the researcher to observe practice and listen to informal conversation both in the nursery areas and coffee rooms. Furthermore in some Units consultants made a point of discussing various points and cases with her which added usefully to an understanding of the mechanisms by which decisions were arrived at, and of practices and procedures in that hospital. In some of the Units there were ongoing as well as very recent cases, where treatment withdrawal was under consideration. The issues were in the forefront of the minds of staff and gave a particular urgency and clarity to descriptions of events and justifications for action taken.

It was interesting to find that a considerable number of staff assumed that there was only one way of proceeding – the way they had seen things done in their own Unit. Many used expressions like 'of course' and 'naturally' and 'obviously', to preface their statements, indicating that they believed these things to be universally practised.

A number of areas germane to the decision making will be described in sub-sections to try to unravel those factors which set a scene for these difficult deliberations. In as much as some factors are closely intertwined it is difficult to describe one without reference to another: thus defining the personnel involved comes after a report of the discussion process but clearly to a large extent this is an artificial divide. However some organization of the material is necessary in order to throw light on what happens. The subsections, then, encompass four themes: the discussion around the decision itself; the involvement of different people; the nature of the withdrawal itself; and the documentation.

Discussion around the decision itself
Initiating the discussion re non-treatment
In most Units it was reported that a feeling emerged that certain babies simply were not progressing well and that withdrawing treatment might be a better option than continuing. Peer groups discussed their feelings together before they were more openly shared. In the university based hospitals it tended to be the consultant who first broached this subject in a multidisciplinary forum although some consultants said they did not do so until they had seen or heard evidence that others were thinking along the same lines. They said they listened to what others told them, watched for reactions at ward rounds and asked certain persons to sound out their colleagues to see if there was general agreement. This could be a fairly subtle process and junior nurses did not always appreciate that the consultants were listening and observing for such cues. From their standpoint it felt as if the consultant acted in isolation and their own views were inconsequential.

A notable exception was one of the DGH Units where consultants were all part-time paediatricians. Here the idea of withdrawing treatment started with the nurses: they were the ones to call the consultant in, alert him to the poor condition of an infant, and suggest that perhaps treatment should be re-orientated towards comfort measures.

Team discussion
Prolonged discussion around these difficult cases was clearly the norm in all Units. Discussion amongst professional staff could take place beside the baby, on ward rounds, in coffee or changing rooms, or in chance encounters. It seemed to be rare for a case conference to be held and at this juncture only one respondent reported such an occurrence.

In some Units considerable efforts had been made to try to integrate the different groups of staff. These included introducing shared coffee areas, replacing a square table with a round one and making it a practice to sit round the table; timing breaks to ensure mixing occurred; inviting all grades of staff to arranged informal events; sponsoring staff on fund-raising ventures. Where there were obvious hard divisions between the staff such as different rooms, or set break times for different grades, there was much less opportunity for informal discussion of troubling cases. It required more effort to actually go and have a discussion with someone of a senior rank and junior staff were more inhibited about expressing their own opinions.

Timing of the decision making

In two of the Units the decision to withdraw was made only rarely and then in circumstances where it was quite clear the infant was close to death. The staff reported going through a process of doing tests to be quite sure that the baby could not survive, before they withdrew treatment. They would withdraw all medication for some time in order to be confident that other symptoms were not being masked by the drugs. Additionally in two of the other Units, one or more of the consultants was reportedly so reluctant to make the decision to stop that a similar situation could arise, unless one of his colleagues intervened. But elsewhere consultants made the decision much earlier and included factors related to quality of future life in the equation.

In general there were major differences between the two disciplines about the timing of withdrawal. Nurses wanted doctors to decide more quickly than they did to stop treatment. On the other hand there were rare occasions where consultants acted in a way which seemed precipitate or premature by other colleagues. If they were not involved in the discussion, more junior staff could be left feeling the decision had been made on the basis of social factors or the consultant's own abhorrence of disability, rather than the illness of the baby. This gave cause for grave disquiet.

Personnel involved

Doctors, nurses and parents were the main people involved in the decision making in all six of the NICUs. Senior medical staff always participated in some way. Junior doctors tended to be involved in the initial treatment of all babies admitted to the NICU, but once serious discussion about stopping treatment began there was a greater tendency to limit the staff involved to a small number and more senior doctors took over the giving of information and instructions about management. The nursing staff were always involved to some extent since they were caring for the baby but the perceptions of the doctors and the nurses themselves varied about the extent to which they contributed to the decision.

It was rare for respondents spontaneously to mention the chaplain or minister of religion at this point even though, when subsequently questioned specifically about his role, they volunteered that his was a very important one. Social workers were cited by only two respondents out of the possible 176. Details about the perceived role of these different professionals are reserved for a later chapter.

Consultants' approach and relationships

Clearly each consultant is an individual and it would seem likely that each would practise in a slightly different way. Since theirs is the ultimate responsibility, the fact that they personally provided insight into the difficulties they encountered was both a testament to their integrity and courage as well as a most valuable contribution to the research findings.

In two Units no one reported any substantial differences between the practices of consultants in their Unit. In a third Unit, the two nurses who did perceive conflicts were in the minority, with a strong sense being conveyed by the majority that theirs was a very united team with the consultants all practising harmoniously even though they were quite different in their personalities and approaches. However, in the remaining three Units differences were great and caused considerable problems. Examples were recounted of open hostility; public confrontation; humiliation in front of colleagues; of an underhand usurping of another's responsibility for a baby; no-win situations where junior staff could not do right because opinions and instructions were inflexible and in opposition; of a consultant switching off a machine without informing either staff or parents and then simply walking away leaving the parents and nurses to find a deteriorating infant.

Where the consultant was seen as autocratic there were frustrations apparent in all other grades of staff. Even very senior sisters felt there was no outlet for their experienced opinions. It was interesting to discover that one such consultant, for defensive reasons, was actually practising in a way that went against his natural inclination and personal philosophy. This personal conflict was not known to his colleagues but seemed to go some way towards explaining his brusque manner.

Medical inconsistencies and perceived delays in making decisions were sources of concern for staff intimately involved with the babies. A sense was conveyed that such conflicts reflected badly on the care of babies and their parents as well as adding to the stress of the staff. If one consultant said to the parents and other staff that it was inappropriate aggressively to treat a given baby but another subsequently recommended that same child should have invasive treatment, the whole team as well as the parents were left bewildered and insecure. Junior doctors found it impossible to please all their seniors. In some cases they were obliged to change their practice daily in line with the consultant in charge at the time. This clearly had a knock-on effect through all grades of staff and to the families.

It was interesting to note that a number of the consultants (or their wives) had had traumatic perinatal experiences themselves (for example, infertility, miscarriage, cot death), or had had experience in their family with impaired children or the death of siblings in childhood. Several observed that they felt they had a special sensitivity in handling parents because they had had such experiences. However, this was not the perception of their colleagues, many if not all of whom were unaware of the personal histories of the consultants. Not one of the consultants who volunteered that they were especially sensitive in this way, featured among those consultants whom other staff rated as particularly good communicators.

The approach of the senior doctors could itself have an effect on the team and their effectiveness. Consultants who were too dominant in voicing their own views and decisions could easily inhibit others from being honest or sharing their concerns. Where they belittled others, shouted at staff in public, slammed doors, or were generally unavailable and unapproachable, more junior staff reported being less able to participate in discussion. On the other hand some behaviours helped staff to feel valued and cared for: the consultant dropping in on staff at all hours; taking the time to sit and listen to how they were feeling and coping both during and after the withdrawing process; being ready to go and talk to parents at the nurses' requests; sharing a coffee and discussion about a junior member of staff's concerns; or explaining the justification for a course of action to an individual or small group of people so that they understood why things were being managed in a particular way. It appeared to be a total sense of caring and sensitivity and a valuing of others which endeared consultants to their colleagues. This sensitive approach fostered a good team spirit and reduced tension.

In one harmonious Unit, the staff had shared a number of traumatic experiences together and appeared to have supported each other and grown closer through the shared pain. Staff of different grades and disciplines had cried together, listened to each other, and offered mutual comfort. By contrast in some Units, the consultants did not confide their own difficulties in other staff and there was a lack of appreciation of how each individual felt. Barriers were erected which prevented them gaining insight into each other's thinking and feelings. Sharing in the decision making, the thinking behind it, the attendant emotions, and the mechanics of the dying, led to closer cooperation and this in turn appeared to lessen resentments, jealousies and conflict.

It was apparent that some consultants established better relationships with their junior and nursing colleagues than did others. In informal discussion, and from observation as well as during interviews it became apparent that popularity, and respect as good practitioners were different factors. In three Units there was no remarked difference between the consultants in terms of ability to relate to colleagues or deal with parents. But in two Units, one consultant was singled out from his peers as the one who cared how the rest of the team felt, who really listened to what they said. Both were also considered to be particularly sensitive with parents. One of these consultants was also spoken of with affection, but the other, though highly respected as a caring and able specialist, was not well liked as an individual. In the sixth Unit, only one consultant would ever make the decision to stop treatment but he appeared to be most unpopular with the team.

Junior doctors' involvement

Junior doctors were variously involved in each of the Units. Much depended on their experience and personalities. But the juniors themselves reported considerable problems in their roles. They were the ones who were closely involved from the beginning. They felt the parents got to know them and were less in awe of them than of senior doctors. But they also recognized the hazards of their own limited knowledge or experience in dealing with potentially volatile situations with inherent legal and moral undertones. Where they felt adequately supported by their senior colleagues they learned through these experiences. But where there was inconsistency, poor communication or inadequate supervision, they felt very vulnerable and stressed.

It is noteworthy, that in the Unit with the least reported tension and the most united approach, junior doctors as well as nurses accompanied the consultant for discussions with parents.

The nurses' involvement

In all except one Unit, there were nurses who believed that the nursing staff were not sufficiently involved in the actual decision making, with a few feeling that the decision appeared to be unilaterally the consultants' with no real reference to other staff. In two Units junior staff reported that only one of the consultants checked their views on a given case. Elsewhere the consultants might well go through the motions of asking for their views, but the nurses felt that their contribution was more nominal than real. As one nurse put it, 'They hear but they don't listen.' Other consultants did not even go through the motions of hearing other opinions, by their own admission as well as in the perceptions of the nurses.

In all Units the nurses wanted the doctors to at least take a nursing representative along with them for discussions with parents. Being present meant they could give consistent information, reinforce what the doctor said, liaise between the different parties, and support the parents as appropriate. But in reality this ideal was not universally practised. In all except one Unit, there were some staff who felt that nurses inadequately participated. In three Units it was usual for the nurse to be involved but in the remaining three it often happened that the consultant went alone to talk with the parents. Some doctors simply preferred to take this consultation alone. Some felt that another person was intrusive at an intensely private moment. During the night or at particularly busy periods nursing staff could not always be freed up to attend. But some nurses felt that doctors did not make the effort to involve them even when there was no reason not to do so.

In one Unit only senior staff were ever involved in these difficult cases and there was considerable resentment reported by experienced junior staff who were the people caring for the babies. In as many as four of the six Units, senior nursing staff sometimes took over parts of the process once the case became one where withdrawal of treatment was a possible option. On occasion this meant junior staff were usurped from their role as key figure for the family. Sometimes the senior nurses who were singled out to accompany the consultant felt that their special role related only to the management of the case not to the decision making; they had not really been consulted about whether treatment should be withdrawn but they were being asked to manage the dying. It could be frustrating to be expected to deal with the consequences of a decision made by other people. In even more extreme cases, a consultant sometimes made a decision, pronounced it and then left the Unit. The rest of the team were left to deal with the aftermath as well as to organize events for the baby and the family, without there having been any discussion about any aspect of this case. Feelings ran high. The nurses themselves pointed out that there was much to be said in favour of their participation from the outset, rather than being asked whether they agreed with a decision which had already been taken.

> 'You're told that a decision's been made: "We're going to make this decision about treatment – what do you think?" Rather than having to wait until after the decision's been made and then say, "I'm not happy about providing this treatment." ... it's a lot harder to try and change the decision once it's been made. But if you're involved in the decision making, [it's like being asked] to plant the seed and watch it grow, rather than having to chop the tree down and start again.' (Staff midwife, more than 5 years experience)

It was, however, common practice for the nurse intimately involved in the care of the baby also to be present at discussions with the family, although some staff reported that this felt like a paper exercise; theirs was a token presence and they did not really contribute to the decision making. In some Units efforts were made to include juniors to some degree so that continuity was maintained and the juniors gained experience but it sometimes happened that nurses who had been intimately involved with families for some time felt usurped by sisters who 'took over.' In the perception of senior nursing staff themselves, such action was a form of protection both of less experienced colleagues and of families. One doctor commented that he preferred to involve the senior nurses, since those who were giving the hands-on care were more emotional and 'start crying or go away.' Permanent part-time night staff were one group who felt they could easily be left out in various ways. A few staff who had been employed in this capacity for many years had rarely if ever been involved in these sensitive cases.

Many junior nurses felt disadvantaged in terms of the information they had about a baby and family when discussions were taking place about withdrawal of aggressive treatment. They felt that they were not in possession of enough facts to really understand what was being discussed. From their position it appeared that doctors held the important discussions behind closed doors, or with only senior nursing colleagues present. A few consultants admitted that they did, indeed, only discuss such matters with senior colleagues leaving the sisters to ascertain the views of more junior staff and report back. More than one consultant hand-picked the staff with whom they discussed such cases since they knew those people who had sufficient experience to really understand the issues. These tended to be senior nurses who had established a relationship with the consultant over many years. For junior staff, this could feel like collusion amongst senior colleagues, and exclusion of their own valid input.

Communication between nurses was also a major cause of concern in two Units. In one of these, strong personalities created tensions which were palpable to the researcher. It was difficult to understand the origins of some of the hostilities but they appeared to relate to territory and status. In the other Unit there was unhappiness amongst the staff nurses and midwives because in their judgement the sisters did not undertake their fair share of the hands-on care and left the more junior group heavily overburdened with work. The reverse situation was seen in yet another Unit: it was difficult to find who was in charge because all staff worked with the babies equally. The nursing workforce was small and frequently overstretched but the different grades of staff worked closely together. In this Unit there was a notable lack of resentment and a very friendly and harmonious atmosphere. Clearly having a basic level of tension and unease amongst the staff, made other stresses, like difficult decision making, more burdensome. Additional stress was superimposed onto already demoralised people.

One aspect of the process was seen to be almost exclusively in the nurses' domain, however. In general it fell to them to manage the dying process. Even in those Units where they were not involved in the discussion around the decision itself, they took pride in ensuring the baby's comfort and dignity, and helping parents to have as positive an experience as they could facilitate.

The parents' involvement

In all six Units there was heavy emphasis on involving the parents in decision making as well as in the management of the dying baby. Indeed a number of nurses reported that it was really the doctor with the parents who made the decision, and the rest of the team simply fell in with their wishes.

However, it usually fell to the nurses to find out what the parents wanted and to tailor management accordingly. A wide variety of activities were reported to ensure that events were orchestrated in tune with parental wishes and needs. Staff talked of waiting until the parents were ready for the next step; of ensuring they were involved in the care of the child before, during and after the dying; of involving other relatives; of slowly weaning the baby off of the ventilator; of putting the baby into another room or ward, into pretty clothes, or a cot; or of giving drugs to reassure the family that the child was not suffering.

A major role for the parents themselves was seen to be ensuring that the baby died surrounded by love and comfort. If they were unwilling or unable to provide this the nurses felt they should substitute for the parents.

> 'If nobody wanted to come to see the baby, I wouldn't want that baby to die without somebody holding on to it. So even if nobody from the family [comes], one of us would cuddle it. Even adults as well, I never liked [them to die alone]. You know how you used to phone the family in the night? And they'd say, "That's fine, we'll be up in the morning. Just do whatever." The thought of, you know, someone just dying ... the thought of dying on your own.' (Staff midwife, less than 5 years experience)

Ensuring parents were quite comfortable with the measures taken was an important aspect of the process. Some staff were particularly concerned to ensure that parents were intimately involved not just to make the experience meaningful but also to reassure them that what had happened was all above board. One nurse commented that doing everything relating to the withdrawal of treatment in full view of the parents, minimized the doubts in their minds. If staff sent them out of the room while the ventilator was switched off and the endotracheal tube removed, and the baby was dead when they returned, they might wonder what exactly had been done and whether the death had been hastened in any way. But others pointed out that parents had varying levels of tolerance for what went on and they should be permitted to decide for themselves the extent of their close involvement.

Consulting colleagues and specialists

In every Unit the practice obtained of consulting others in the decision making. This might be the baby's consultant asking for the opinion of his fellow consultants. It might be inviting other specialists to offer an opinion. A few consultants volunteered that they would always consult with a more well known neonatologist before withdrawing since this was not only a personal reassurance, but would carry greater weight in the courts. Two always ensured that they had a 'backstop' to protect them, and never set themselves up as the final arbiter even though they had many years of paediatric experience at a consultant level.

There was comfort to be obtained from having others involved in the decision. Where it was taken without the benefit of others' counsel, it produced a degree of isolation.

> 'I think I'm lucky in having two colleagues that are very cooperative and very nice to work with, so that we do share our problems ... and it tends to be a collective decision ... I do work [elsewhere] where I don't actually work single-handedly, but where my other colleague perhaps isn't there a lot of the time because he has other commitments. And I have found myself on one or two occasions with a position to take, that I've taken single-handedly. I haven't got any regrets about any decision – I think, as far as I know, those decisions were correct. But I've always found myself feeling a bit lonely. There's just a bit of insecurity in being there on your own taking that decision, whereas if I'm here I know that I've got my other two colleagues here, and I can draw on their back-up.' (Consultant, more than 15 years experience)

The actual withdrawal
Actually discontinuing treatment

Even within each Unit there were differences of opinion about just who switched off the ventilator and withdrew the endotracheal tube. Some consultants said that they believed it should always be their task since it was they who ultimately made the decision, who carried the responsibility and who would follow up the parents subsequently. For their babies then it was a consultant's task. Alternatively some nurses welcomed the chance to do it themselves since they could be more leisurely about it, do it at the right moment for the parents, and even involve them sensitively in the act of disconnection if they wished it. A number of the nursing respondents had withdrawn the life-supporting equipment from babies they had cared for, and a few commented that they were more gentle than the doctors in this regard. Others said the identity of the person doing the disconnection was unimportant: doctors, nurses or parents might do it.

One consultant was quite adamant that parents should never actually disconnect the machinery because of the potential legal and emotional consequences, but even in his Unit other staff said parents did do so on occasions. Presumably these were the babies who were cared for by the other consultants. Much appeared to depend on the cases each respondent had been involved in but there seemed to be little open discussion about these practicalities since beliefs were quite divergent in each of the Units.

Specific acts

There were two aspects of the actual withdrawing of treatment which require a special mention: the use of drugs and the practice of withholding nourishment.

THE USE OF DRUGS

With the known sensitivities around the use of drugs in terminal care, caution was exercised in questioning respondents about their practices. This meant that some spontaneously offered information about this topic; some were gently probed; others did not offer an opening for such questioning or the interviewer considered it was unwise to pursue such a delicate area of exploration. However, sufficient data were obtained to make it apparent that opinions differ about the use of both pain relief and paralysing agents.

Drugs are widely used to ensure pain relief and to control dying. However, for one doctor who had had some experience in a Unit providing ECMO, there was a difference in the treatment of premature infants and other larger babies. In his judgement there was sometimes an element of uncertainty with premature infants so they should not be paralysed to take away that chance. By contrast, with the relatively big babies on ECMO, death is certain if the ventilator is withdrawn, but it is potentially much more traumatic. For him in such cases it was essential to minimize that trauma.

> 'I would not only give [babies on ECMO] morphine but I would give them pancuronium so their death is quick. Because we know this baby is not going to survive. We're sure, 100 per cent. Why give them a transitory period of coming off the machine gasping and moving? ... now if that period is taken over by a struggle by this baby who's writhing and pushing and shoving and gradually becoming bluer and coughing – and even with a good dose of morphine, sometimes you can't control it – I think that's inappropriate. But for the baby who has been extubated, whose breathing is shallow and relaxed and who's dying, then I think that's acceptable. But the baby who is going from pink, eyes open, looking around, sucking, doing everything, to being writhing, blue, horrible, I don't think that's appropriate. And that's not in the best interests of the baby or the parents or us.' (Consultant, more than 10 years experience)

Other consultants however applied the same principle of orchestrating a 'good death' and reducing to a minimum the distress of the family, to premature babies in the NICU. They would both sedate and paralyse such infants to ensure the dying happened as predicted and was dignified and calm. In only one Unit in this study did staff volunteer that paralysing agents were used to manage dying with premature infants. In this centre pancuronium was given to infants on mechanical ventilation fairly routinely. If the decision was made to stop treatment, and there was the usual dose of paralysing agent still in the system, this meant that the baby died swiftly after the withdrawal of the endotracheal tube and ventilator because the muscles could not prolong spontaneous respiration. Staff spoke of the advantages of being able to control and predict the sequence of events. There was, they felt, enormous distress for parents in watching a baby gasping for hours even though they had been reassured that he was not suffering. With pancuronium on board, this distress was minimized since the parents could be advised of what to expect, and it would happen as predicted.

> 'First of all you want to be sure, and this is the most important thing, that what you said was going to happen, was going to happen. What you don't want is

for that baby to *not* die. You don't want the baby to be thrashing around looking blue and horrible, and struggling for breath and not dying. So you have to be careful about when you take the baby off the ventilator. I'm not saying you should pump the baby full of drugs so that it has no choice. But you shouldn't be taking the baby off at a point when you feel it's going to carry on breathing. You should be taking it off at a point where there's going to be a few breaths and the heart rate will continue but basically it's going to die anyway. So you've got to time that.' (Consultant, less than 10 years experience)

Some consultants in other Units when specifically asked about the use of such blockades, were not in support of such a practice. Others asked directly if other consultants practised in the same way and were astonished to hear that there were substantial differences between Units.

However, only one respondent suggested that opiates were unnecessary for neonates, although one other person, a nurse, did volunteer an opinion that sedation was sometimes used to compensate for staff inadequacy. She instanced cases where in her judgement babies had really needed cuddling or pacifying, but staff were too uncomfortable in the management of a dying baby, or too hard pressed to meet these needs and instead administered sedative drugs to quieten the child.

As has already been described, in two Units all drugs were withdrawn from infants once a decision had been made to stop treatment: this included opiates. The majority of doctors, however, continued to administer opiates with a small number volunteering that they were prepared to give additional doses to hasten death once it was clear that the baby would die. It was neither expedient nor possible to gain any accurate sense of how many people supported this practice or how many actually did speed up the dying process in this way.

In the two DGHs a sense was given that they were extremely cautious about withdrawing treatment. Staff reported that certain individual consultants would never make such a decision. Overall doctors in these Units appeared to be guided by more concrete evidence. Some nurses as well as doctors clearly assumed that specific criteria had to be met in much the way that they do for brain death in adults. They carried out various tests, tried reducing ventilation on a trial basis, and withdrew all drugs before establishing a prognosis and withdrawing treatment. By the time all these procedures were finished the baby was near death anyway and some respondents appeared not to know that other Units practised differently or that treatment was ever withdrawn at an earlier point.

WITHHOLDING NOURISHMENT

The problem of severely birth asphyxiated infants was raised spontaneously by some staff. As with the question of administering opiates, great care was taken in probing this sensitive area of practice. As a consequence, not all respondents volunteered what the practice was in their experience.

Where the damage is so severe that the infant has no sucking reflex, decisions have to be made about whether and how they will be fed. Sometimes they are tube fed but some clinicians believe that the most acceptable method of dealing with such a situation is to offer a bottle feed as would be normal practice with babies; if the child does not suck he will obtain no nourishment and eventually die. In only one Unit did a number of staff cite this practice of withholding fluids and feeds from an infant as one with which they were familiar. In this Unit there were nursing staff who refused to be party to such a practice, but others had been involved. A number of them were openly distressed reporting it. However, one of the consultants who prescribed this kind of management had a different perception of this practice:

> 'I manage [these babies] by speaking to the parents, saying, "A basic function in a baby – and a term baby in particular – is the ability to feed, and to suck, to sustain life, grow and such like. And we don't know if your baby will do that. If the baby's unable to do this, I don't think it's wise for us to interfere by putting tubes in. What I would do is I would offer your baby bottle feeds, and I would let your baby feed as much as he or she can take. That might be nothing. This will inevitably mean that the baby will get weaker. The baby might start to get distressed. Once your baby starts to feel uncomfortable, I would then relieve any pain of the baby." Those are the bad asphyxias, who come off the ventilator ... some of them'll last for anything up to three months, hopefully less than that.' (Consultant, more than 20 years experience)

It sometimes happened that these infants died more quickly than would be expected from starvation.

> 'My impression of the ones we've had here, they've not actually died just of starvation as such, because they've died quicker. They've usually died within two or three days ... I don't know if it's poor respiratory drive because the brain stem's been damaged or if it's in some cases an aspiration pneumonia because they've maybe inhaled. I think that may be the cause in a lot of them ... Another thing I thought about was, I wondered if some of the babies actually die from a prolonged convulsion ... because a lot of them tend to have cyanotic episodes, and some of these cyanotic episodes may actually be convulsions.' (Registrar, less than 5 years experience)

Elsewhere babies who could not suck were given tube feeds and died from additional complications such as infections, or failure to resuscitate in an emergency. In some instances increased doses of opiates eased the baby's dying.

> 'That's often a very difficult situation when you know the baby won't suck and then they've got a tube, and I think – well, certainly in my experience, we have refused to remove the tube for feeding ... you feel you can't starve a child to death, but they have often then decided to put up an infusion of an opiate so that the child will just gradually slip away, but I've only had a few experiences of that ... I kept offering the child feeds and holding him and things, and – it's so much easier just to stop a ventilator and you know that the child's dependent

on that, but I find it very difficult to sort of just withdraw ... it's not cut and dried in the same way that a baby's dependent on ventilation ... I feel then that I'm killing that child by giving opiates. I can't deal with that.' (Staff midwife, more than 5 years experience)

It was clear that the severely asphyxiated infants were a group who gave great concern.

Documentation

Although the importance of careful documentation was clearly recognized it was noteworthy that in each Unit there were staff who were unsure of the adequacy of the system in their Unit. Documentation was seen to be important for two reasons: communication amongst staff; and for legal purposes. A small number of consultants themselves reported that they were personally bad at recording these things.

A minority said they would be selective in their reporting; for example, recording the decision to stop aggressive treatment but not their use of opiates to hasten death.

'We would have some nice socially acceptable term like, "Care will be re-orientated to make comfort the prime consideration," or something. Which means that we're going to give the child lots of morphine to make sure the child isn't suffering while we allow the child to die. But we're not going to actually say that we know in doing that we're going to suppress the child's respirations; we're going to take the child off the ventilator in association with that, in the certain knowledge that the child won't breathe and will die and in that respect that we're actively contributing, knowingly, to the child's death.' (Senior Registrar, more than 5 years experience)

Others recorded everything in such a way that those who were entitled to know what had been done could find the information but it would not be overtly clear to other people who might simply misinterpret things.

'I don't put down the details – did I hurry it along – did I make it more comfortable, or whatever. You could find traces of that if you were clever. They're there – in the pharmacy, the prescription, the DDA book. But I wouldn't document it.' (Consultant, more than 15 years experience)

However others said that the whole key to good team work lay in accurate and comprehensive documentation so that each person knew exactly what had been said and what measures to pursue: they recorded everything plainly. A notable viewpoint was expressed by one doctor: this senior registrar did not think these decisions and the consequent practices were documented at all but had no misgivings about such a situation.

Where the decision was made late on and only hours before the baby would have died anyway, as was the case in two Units, there was little controversy about what was recorded. But where practice was more debatable, consultants were alive to the legal ramifications of their reporting, sometimes selecting what they would leave out or how they would phrase things. Since a number of the consultants had actually been involved in legal cases it was interesting to hear how they dealt with this whole area of reporting. Where the whole team were involved in an open way in procedures and practices, there was apparently less difficulty in reporting – everything was accurately documented. But there was a potential conflict if the consultant did not want everyone on the team to be aware of exactly what was being done. Here practice varied. Inadequate documentation could however, increase the uncertainty and confusion of junior staff.

A small number of consultants bemoaned the current way that junior doctors were trained. They were not taught to record well. In the judgement of these doctors, nurses' notes were much more useful and comprehensive. They themselves frequently referred to what the nurses reported and obtained a better sense of how a baby was progressing.

The nurses largely took their own careful record-keeping for granted but regretted the doctors' more sketchy notes. Inadequate documentation could put them in very difficult positions. As one nurse said, a note to the effect that treatment was to be wound down, for example, could be indicating gradual withdrawal over hours or days or weeks. What did it actually tell people? Knowing that was germane to the management of the baby and the parents. But on occasions the nurses felt that extra vigilance was needed in their own reporting, too.

> 'I find it a bit more difficult because the way that the care plans are worked out here, you don't have easy access to just jot down: "At 2.30 total parenteral nutrition taken down." And they just put: "As discussed with [so and so], withdrawal of treatment". Perhaps that day I should have been more on the ball, because I think now, if someone had said: "What were your actions at 2 o'clock? What were your actions at 3 o'clock?", if there's nothing written down, I wouldn't have any recollection at all, which isn't a good situation to be in by any means. No matter how certain you would be that you had done everything correctly and the parents felt you had done everything correctly, in the end it's your head on the block if they decide that you didn't.' (Staff Midwife, less than 5 years experience)

Satisfaction with procedures and practices

Gaining any picture of satisfaction is time limited. As one consultant remarked,

> '[Is it working satisfactorily?] Yes, as well as it can at the moment. But in ten years time I hope to look back and say, "No, it wasn't." Just as what we were doing ten years ago wasn't as good as it is now.' (Consultant, more than 15 years experience)

Overall the majority of the staff in three of the Units felt that their practices were generally satisfactory although it naturally depended on the circumstances and personnel involved. Occasionally things were not well handled due to a variety of circumstances. Sometimes tension or conflict appeared unavoidable, such as when parents held entrenched views which did not permit the staff to manage a case as they would have liked. In a fourth Unit, there was so much tension between the various grades of staff that an underlying unhappiness pervaded all their opinions. In the remaining two Units internal differences between the consultants made it difficult for junior staff to feel at ease with what was being done.

In order to get a picture of those things which respondents felt caused the problems, they were asked what it was that made the practices unsatisfactory. Responses fell into four main categories: the timing of events; communication and team work; the environment; and the actual management of the dying.

The timing of events

The timing of events was the single largest problem area for both doctors and nurses. Respondents recognized that it was extremely difficult to get the timing right for everyone. Junior medical staff and nurses in general felt that consultants were too slow in deciding to forego treatment. Nursing staff felt that the decision was too often not right for the parents. But the nurses recognized that their own close relationship with the families gave them an emotional involvement which made it harder to stand back from the case and make a dispassionate assessment. They were listening for long periods to the parents, taking on board their distress and also worrying about the effect on the infant of prolonged treatment when the prognosis seemed so bleak. Delays appeared to them to represent indecision. Furthermore sometimes the decision fluctuated and they received mixed messages making it very difficult to communicate consistently with parents. When they were already distressed by the deteriorating condition of the baby, such confusion seemed hard to contend with.

Senior doctors were sometimes aware of the impatience of other team members but some felt this was something they had to tolerate; a burden they carried along with the responsibility for the final decision. In their judgement it was a feature of the inexperience and peripheral involvement in the discussion of these other people. Others, however, went to considerable lengths to reassure staff that they understood their feelings and to give a rationale for the delay.

Communication and team work

The way the team operated left room for improvement in the eyes of a considerable number of the nurses but only a tiny minority of doctors. Factors here related to the consultant's approach, the involvement of junior staff, and the way information was relayed through the different grades. The nurses found it difficult not being fully acquainted with thinking or intentions. This left them unsure whether their own feelings about this baby were shared and also unsure how to communicate and deal with parents. Having ideas of their own and having no opportunity to express them was a source of frustration. But sometimes sharing them felt like a token involvement since there was no evidence that the consultant took any real notice of what they said. Furthermore, acting, as they often did, as liaison people between the doctors and the parents, they felt particularly vulnerable when they were not totally in the picture about plans for this child. For example, they felt that parents were not always aware of the options available but if they were not present at discussions with the parents they could not be sure of just what had been said.

However, a very few nurses additionally expressed doubts about their ability to think rationally when they were so closely involved with these families. Their emotions were engaged in a way that the doctors' were not. The medical staff left the baby in question and had other tasks to distract them whereas the nurses were 'trapped' with that baby and those parents with little reprieve for long periods of time. This could distort their judgement.

The environment
The facilities available caused considerable concern to nurses but was not mentioned as a cause of suboptimal care by the medical respondents. Providing privacy was difficult.

> 'I think when a baby's for terminal care or a baby's having treatment withdrawn, it's very difficult if they're in the same nursery, to start putting screens round, and having parents going in and out, when they probably know that everybody's looking at them quite pitifully ... I think it's difficult here that at times there isn't anywhere to move the baby if we're busy – to have a quiet corner where they can just let out their grief without being aware of lots of listening ears. I think it falls down in that respect.' (Staff Midwife, less than 5 years experience)

In most Units much of the time there was a great pressure on beds and rooms and a shortage of staff. Even where rooms had been allocated for this type of circumstance, it was not always possible to take the baby along to that area since there were inadequate staff to allow one person to be freed up to leave the nursery area. On occasion the Unit was just too busy for them to have the time adequately to deal with the families or spend time exclusively with a grieving parent. This sharing of themselves created tensions for the nurses since it was difficult simultaneously to be cheerful with parents whose baby was being treated and be quiet and sensitive with those whose baby was dying.

Another particular anxiety was that terminal care was sometimes left to inexperienced staff. A case in point was a birth asphyxiated child who was not dependent on mechanical ventilation. Requiring no expert techniques such a baby tended to be nursed in the area reserved for babies who were fattening up, or who no longer needed close monitoring. These nurseries were often staffed by the less qualified nurses. Some respondents considered that they should always be cared for in the intensive areas to ensure they were given the best possible care in their dying hours or days. But such a practice was logistically problematic.

The actual management of the dying
The way each case was actually handled was an additional cause for concern for the nurses although no doctor expressed misgivings about this aspect of withdrawing treatment. Some comments related to the general context for these cases. Respondents

wanted such babies to have continuity of care and to have the best care available. In some Units the nurses commented that cases were too rare for many staff to gain much experience so they were always learning.

Major dilemmas surrounded the administration of drugs and the question of feeding. A considerable number of nurses in one Unit reported that babies who were birth asphyxiated and severely impaired and who had no sucking reflex, were offered bottles but no other means of obtaining fluids or nutrition. As has been reported, they found this profoundly distressing. The common practices elsewhere were to tube feed and wait for an infection, or not to resuscitate the baby in a subsequent emergency, but this appeared less distasteful than watching a baby die of starvation. Other nurses were disturbed by the level of opiates given in some cases which in their judgement hastened death unacceptably. None of the nurses questioned more closely on either of these issues had expressed their misgivings to the consultants.

Recommendations for change

When respondents were asked how things could be improved almost all their responses related to better communication and collaboration. They looked for much more team work, with consultants listening to and respecting the views of other team members. In this way they felt that such cases would be handled more sensitively, the timing of discussions and events would be more in tune with parental needs, and there would be an overall consistency and clarity.

A minority recommended that the whole business of managing severely asphyxiated babies should be reviewed. Some suggested that if decisions were made at an earlier stage while the window of opportunity was open which permitted withdrawal of treatment leading to death, these lingering distressing cases would be avoided. Others, recognising the difficulty of being sure of a prognosis early on, advocated a form of euthanasia in these extremely difficult circumstances.

Discussion

Practice varies between Units, between doctors and between nurses. However in all NICUs parents and consultants are key participants in decision making, both sides consulting others to enable them to reach an appropriate conclusion. While parents may seek the advice of family members or their GP or religious leader, consultation as far as the medical staff are concerned involves seeking the opinions of other team members or other consultants and specialists. There is comfort for consultants in having confirmation from their peers that they have made the right decision.

Dissatisfaction with nurses' involvement

There is, however, considerable dissatisfaction among the nursing staff about their own level of input into decision making. They perceive themselves as having unique insights into the lives of this baby and his family and a special role in providing hands-on care. Yet they frequently feel left out of the important discussions. Even those who accompany the consultant to discussions with the parents feel sometimes that theirs is a token presence, as a witness more than an active participant. One nurse who had been the person most intimately involved with a baby's family over a prolonged period was taken to the discussion about withdrawing treatment. She was astonished to hear the consultant say, 'The nurses and I feel ...' when she knew that no one had ever asked for her opinion.

Responsibility usually devolves to the nurses, however, to actually manage the withdrawal of treatment and the dying in line with parental wishes. Indeed a number of consultants paid tribute to the special skills of the nurses in handling these difficult terminal care situations. It is a source of tension and sometimes of conflict when they are left to deal with the consequences of a decision when they either do not understand how such an irrevocable option was chosen, or when they actually disagree with the course of action being taken. For sometimes, apart from not having been involved in the discussion, they feel they are inadequately informed about what is known, what has been said and what decided. Neither verbal communication nor written documentation appear to be satisfactory. In the perceptions of all grades in some Units, communication at all levels is inadequate. Consultants do not share their thinking with other team members, senior nurses do not faithfully seek out or represent the junior nurses' opinions, junior nurses themselves complain among themselves but do not convey their dissension to grades of staff who might be able to do something about their grievances, and written reporting leaves much room for improvement.

But there are examples of good communication. In one Unit in particular all grades of staff share their feelings in a variety of ways. Together they address the powerful emotions engendered by these difficult decisions. They support one another because they understand how their colleagues feel. The consultants work closely together and they are open and comprehensive in their discussions with the rest of the team. This seems to be the key. If the consultant lets his colleagues know exactly why he thinks the time to withdraw has not yet been reached and they understand his reasoning, they will be more likely to accept the necessity for the delay. If they, in turn, share their own feelings of distress at the prospect of another eight hours looking after a baby whose every breath is painful, or whose parents are so distressed they exact a high price in terms of support and answers, their voice too has been heard and efforts can be made to offer them support and perhaps relief from the relentless drain on their emotions. For more junior staff, there is added relief in simply having had their say since they are mostly very aware that the responsibility does not rest with them. But if each does not know how the other feels, a situation develops which is ripe for misunderstandings and resentments.

Communication in relation to the timing of withdrawal
Without question the single factor giving the most widespread cause for concern is the timing of the decision to withdraw. In some Units treatment is only ever withdrawn when death is certain and imminent, and here there is disquiet about the protracted nature of the experience imposing prolonged stress on parents and nursing staff. Where the decision is made much earlier on, anxiety relates more to the reasons for the withdrawal and the means by which death is facilitated. Listening to the perceptions

of each side in these conflicts it became apparent that a failure to understand the peculiar burdens carried by the different participants in these painful situations was a major contributing factor. More will be said on this matter in the chapter dealing with conflicts. But much appears to hinge on the sensitivity and approach of the consultants. If they present a united front, work consistently and openly and communicate well, they set a pattern for the Unit which results in markedly less tension than where the consultant is perceived as autocratic and arrogant and out of touch with the feelings of colleagues. Practices are reported within given Units which are mutually exclusive: all informants cannot be right in their perceptions of what goes on. There is then every indication that there is much work to be done in helping people to communicate well. And when it comes to documentation, which is known to be crucial to good team work, and for legal protection, it is clear that present practice is also inadequate.

Current constraints

It is important however, in presenting any deficiencies in present working arrangements, to draw attention to the constraints under which staff are labouring. A recent survey of NICUs found substantial discrepancies between recommended levels and actual staff numbers of both nursing and medical complements.[158] All the Units studied in this present enquiry were reported as working with less than the full establishment of staff. If there are not enough people to do the work then clearly some refinements will be jettisoned in order to give basic life-saving care. Giving good quality care to dying babies and to their families is a time-consuming and therefore costly occupation. Not being able to provide it is a source of great frustration and distress to staff. This conflict between delivering high quality care to a limited number as against lower quality care to a larger number is a real one which is known to cause considerable friction in NICUs in general.[159]

The mechanics of deaths

Considerable and vigorous debate has centred around just how babies who are not for treatment will die. Doctors themselves have argued forcefully about the legitimacy of using sedation or other drugs which may hasten death by suppressing various functions.[30] Differences of opinion were clearly seen in this present study. Whilst employing paralysing agents alongside sedative or analgesic drugs is a practice amongst certain neonatologists, there are uncertainties in the minds of many practitioners about the wisdom of using drugs to orchestrate the dying. Pain relief is almost universally accepted as good practice. But the use of larger doses of analgesics and of paralytics raises serious questions relating to intent. Is it a form of euthanasia? Is it really being carried out in the best interests of the baby, or is it rather for the comfort of the parents or staff?

One group of babies who engender grave concern are those who have suffered severe birth asphyxia. The window of opportunity to withdraw treatment from them has often closed by the time a firm prognosis is reached. Opinion and practice varies considerably in the management of these cases. But one option in particular, the withholding of feeds which results in the baby starving to death, is a practice which produces enormous distress in nurses, a distress which has been recognized elsewhere.[160]

The moral permissibility of discontinuing feeding a patient has gained public attention and been vigorously contested in recent years. Notable landmark cases have been referred to already: the Hillsborough disaster victim, Tony Bland, in England; and in Scotland, Janet Johnstone who took an overdose of drugs, both of whom ended up in a Persistent Vegetative State. The courts were applied to for legal sanctioning of the withdrawal of feeding, both the families and the medical teams being persuaded that further treatment was futile. Feeding was withdrawn from Tony Bland in 1993 and as this chapter was being finalized, doctors had just been given permission to allow Mrs Johnstone to die in this way. The plight of a young child, Thomas Creedon, severely brain damaged, blind, deaf, suffering fits and believed by his parents to be in constant pain, also raised the issue of feeding since Mr and Mrs Creedon were requesting that his gastrostomy tube be removed. In this case however, medical opinion was not wholly in agreement with the parents' wishes, although some outside experts believed they were right. However, Thomas died of natural causes at the beginning of this year (1996) before the court's response could be tested. When feeding is continued in spite of the apparent futility of treatment, questions are raised about bodily integrity and privacy, exacerbation of the suffering and distress of both patient and relatives, and the allocation of resources. Yet some fear that a liberal interpretation of the law would lead to the most vulnerable being put at even greater risk of abuse.

Many people rely on the simple distinction between acts and omissions to distinguish the morally acceptable from the unacceptable. But to do so is to over simplify a complex issue. The acceptability or otherwise of different courses of action turns rather on other significant considerations such as the balance of harms and benefits, the futility of treatment, the degree of suffering, the duties owed by the various people to the patient, the risks and potential repercussions of committing various acts or omitting others, and the certainty of the prognosis.

The provision of basic commodities like food and water has a particular meaning to both nurses and families when it comes to caring for the sick and vulnerable. It is apparent through the letter pages of a number of reputable professional journals that there is considerable disquiet about court rulings and official statements in this area. In the minds of many, basic feeding and hydration is not equivalent to mechanical ventilation. Although much has been said about dying as a result of the withdrawal of these essential items being difficult intellectually for the observer but not physically uncomfortable for the patient, there are those who question the suggestion that dying of thirst is not uncomfortable.[161] But the main objection to withdrawing feeding and hydration appears to be a psychological one. Many people cannot accommodate this withdrawal of something which so essentially represents caring and nurturing.

Less emotive and more accepted now is the doctrine of double effect. Treating pain and suffering with medication in sufficient dosages that death is hastened, but only as a side effect of the relief of suffering, is a practice widely adopted and accepted in medicine. Indeed, so commonly understood is this course of action even outside the confines of the health care team, that respondents said parents were sometimes suspicious of their motives when they advocated sedation for a baby. They had frequently to emphasize that the dosage was only sufficient to ensure the child would not suffer discomfort from noxious stimuli, and was in no sense for the purpose of ending his life.

Internal policing

Nurses have a duty to question instructions to administer doses of drugs which lie outside the margins of safety and examples were given by both doctors and nurses of individuals challenging prescriptions or verbal orders for doses out of the normal range, and in some cases refusing to participate. Some doctors always give these larger doses themselves, although the extent to which they document their actions varies. Other senior doctors proceed cautiously and negotiate with trusted colleagues a level which all can accept without infringing their moral scruples. This internal policing appears to be a healthy safeguard against idiosyncratic violations.

Alternatives to drugs

High on nurses' lists of priorities come measures designed to minimize suffering and distress, the so-called 'comfort measures'. Sensitivity to the specific likes and dislikes of individuals is the essence of this art. These alternatives to medication form part of the armamentarium of the nurses' repertoire and they clearly take pride in exercising these particular skills. The nursing respondents in this study gave many examples of the kinds of activities which were intended to facilitate the comfort of both the baby and the family. Some fear that sedation is sometimes resorted to too precipitately and to save time and resources. Sitting cuddling a baby, soothing his distress or massaging his body are seen as preferable in certain circumstances to simply pumping him with opiates, but time often does not permit such attention to an individual child.

Clearly in these matters too there are environmental and organizational constraints which limit what doctors and nurses can and cannot do. But it is important to understand current practice with all its limitations if we are to move forward in improving the management of these most difficult cases.

Conclusions

These are rightly team decisions. Excellent communication is essential if all views are to be properly respected and taken into account. The limits of exactly what means to employ to facilitate a death in some circumstances are open to question but the involvement of the different members of this expert team should ensure that abuses are prevented and matters are dealt with sensitively and within both legal and professional boundaries.

---

*For the purposes of the present discussion, pain is taken to mean a distressing, hurtful sensation in the body; and suffering to mean a sense of anguish, vulnerability, loss of control and threat to the integrity of self.[162]

CHAPTER TEN

Roles and Responsibilities

In the past when doctors' decisions went unchallenged, roles and responsibilities appeared clearer than they are today. There was less threat to the medical staff, and relatives were unburdened by the responsibility of weighty decisions. With the development of the nursing profession and the advent of parent participation in decision making, demarcations are much less obvious.

> 'In traditional hospitals, doctors are at the top, nurses and other health workers in the middle, and patients at the bottom in terms of knowledge, autonomy, and control over resources. There are also clear vertical orders of seniority within and between the professions. Yet informed consent is a horizontal, democratic approach, with doctors supposedly on equal if not deferential terms with patients and their parents. Introducing the new equality of consent between doctors and patients challenges traditional hierarchies; it is like new wine in old bottles.'[24]

It seemed germane to this investigation, to explore the perceptions of staff caught up in these changes, of the relative roles of the different professionals who might be involved in cases where treatment was being withdrawn or withheld. But in order to set a context for staff responses, it is first necessary to understand that there were essential differences in the study Units in terms of organization and work remits.

Essential differences in the Units

A range of factors could well have influenced the respondents' perceptions of an ideal. The clearest picture would have been given by a sketch of each Unit but that would have made it relatively easy to identify them. Consequently, only general illustrative material is included in this brief summary statement.

Career structures

Promotion was more likely in some Units than others. In one Unit, for example, some midwives had remained at E grade level for up to six years even though they had an additional neonatal qualification. Elsewhere simply holding this qualification helped them up the promotional ladder.

Tasks outside the Unit

In several of the Units the nursing staff were required to attend deliveries of infants who might require admission to the NICU, while in others it was only the doctors who took on this responsibility. Whereas in some centres the nurses who went were always senior staff, in other places very inexperienced midwives were called and they described eloquently their horror of being on call for this role.

Transferring babies either to other departments for investigation or to other hospitals for specialized treatment, necessitated at least one escort being removed from the workforce. Flying Squad calls further depleted numbers. Some Units were dependent on only a skeleton service to start with and staff were stretched to the limit by this reduction. When respondents were asked how such a situation developed, they replied that senior administrative figures determined staffing levels. Provision was rarely made for these emergencies. Managers who had no experience of this specialty, simply failed to understand the work involved. They saw only small numbers of babies and a high ratio of nurses to patients. It was interesting to note that in the Unit under most pressure in this regard, there was a high degree of team work and a great spirit of friendly tolerance. Staff appeared cheerfully to take on a colleague's work as well as their own. By contrast in the Unit with the highest numbers of staff on duty, and with a capacity for sisters to do little hands-on care, there was the most grumbling, and widely reported and observed inter-professional tension.

Medical selection

Staff in the DGHs remarked that they tended to attract a different type of doctor. The fast tracking doctors who were perceived to be the brightest and most able, mostly went to university based Units. DGHs were largely staffed by foreign doctors who often had language difficulties as well as cultural issues to contend with. Nevertheless some of these doctors from abroad came with a vast amount of experience. Their expertise was not, however, always recognized in Scotland where people who had held very senior posts elsewhere were sometimes employed at SHO level and obliged to undertake the menial tasks, and take regular on-call nights, with little opportunity to teach or share their own knowledge.

Doctors' hours

In some Units junior doctors had adopted a system of shifts which allowed them to sleep after a night on duty. Elsewhere the SHOs worked with the more traditional system of following nights on call with a full day's normal work. There was a strong feeling of resentment amongst a few SHOs in the latter group but it was interesting that they appeared more ready to participate in the study in spite of being extremely tired whereas those who could go home to bed in the morning guarded their sleeping time more vigorously and did not volunteer to stay on at the end of a shift to be interviewed.

Awareness of differences

It sometimes happened that respondents asked the researcher a specific question about what was done elsewhere. A balance had to be struck between maintaining an easy relationship with the individual which encouraged honest and full discussion, and attending to the scientific rigour of the enquiry. Where a sense was gained that offering a response was the correct way to proceed and would not affect the respondent's own contribution, an honest answer was given. Sometimes the respondent was told a response would be given at the end of the interview. In this way it became clear that the range of practices which exist is not generally appreciated.

One very senior consultant expressed his disbelief that any paediatrician would withdraw treatment any sooner than in circumstances where death was only a matter of hours away. Some consultants were horrified at the idea that babies were sometimes paralysed at the time of withdrawal. Sisters who had had some brief encounters in other Units, said they had been shocked to discover that some large centres did not go through a rigorous process of withdrawing all drugs and performing tests of brain activity before stopping treatment. It had been even more alarming to find out that in some places they actually increased the medication before withdrawing ventilation.

Some staff in the DGHs commented that they were themselves in a difficult position. Not being acknowledged authoritative experts, they felt that in the event of a legal action their opinion would not be as powerful a voice as 'Professor So-and-So's.' They tended to defer to the judgement of these 'eminent' colleagues before taking action which might have repercussions.

In some of the Units there was no opportunity for nurses to go elsewhere to undertake the Neonatal course, whereas colleagues in other places could do so. The nurses themselves regretted this since they said it made them very insular. There was much to be gained by seeing practice in other centres.

The question

Respondents were invited to give their own assessment of roles and responsibilities with no attempt being made to guide their thinking. They were asked to imagine their ideal NICU, free from the constraints of their present environment, and to identify the roles they would allocate to each group of professional staff: consultants, junior medical staff, nurses, social workers, and chaplains. They were then asked to cite any other people who might have a role to play.

Tables of raw data on this topic would be of limited value, since it is highly probable that some of the more obvious roles were taken for granted and not listed by staff familiar with the organization of a NICU. In addition staff offered a number of suggestions in each category so the number of comments would not equate with the number of respondents who considered each broader role an appropriate one. There is more value in an overview of what each role should encompass.

Consultants

A number of roles were identified for the consultant. To some extent it would have been quite possible to subsume all of them within the broader roles of leadership and communication. To do so would have been to lose something of the detail of what their task encompassed.

Leadership

The leadership role for consultants is clearly an important and well recognized one.

> 'Not only is it your decision but it has to be *seen* to be your decision so nobody else is left feeling responsible for it. If you've got a problem with that then that's something you have to share with your senior colleagues.' (Consultant, less than 10 years experience)

Another part of the consultant's leadership role lies in ensuring that the right decision is made based on a sound assessment, making sure that the baby is not suffering or distressed in the meanwhile.

Decision making

The burden of the final decision was placed squarely in the consultant's domain by the vast majority of the respondents in this study. It is seen to be a task which goes with promotion to this level of seniority.

At this point it seems appropriate to comment on the reality of this role for consultants. Medical respondents were asked specific questions about the task and burden of decision making. Just under half (26, 46%) of the doctors interviewed had taken responsibility for the final decision about withdrawing or withholding treatment. Most of these were consultants (20), so only one consultant had not ever made the decision. It is important to remember that the sample was skewed in the direction of senior medical staff since all consultants were included in the population but only a proportion of more junior doctors had opportunity to participate. Only one senior registrar and five registrars said they had at some point been in this position also, although a further four doctors (7%) had made the decision at the point of resuscitation in Labour ward.

> 'Indirectly [I do take responsibility]. If you have a baby – resuscitate a new born – if it was moribund – the way you present the information to your consultant on the telephone at home influences the decision. So indirectly you are making the decision ... In the notes you write down, "Dr So-and-So says stop resuscitation." But they're basing that on your evidence and your decision, because you're the one there, and you're the one that's going to say this baby is not going to be resuscitatable. [It is still burdensome], yes, very much so ... it weighs heavily at the time, I think. I think for me to make the decision I have to be beyond any possibility of doubt that this baby is not [resuscitatable] ... I think the more experience you have, the less you keep going because you can see – and you have the authority.' (Registrar, less than 5 years experience)

The frequency with which such decisions had to be made varied. Seven had accepted the responsibility only once or twice. At the other end of the scale, seven took this kind of decision once a month or more; the remaining respondents between one and four times a year.

But interpretations about exactly what it means to accept the final responsibility vary. One consultant was quite definite about the limits of his responsibility.

> 'The *family* decides in a situation where there is severe impairment but short of death. *I* decide when I know [it's incompatible with life].' (Consultant, more than 10 years experience)

For others, things are a lot less clear-cut. One senior doctor explained how he got a feeling for the right course of action by leaving the information to settle on his 'mental back burner'. It requires patience and time to adopt this method. But he was so persuaded of its success, that he tried to help parents to rely on their own feeling in the same way.

> 'I don't know how this decision making process is done. But I know I come to a point where I get a gut feeling that all is right. And I often say to parents too, "You've not to think about this too deeply. Talk to each other and a point will come where you feel the decision will be made on its own." So, in some sorts of ways, you feel your brain has gone into neutral with all the information put into it and coming out with an answer ... By the time you've arrived at that decision you just know it's right for this baby in these circumstances.' (Consultant, more than 15 years experience)

Although on first reflection it could be thought that this technique might well engender frustration in colleagues who were looking for a swift decision, but were unable to see the consultant's brain in neutral, it is noteworthy that this was one of the consultants whom colleagues singled out as especially sensitive with both staff and parents. His calm approach, coupled with his ability to really listen to what people were saying and to pick up cues from a variety of sources, gave staff confidence in his judgement. In his own assessment, this way of operating gave him personal confidence: 'the fear of recrimination doesn't come into it because by the time you've arrived at that decision, you just know it's right.' He was asked, could such a method of working be taught: he did not think that it could.

To return to the question of the ideal role, the respondents believed that the consultants' position as final decision makers made it imperative that consultants listen carefully to all concerned, consult with their peers and specialist advisers, and communicate effectively with both staff and parents.

Communication

Communication is an important function of the consultants' role in the thinking of proportionately more nurses than doctors. It is a two-way street: the doctors need to be as adept at receiving cues as at giving them. To this end junior staff and nurses look to the consultants to be available and approachable, otherwise it is difficult to establish an open relationship which allows free expression of their beliefs, wishes and worries. Seniors need to share their own thoughts and opinions with the team, as well as listen carefully and deal appropriately with the views of everyone else. Experience can substantially influence the quality of such communication.

> 'I would listen very carefully to their prognosis on the baby – to their clinical judgement on a baby. I would expect it to be *fully* explained to me not just a case of, "This baby is incompatible with life." But perhaps to hear from them, "Because I have seen myself ..." or "This happened ..." I think as soon as they start sharing *real* things with you rather than sounding as if it's out of a textbook, that you can start to relate to that, and perhaps lose some of your own preconceived ideas [that] the [doctors] don't seem to be doing very much ... if you actually begin to hear *why.* So I think they have a responsibility because of that knowledge to, in as plain as possible terms, make sure that the junior staff, whether it be medical or nursing, actually understand why they have decided to make the judgements on a clinical basis rather than just saying we are going to do this.' (Staff Midwife, less than 5 years experience)

Communication with the parents too, requires a high level of skill if the exchanges are to be sensitive and productive. Some consultants were singled out as expert communicators. Probing for clues as to what constituted expertise in this area, elicited a picture of sensitivity to people's feelings, genuine interest in their opinions and wellbeing, a non-judgemental approach, warmth and compassion, skill in listening, and an ability to pitch and pace appropriately the language and content of a discussion coupled with the patience to repeat information over and over again without irritation or condescension.

Close involvement

Certain consultants were singled out for special commendation by nursing staff. They were the ones who became closely involved in the lives of families, appearing at all hours to support, inform, listen or assess. Even where these doctors were not personally popular, staff admired their dedication to the comfort and wellbeing of babies and families in their care. A considerable number of respondents criticized other consultants for being too remote from events in the nursery. By demonstrating a strong commitment to the families, senior doctors supported both the rest of the staff and the families. Where they appeared just for ward rounds or to give instructions over the phone without coming to see the baby, staff were left feeling that they did not really appreciate the impact of such traumatic events on the rest of the team or on the families. It was difficult for other team members to believe that the decision was soundly based, to communicate their own views or queries, or to reassure parents. In order to fulfil such a role it is recognized they need to be dedicated neonatologists, able and willing to be in the Unit as necessary.

Active participation in treatment withdrawal

A number of the consultants themselves volunteered that they thought it essential that the consultant him or herself should be the person actually to discontinue aggressive treatment: this was not something to delegate to others. In their judgement it is inappropriate for the senior person to decide to withdraw treatment and then leave the actual 'deed' to others. But one consultant suggested that the more he thought about it, the more he wondered if the staff caring for the baby might not view his sudden practical involvement as an intrusion. He was resolved to find out how they felt before continuing to do this. In the perception of junior and nursing staff, however, the actual switching off is not so important. The consultant's general ongoing support and presence is what is needed in all parts of the dying process.

Information

The burden of supplying information to parents when treatment is of dubious value fell to the consultants in all the study Units. However, there are so many different options sometimes that the effect of absolute honesty can be bewildering. Judgements have to be made about what to select and how to present the facts. It was deemed best to inch forward testing out parents' reactions along the way, when tackling these very sensitive issues.

> 'If the parents said, "Well, you tell me what exactly [we] would be facing," and I said, "Well, you would maybe have a child in a wheelchair. They might never talk. They're never going to be able to feed themselves. They're going to need help to get around. [Impaired] hearing and vision. They haven't got very good sensory awareness – these are the sort of things we're looking for ... At this point, you know, we will not be doing anything more active, but we won't be withdrawing anything." [Then you see] what the parents' reaction is. And they'd then be in a position of saying to me, "Well, what more will you be doing?" And then we decide – well, if the child gets a chest infection, would we do any more than we're doing right now? Or if the baby can't be fed by tube, would you go back to putting up drips? And so on.' (Consultant, more than 20 years experience)

Consistency

A considerable number of junior staff appealed for consultants to be consistent. It is profoundly disturbing if the decision keeps changing because the consultant keeps changing his or her mind with every slight change in the baby's condition. Junior medical staff and nurses are at the sharp end, constantly having to discuss the situation with parents. It is impossible to justify repeated changes of opinion. Furthermore, as well as making it increasingly difficult to support the consultant, their own position is jeopardised, since parents stop trusting them too.

Distress is added to stress if the different consultants all hold different views and expectations. Everyone else is bewildered by fluctuations in orders or decisions, and those expected to carry out such orders can be caught in a Catch 22 situation of pleasing no one. Awareness that their future careers depend on references from these consultants, superimposes further burdens.

> 'I think initially most of the junior doctors feel happier with protocols. They know where they stand. I think, in fact, that it actually doesn't make life so

rigid. Because once you have protocols and once you have junior staff who know where they stand, it's actually easier to take decisions. And it's easier to take the next step. It's when every single time you do something it's wrong, because there's a different person in charge who doesn't agree with it – that kind of thing actually makes it very difficult to make any decisions at all. Because you're so busy thinking, "Right, who's on? What are they going to say about this? Should I have done more? Should I have done less?"' (SHO, less than 1 year experience)

Junior medical staff

There were mixed feelings about the role of junior doctors.

Learning

In the minds of most people in NICUs, theirs is essentially a learning role and they should simply carry out instructions. Others qualified this by saying that it depends a great deal on the individual and their background and attitudes: they should become involved as much as they feel ready to and as is considered appropriate. There is a wide range of experience amongst junior staff as well as degrees of empathy and skills in social interaction.

Involvement in management of the baby and family

It is well recognized that this is an extremely sensitive time for families and that introducing extraneous people can be intrusive. As one respondent put it, care of the dying is 'not a spectator sport'. But some respondents commented that the parents actually often know the junior staff better than the consultant, and even the most inexperienced doctor can offer human support and warmth, and a sense of continuity. The integration/intrusiveness factor depends in large measure on the sensitivity of the junior doctor concerned.

A few junior staff themselves noted that parents sometimes feel more comfortable with staff who are closer to their own level of understanding, speak a language more like their own, and are themselves rather insecure and unsure. As they commented, it is always possible for junior doctors simply to say that they do not know something but that they will find out. Sometimes indeed, parents shop around for information and it is not helpful for doctors to be unresponsive to parents' needs. One staff grade doctor observed that parents not uncommonly look to middle grade staff for confirmation of their fears or the consultant's prognosis. Research staff can on occasion be much more intimately involved with particular babies and some doctors felt that they then develop a relationship more akin to the nurses' closeness to the baby and the family during these intense periods of data collection. It seems natural and appropriate for them to talk with the parents and share in the communication in all directions. Furthermore junior doctors will never learn how to deal with these situations well if they are always excluded. There is clearly a fine line to be drawn here and much depends on the skills and personalities of all those involved.

Senior colleagues however, are all too aware of the potential for misinformation. Some instanced examples of junior staff wrecking days of careful negotiation by a chance ill advised comment. When they are themselves treading carefully to avoid conflict or recriminations, they do not need junior staff, no matter how well intentioned, inadvertently misleading or clouding the picture. There is clearly considerable margin for misunderstanding and conflicting information in this most delicate area of communication.

Many senior nursing staff have helped successive generations of junior doctors to learn their way around neonatal care. For them there is a degree of irritation in situations where a junior is at one point dependent on them for assistance with even the most basic of tasks, and a few weeks later adopting a superior tone or approach. It could well have been this factor which made most nurses give a very minor role to junior doctors, or at least limit it according to their experience. Whilst it is perfectly appropriate for them to put their views to the consultant, and to input information about the baby's general clinical condition in an environment where others are protected from their inexperience, they should not be put into situations of responsibility for tasks or communication beyond their competence. A few went further and suggested that it was the nursing staff rather than the junior doctors who should have a much more active role in these sensitive situations.

Technical role

The principal role in general of the junior doctors is seen to be a fairly technical one – taking blood and running tests. However, it can be traumatic for them still to be carrying out invasive procedures on infants who are not going to survive, especially when they have got to know the baby and the family over many months.

> 'Maybe the junior staff feel, once the decision has been made that ... "I don't want to inflict any more pain or distress on this baby and why the heck am I going to be doing more blood gases or ... Why should I be putting up a drip?" ...The SHOs run around quite often being mainly technical and they're seen as the baddies, there's certainly no doubt – certainly in the bigger kids. They're the baddies going round stabbing the children ... I think, maybe I don't do this enough, actually involve them both in providing comfort to the child, and one of the helpful injections they can give to babies is morphine. And they can learn from the experience if it's done properly. They can continue to act, if you like, socially, as a member of the team, and if it's a long drawn out thing, not feeling left out and feeling they have to avoid the glance and questions of the parents ... what I say to them is, if the parents ask questions that you can't answer, just say you can't answer them, but certainly don't avoid the family.' (Consultant, less than 10 years experience)

A few junior doctors themselves admitted that they felt distressed when they lost babies. But some felt that they could not let it be seen that they were upset. They had a position to maintain and others to support.

'You've obviously got to be there to support the nursing staff that are looking
after the baby when this happens. Because usually they're in floods of tears and
you're left trying to not be like that. And the parents are in tears. And it's just
you that's got to keep going. And I think that can be very difficult because then
you're made to feel that you're not a human being, because the nurses can cry
and do what they want, but you can't. You can't do that. You've got to take
charge of the situation. I think somebody has got to remain [calm]. At the actual
time you have to be the doctor. I think afterwards you've got the opportunity
then to be the human being. But I think it's very difficult to do both. It's very
sad and I think a lot of nurses don't realize that they do have an outlet, and they
can [cry], but if a doctor started doing that, it wouldn't work. So I think that's
hard for the juniors because you've got to look after your nurses as well.'
(Registrar, less than 5 years experience)

It is noteworthy in this context that there were far more examples of the nurses feeling
that they supported the junior medical staff than the other way around.

Nurses

There was a clear consensus in both disciplines that the nurses' role is a key one.
Being intimately concerned over long periods of time with both the baby and the
family, their very closeness gives them unique insights and responsibilities.

Care of the baby and family

Their principal role is to care for the baby and support the parents. Close involvement
over long hours gives them a special relationship with the family. On the surface this
might appear to be a straightforward role. In reality this is not always so. Being unable
to escape from the parents carries its own burden.

'[The nurses] are going to be there 24 hours a day, sitting beside the parents.
And their role is to support the parents. It's sometimes very difficult as a nurse
if you are trying to help parents who've got very different views from you. I can
think of parents who're sitting there going on about how could God let this
happen ... or if you've got parents who are, say, blaming the medical profession
for the state their child is in. And let's face it, 99 per cent – or 95 per cent of the
time – if it's happened shortly after delivery we really don't know what's happened
... but whatever is the case, you cannot either agree with them or disagree with
them about what they're saying, but you have to still be there and be sympathetic
to them, when they're saying, "That bloody doctor's killed my baby" ... Very
difficult to know what to say. So you end up being a total jelly fish in that you're
... trying to give support to the parents, listen to them, not have them feel you're
disagreeing with them.' (Sister, more than 15 years experience)

The nurses consider it is important to recognize the limits of their own competence
and tolerances when it comes to these stressful cases. Because the management of
such families tends to devolve to fairly experienced staff, it can take a long while for

nurses to amass enough experience to feel able to deal with a fami'
worker if they have no natural aptitude for the task. Furthermore, ever.
grounding in experience, everyone can have days where they are less roʋ
other times. As one senior nurse put it:

> 'I think we have to recognize that, when we're dealing with parents in this
> situation, they have the right, first hand, to somebody that is skilled, that is
> competent and that is able to give what they need – support, information – in
> the right way. And that that professional is comfortable in her role ... I think
> we're not good at recognizing – if this isn't something that you feel able to
> handle today, or that you don't feel you have the skills, accept that. There's no
> shame in that.' (Senior Sister, more than 5 years experience)

Contributing to the discussion

There was widespread agreement that the nurses should also input into discussion
about treatment decision. They have a unique role to play.

> 'The best nurses are all good communicators. I depend on them to tell me
> when they feel a child is getting worse, and often that's not from numbers but
> just their feeling ... I depend on them to tell me when a child is sore or distressed
> or restless. And I depend on them very greatly to relay what the parents are
> feeling ... they're extraordinarily insightful as to whether there are paternal/
> maternal conflicts – as there sometimes are. Whether the granny is an absolute
> rock or an interfering old biddy. Where the constructive, destructive influences
> are in the families. And the nursing staff are the people who are easily the best
> at that. They can suss out very quickly what's going on ... I mean they have a
> multitude of different things [to do] – they have to provide obviously the excellent
> clinical care for the child, communicate with me, with the parents – bring us
> together if they feel we are apart in our thinking ... and then around the time of
> withdrawing from the intensive care, they must be involved in the decision and
> to make their feelings known ... and then, of course, they do all these fantastic
> things ... the little touches are extremely important. All these things are essential
> and they also have a strong administrative role too.' (Consultant, more than 15
> years experience)

Furthermore, there was a peculiar stress reported in having to care for a baby and
support parents where the nurse doing so does not agree with what is being done.
That individual might not have been on duty when discussions took place. Or she
might simply not have been asked what she thinks. Either way it is traumatic to be
caught up in such an event when the nurse herself has strong feelings about its
rightness.

Opportunities to contribute to the decision do not happen to the nurses' satisfaction in
most Units at the present time. For them there is a profound difference between those
consultants who go through the motions of listening to them, and those who really
hear what they are saying and take due account of their opinions. The latter are

thought to be in a decided minority. And yet it is recognized that nurses can provide unique insights because of their intimacy with the baby and parents. Some experienced nurses went further and spoke of an intangible quality which they could provide: an 'intuitive' assessment of outcome which they considered almost invariably turns out to be sound and is subsequently verified over time and with hard evidence.

Being involved in the discussions not only gives the nurses opportunity to provide valuable information about the parents' circumstances, wishes and reactions, but it also better equips them to provide appropriate information to the parents. Theirs is an important role in liaising in both directions. Indeed in some circumstances they feel they have a special role as advocates for the baby and/or the parents. It is widely appreciated that parents often do not take in all that is said to them under these trying conditions. Furthermore the nurses in this enquiry considered that the language doctors use and their perceived more exalted status make it difficult for parents to develop an easy relationship with consultants. The parents see them relatively infrequently and in some cases only when things are going badly. This in itself erects barriers. Sometimes too there is opportunity for crossed wires simply because the doctors do not know the parents well. As one nurse explained, a mother had told her categorically that she did not 'believe in heaven' and was concerned about what would happen to her infant daughter. When the consultant said to her, 'Baby N is going to die. I think it's time for her to go to heaven', the comment appeared to the nurse to be singularly inappropriate although she realized that it was an innocent remark since the doctor was ignorant of the mother's views.

Support of colleagues

The nurses themselves felt they had an important role in supporting the other staff. Some limited this to nurses supporting each other through difficult experiences.

> 'You just see them about to slither down the walls and you go and you pick them up and give them a big box of hankies and send them somewhere nice and quiet like the sluice, for instance ... because we don't get used to it, because you never get used to it.' (Staff Midwife, more than 5 years experience)

A few instanced specific forms of support such as allowing juniors to opt out if they found the situation more than they could handle. Senior staff have a particular role in being alert to the needs of those actually engaged in handling these difficult situations.

> 'I think you need the support of senior nurses – but you don't always get it. And I think it's really important because if it's a one-to-one nursing situation, it can be very stressful, if you're with that baby all day in one of these rooms. And you need to know that you've got the support of the nurse in charge and you need to know that if you've got to leave the baby in Intensive Care, that you're going to have the backing. And that if you need anything they'll be there for you, and even to get a break from such a situation. Sometimes you need just five minutes and it's the nurse in charge that can let you out.' (Staff Midwife, less than 5 years experience)

Others extended the supportive role to include the medical staff. These respondents were aware that almost everyone is stressed by these peculiarly troubling decisions and they considered that the nurses, who feel the pain acutely because of their intimate involvement, can empathize with the suffering of others and offer comfort and sympathy. The bewilderment and insecurity of the most junior doctors, experiencing these things for the first time, unsure of their role or their own opinions, make them a particularly vulnerable group. But the burden of the final responsibility resting on the shoulders of the consultant was appreciated by some senior nurses who felt that, having known the consultants for years and having been through numerous such events with them, they were in a position to offer support to these senior medical colleagues too.

Obeying instructions

Although an active role at the centre of events is seen as appropriate for the nurses by almost all respondents there was one doctor who expressed a different view. He saw the nurses' role as doing what they were told to do by the consultant.

Chaplains

There was overwhelming agreement amongst all grades of staff in both disciplines that the chaplain or minister of religion had a very important role to play. But it was interesting to find that almost no one saw a role for the chaplain in the actual decision making. Talking things through with parents or staff to help them to come to a decision personally is certainly within his remit, but not directly contributing to the decision making discussion. His role is much more a supportive one.

Support of families

Very many staff spoke glowingly of the contribution of their own hospital chaplains who seemed to know what to say and how to listen even in the most difficult of situations.

> 'I think they often – because they have much more experience of life and death than many people who actually work here – they often are the best ones at knowing what words to say, when to say them, when not to say them.' (Staff Midwife, less than 5 years experience)

> 'A communicator and as a vehicle for parents to express grief and anxiety and everything ... because he's really good, so I'd have him. Because he's got so much time for people and he lets them talk, and he doesn't give them advice. He lets them express their emotions and their fears and anxieties, and just lets them talk. He provides a service that we can't always provide because we don't have time – too busy sometimes. As much as you would like to spend lots of time with people, it's impossible.' (Staff Midwife, more than 10 years experience)

Spiritual support

Offering spiritual support is another area designated as the role of the minister or chaplain. He is in a position to answer some of the deep questions in life, offer a moral view, and give hope in difficult situations. One consultant said that the chaplain gave an authentic air to proceedings in the Unit which was reassuring to staff and parents alike.

> 'Although, as he says himself, only a minority of our population are church-going, 90 per cent of those who are not church-going like to have some sort of blessing for their child, or some sort of religious symbolic moment. And he provides that. He's enormously experienced and is a very friendly, reassuring presence in the ward. And it's almost as though there's a stamp of authenticity to the whole thing when he comes in; I suppose it kind of emphasizes that everything's above board.' (Consultant, more than 15 years experience).

It is noteworthy that a considerable number of respondents commented that parents need something to cling on to at these traumatic points in their lives, even those who are not at all religious normally.

> 'Many parents regardless of what religion they are or their religious convictions ... I think deep down, nobody wants to think of their baby's going somewhere terrible. Even if, say, you're atheist, nobody wants to think that this little child – that was all his life meant and then he's going into a box in the ground and that's going to be him. I think people need some hope that somewhere there's a rest. And I think to see a minister in the flesh makes them realize, well, this innocent little being probably is going to go somewhere they can have some rest. And I know I've seen lots of families who've been terribly upset, when the minister comes just cling on and ... baptisms and christenings and ... to have them blessed and given a name at those times, is a great comfort.' (Staff Midwife, less than 5 years experience)

In addition, a few staff said that they were themselves indifferent or antagonistic towards organized religion but when these stressful situations arose they found comfort in being with the chaplain and talking things through with him.

Ceremonial rites

Functions which were almost exclusively in the ministers' domain were the ceremonial rites: spiritual blessing, christening and burial. Although in certain circumstances staff did undertake to perform a baptismal ceremony of sorts, this appeared to be in the nature of a stop gap. However, in one case a nurse admitted that she had on occasion baptised a child when parents had declined such a service because she considered it was important for the baby. It was not right, in her judgement, that a baby's spiritual welfare should be jeopardised because his parents failed to appreciate the significance of such an act. When asked, she confided that she did not confess to the parents that she had done so.

The seriousness of the ritual of baptism could serve an additional function. Many staff made reference to the fact that simply suggesting baptism could help to alert parents to the gravity of their baby's condition.

When it comes to a funeral, some nurses commented that there is a difficulty in asking a minister from outside to conduct a service for an infant he has never seen. By contrast, introducing parents to the hospital chaplain who is familiar with life in the NICU, and who has seen their baby, enables them to approach him for this service subsequently if they want to have a more personal ceremony. And for those parents who do not attend a church, this choice avoids the embarrassment of approaching their local parish minister who, staff felt, might ask awkward questions or make them feel guilty or substandard.

Bereavement counselling

Ministers are seen to offer a valuable contribution in terms of bereavement counselling and care both during and after the dying. Coming from outside the immediate care giving team is a positive asset in this regard, as is their ability to follow progress and be an ongoing support both in hospital and in the community. They can also operate as resource people, putting parents in touch with individuals and organisations who might be of some help. Being closely involved in the rituals around death, ministers additionally have a role assisting in the practical arrangements.

Support of staff

Many commented on how supportive their chaplains were to the staff themselves. Most welcomed their quiet involvement not just when acute situations arose but in an ongoing way. Having them just put a head round the door to ask how everyone is can be enormously heartening and reassuring.

> 'He also recognizes that we as staff feel a sense of failure and guilt when a baby dies, whether the [staff] recognize it or not. We do feel low, morale of the Unit drops. The post-breakfast ward round [next day] is usually a pretty turgid affair because people care and that's good. So [the chaplain] often will wander around looking casual as though he just happened to have got here because he strayed from his path, but in fact he's there just making sure that people are not falling apart or having too hard a time.' (Consultant, more than 15 years experience)

When things become tense and hard questions are being asked ministers can act as confidants who bring an outside perspective and whose discretion can be relied upon. As we have seen, even declared atheists who had little time for religious matters said that they found the chaplain a great source of personal support. Some staff did qualify their comments by singling out specific individuals who were particularly skilled in this work but only one junior doctor had nothing good to say about ministers of religion in general. She had had a number of bad experiences with chaplains who had behaved in her view ghoulishly or intrusively.

It was not intended in this project to interview anyone other than doctors and nurses. Nevertheless there was opportunity to speak informally to members of other disciplines during visits to the study Units. Chaplains who discussed things with the researcher were divided about what they offered. Some felt their strength lies in what they represent; others felt their very outside-ness makes them unthreatening and therefore endears them to medical and nursing staff as well as parents. Yet others considered that they can appear calm and unhurried, not caught up in the frenzy of ward activity. This sense that they have nothing in particular to busy them, gives them a peaceful aura which encourages people to unburden themselves. One specific supportive function they can offer to doctors and nurses is to alert them to rituals and practices of certain religions or denominations to prevent them from infringing taboos or offending sensibilities inadvertently.

A minority of the staff (1 doctor and 3 nurses) considered that the minister must be someone known to the parents in order to fulfil this role. For the majority, hospital chaplains appeared to meet requirements more than adequately, although one doctor admitted he had no idea what chaplains actually did.

Social workers

Social workers were less highly commended. A considerable number of the nurses observed that these people are viewed with suspicion by parents in general: they are women who take away children and are only involved with families who have problems or criminal connections. In fact the professionals in NICUs appeared to perceive them rather negatively too.

> 'Social workers as such have an image which people don't equate with support around death. They do equate them much more with information and money and all this sort of thing.' (Consultant, more than 10 years experience)

Even those who felt they might have a role, tended to qualify their suggestions with statements to indicate that they should only be brought in if they are already involved, or where families have particular difficulties in coping.

Support of families

Their role is principally to support the family in whatever way they need, largely in relation to practical matters like finance and housing. If they are involved throughout, they are in a position to provide a degree of continuity between hospital and home, a factor which is particularly helpful when it comes to bereavement counselling. As with the chaplains, they are outside the immediate care giving team so if a good relationship can be established they provide a useful listening ear.

Contributing to the decision

In cases where families are not coping well and do require extra support, the social worker can then supply inside information to the NICU team. They are therefore seen by a few staff as having a role contributing a useful dimension to the discussion about treatment withdrawal but the boundaries of their role are clearly circumscribed.

Other personnel

Having asked specifically about these five categories of staff, the interviewer then gave respondents an opportunity to nominate other people who in their opinion should be included.

Whoever parents find helpful

A number (7 doctors and 26 nurses) gave a fairly blanket response to the effect that anyone who could help either the parents or the staff should be included: this would vary from case to case. The point was made that a variety of people encounter the parents during this stressful experience. Whether they meet them in the corridor or serve them meals or clean their rooms, it helps to know enough of the circumstances to be tactful and sympathetic to their needs. In the interests of providing a consistently supportive environment, a range of people might need to be involved to a limited extent, although those making the decision should be kept to a minimum.

Only four groups of people were repeatedly cited: community staff; support groups; extended family and friends; and counsellors.

Community staff

The importance of follow-up work was emphasized and the role of GPs, health visitors, family care sisters, liaison health workers, and community midwives recognized.

> 'There should be somebody from the community involved. I feel there's a big gap there, that these parents are going home and they've lost our support. They look on us sometimes as aunts and uncles of the baby, particularly if the baby [is with us for a long time] ... surrogate parents almost. And suddenly that link is broken and they go home to a community that's never known this baby.' (Staff Midwife, more than 5 years experience)

Support groups

Parents are very vulnerable at these times and access to specific groups is seen to be an appropriate adjunct to the support available from staff in the Unit. Particular cases might need special attention. For example, some parents benefit from contacting a society specializing in a specific condition, or perhaps input from a parent who has been through a similar experience. Organized groups or named individuals can facilitate such a meeting. In addition there are certain needs which are specific to a given parent: language problems might be helped by reference to an interpreter; mental disturbances to a psychiatrist; or religious dilemmas to a church leader.

Extended family and friends

Gaining support from lay people is a very individual matter. The people who offer the best service at one point may not be the first choice later. Those who have previously been a source of valuable sustenance in other circumstances may prove unequal to this specific task. Emotions run high and may render hitherto strong strategies immobile.

It is only through the real life encounter that mettles will be tested and their adequacy known. Some families cast their net wide. Others retreat into a very isolated place. Each coping process has to be respected.

> 'The family – grandparents or aunties and uncles as much as the parents want them to be. You have some families that want everybody and their aunty round about them. And you have other people that want it to be very private and just Mum, Dad and baby, sort of thing. And I think you have to abide by the parents' wishes in that respect.' (Staff Midwife, more than 5 years experience)

Staff did, naturally, have their own perceptions of general advantages in involving other family members. For example, one senior consultant felt that the grandparents in particular have a very special role to play:

> 'Perhaps this is a function of age, but quite often the grandparents' perception of the quality of life and its likely effect on their children, is much more in line with mine ... obviously this is a disaster in the family – a period of nine months of expectation of happiness, in whatever week, is turned the other way round, and I think that it's probably easier for them to share this together rather than the parents have to [deal with it] themselves and then sort of mediate the grieving for the next generation up ... again, this is guesswork, but I suspect that parents, even though they can accept the logic of the situation that you're putting to them, have difficulty with the emotional concept of killing their baby and the presence of the grandparents who can say, "No, that's not what you're doing," [can help] ... The doctor has to be logical ... you give them the logic, but it's not a logic they're looking for, and it may be that the presence of the grandparents may be that buttress.' (Consultant, more than 25 years experience)

But most were content to leave the choice to the families themselves.

Counsellor

Considerable stress is generated during the period of decision making as well as around the time of death, and some staff felt a need for adequate counselling and support for themselves as well as the parents. Ten doctors and 24 nurses specifically suggested that a counsellor or psychologist should be available for this purpose.

> 'It would be very good if we had a counsellor that the nursing staff and medical staff could go to talk to, to get the absolute furious anger out of them. But it may be the parents you're angry with because they're being so awful about this poor child. Or it may be your colleagues you're angry with, or upset with. It would be very good if there was somebody that you could speak to in utter confidence and get it all resolved, because ... all of us have at some time gone into a room and just cracked up.' (Sister, more than 15 years experience)

However, some staff had previous experience of psychologists and psychiatrists specifically appointed for this purpose and had reservations about their inclusion. This subject is expanded further in Chapter 13.

Outside advisors

Sometimes peculiar difficulties arise with certain families. A small number of respondents suggested that a variety of people might be drafted in for such situations. The identity of the appropriate person would be to some extent determined by the nature of the conflicts: other medical specialists, ethicists, legal people or other outside arbiters. Far more, however, were vehement in their dislike of the suggestion that such bodies might be involved where they had no real medical knowledge.

'I'm very much against the idea of there being any more regulation than there is. ... I've never seen any sign of anyone trying to do anything that is legally or morally wrong, and the more legislation or the more words on paper that get involved, I think, the more our hands are tied.' (Sister, more than 15 years experience)

Discussion

As we have seen these are momentous and agonising decisions. Relationships, roles and aims change over time and with circumstances.

'there comes a time when to cherish and respect life means to care but *only* to care for the dying, no longer to oppose death, to accept its coming, to comfort and to keep company with the dying, not to prolong their dying but to make human presence in that solitude, never to desert them, to ensure as much dignity as possible to the dying in their passage.'[163]

There are various and sometimes competing needs to be catered for. The baby is at the centre of concentric circles of protection[24] and it is important to understand where role demarcations begin and end.

'One of the marks of a morally healthy society is its ability to differentiate roles and tasks for the care of its members. Medicine as a moral art is dependent on such differentiation of function to create the forms and limits of the care doctors should provide.'[23]

Overall it is apparent that doctors and nurses working in NICUs feel that the team dealing with a family in these delicate circumstances should be kept as small as possible. There is enough for parents to grapple with without introducing layers of confounding advice. In general the relationship built up with the immediate medical and nursing staff is a special one. Outside influences can potentially complicate things since few others really understand the issues or medical details which are germane to the decision. Nevertheless parents should feel free to consult anyone whose opinion they value. Similarly staff should be free to consult in whatever way they consider appropriate to be sure of the right course of action. Outside of the actual decision making the contribution of anyone who can support in any way is to be valued.

Doctors' roles

Consultants occupy a key position in NICUs. They have not only to make personal decisions based on available evidence but they have also to deal with the tensions and uncertainties within the rest of the team and of the families. As an august international group concluded,

> 'Part of the doctor's clinical wisdom consists of responsibly weighing interests and creatively resolving apparently irreconcilable conflicts.'[164]

But as has been said, it is not a doctor's job to make everyone happy.[23] Indeed it is a fact that care designed to cure often involves a fair degree of suffering and sometimes an inability to cure inflicts great suffering on relatives. Thus, neonatologists are not expected always to spare parents' suffering. Rather their task is first to attend to the health and wellbeing of the baby. Limiting the parents suffering wherever possible is a secondary concern.

Within the NICU as in other areas of medical practice, doctors are the responsible moral agents,[165] legally and professionally accountable for the decision, although they may share the final decision closely with parents and others. Indiscriminately and aggressively treating all babies in their care is neither good practice nor is it required of them. The art of caring has to be mixed generously with the science of medicine.

> 'An approach based on sympathy and shared humanity is much to be preferred to one which stems from a "paralysing injunction" not to harm: "Seeing the world comprised of relationships rather than of people standing alone, a world that coheres through human connection rather than through a system of rules".'[166]

To effect this balance they need qualities of leadership, sound judgement, good communication, active, sensitive involvement in the lives of the families concerned. To be sensitive they need to be as skilled in listening and watching for cues from others as in conveying information and offering guidance to colleagues and parents. There are consultants in the Units in Scotland, albeit perhaps a minority, who manage to combine all these qualities, although staff are hard pressed to define exactly what it is that makes them so special. A certain intuitive skill combined with a genuine compassionate understanding of people seems to underpin the way they operate. Consistency and an ability to use appropriate language and to pace discussion and activities in line with needs add to the overall impression of sensitivity created. All such consultants command great respect from their team and this does much to create a spirit of harmony.

Junior doctors

It mostly falls to junior staff to attend deliveries in Labour ward. But as has been pointed out, the delivery room is no place for snap judgements about whether a baby lives or dies.[34] It is therefore common practice for junior staff to initiate resuscitation until such time as considered judgements can be made by more senior experienced colleagues.

Junior doctors come to neonatology with varying amounts of experience of life and or medical practice. In order to encourage continuity there is a case to be made for including them in ongoing contact with the family although there are very real dangers of misunderstandings developing if they are not guarded in what information they take it upon themselves to convey. Sometimes weeks of careful negotiation by the consultant can be overturned by a chance innocent comment by another person not aware of the fine nuances of communication in such a sensitive area of practice.

Doctors can bring to their practice certain preconceived ideas about what is expected of them. Two such ideas were mentioned by respondents in this study: one relating to the show of emotion and one relating to their place in the power structure. Some doctors thought it did not become them to show emotion, this was something reserved for the nurses. Indeed one SHO thought that the entire fabric of the NICU would be undermined if doctors started being overtly emotional. They were the ones who kept the team functional, she believed. But there are senior doctors who admit that they are not afraid to let colleagues and parents see that they are hurting too. There is some evidence that sharing grief openly can have a positive effect on families.[167,168] Demonstrations of compassion and real feeling help to give the baby worth. If the staff care enough to be upset when the baby dies it shows that the child was special to them too and they grieve with the parents.

When raw inexperienced doctors first enter a NICU they depend to some considerable extent on the wise guidance of the nursing staff. But some clearly have an idea that they are above the nurses in the hierarchy and must adopt a more superior role once they have found their feet. A lordly overruling attitude is a source of great irritation to these very experienced nurses and leads to resentment and sometimes deliberate actions to circumvent involving the offending doctor or to undermine his authority. The gentle but often undervalued example of secure consultants who pay due respect to the complementary skills of their colleagues is in stark contrast to this behaviour of people who are so unsure of their position that they are threatened by the competence and expertise of others in the team.

Nurses' role

Nurses are seen to hold a special place in relation to the baby and his family by virtue of their close involvement over long periods of time. Their skills in comforting and caring for infants in trying circumstances, and in saying and doing the right thing to help parents in distress are beyond measure. But even with their unique insights they feel seriously undervalued when it comes to input into decisions. This troubles them greatly since they feel they cannot then adequately defend the best interests of their infant patients.

Since the 1970s there has been much attention given to the idea of nurses as patient advocates, but before that idea gained credence, nurses believed their primary obligation was to obey doctors and maintain order in hospitals.[169] Advocacy involves the protection of patients' rights and interests. It carries with it certain connotations of assertiveness and conflict with others who might not be making the patients' rights their prime objective. But there are certain difficulties with the image of the nurse as moral guardian and Bernal has suggested a better model might be a covenantal one which leaves the different parties free to enter into agreements, establish moral principles and keep promises.[169] It is a less combative and more cooperative approach to nursing's role. (It should be noted that the idea of a covenant has also been applied to medical practice.[170])

Nurses for many years have stated forcefully that, though they have unique insights into the condition and reactions of the infant, their voice has not traditionally carried much weight in ethical decision making, although it has to be said that the cries from the States are more numerous than those from the UK.[171-79] It is the case that nurses have in some respects acquired more responsibility, but they sometimes lack a corresponding authority within the health care structure. This lack can make them reticent about promoting their views and many nurses in NICUs confess that they rarely confide their opinions in anyone other than their friends at work who tend to be amongst their own peer group. A variety of reasons have been promoted as causative factors in making nurses reluctant to express opinions or challenge decisions on ethical issues: a sense of powerlessness, a tradition of obedience, lack of support, institutional restrictions, job insecurity, limited practice in ethical decision making, inability to articulate an argument, and conformity to the 'doctor-nurse game'.[180] All these can be applied to neonatal nurses.

But perceived powerlessness can render nurses ineffective in situations which are medically dominated, and circumstances where life or death decisions are being made is one such. Power is necessary to fulfil a role effectively. One source of powerlessness can be an inability clearly to articulate a defence of one's viewpoint and many respondents said at interview that they had never before thought through the issues logically or looked behind their 'gut feelings'. Such indecision and uncertainty may be conveyed to a peer who shares a similar stance without threat, but render an individual disadvantaged in the face of more articulate seniors who can communicate a clear argument for their own position.

Although a large number of studies (most of which have been based in the States) have explored nurses' ethical reasoning, these enquiries have not been built one upon another and understanding has not therefore been cumulative.[181] Furthermore the literature on nurses' moral reasoning ability is fraught with methodological problems.[182] Whatever the reasons for their reticence, the effect on practice is serious. Many nurses admit that they do not, and would not, challenge medical decisions even when their consciences are pricked. If they feel something morally wrong is happening to a baby and they keep silent, it is difficult to think what might spur them to vocalize their objections. It has been suggested that nurses are not free to be moral agents because they lack a strong sense of professional autonomy and perceive themselves as putting their jobs and reputations in jeopardy by stepping out of line with prevailing opinion.[183] Certainly some are reluctant to draw attention to themselves. Others are anxious about their future employment if they 'rock the boat'. Some also believe that the decisions of experienced consultants must be right and in some way their own perceptions must be flawed. But others are able in unthreatening and protected circumstances to offer a rational argument for their own choice which is diametrically opposed to what a consultant determined to be right. Yet hardly any of these people went further than grumbling to their friends.

Clearly the background and experience of staff can influence their preconceptions and attitudes[184,185] but a desire to act always in the best interests of the baby should compel nurses to protect their patients. To do this, collaborative decision making is required[176,178] with nurses actively adding their perspective to that of their medical colleagues whose training and role may well predispose them to see things in a different way.

Chaplains and ministers of religion

The role of the chaplain is a rather ill defined one and it seems likely that as health care professionals become more conversant with the ethical arguments there is scope for a degree of role confusion.[186] In as much as they are engaged in profound discussions about life and death, doctors and nurses may well attempt themselves to address some of life's deep questions rather than simply referring these issues to a minister of religion.

It is clear however, that nurses and doctors greatly value the input of the religious representatives. Even for the staff or the families who hold no religious convictions themselves, there is comfort in talking with such a person and perhaps having some form of ceremonial blessing or rite. For the true value of the minister is in more than his authority to perform baptisms or funerals: rather he brings a reassurance and an air of calm which is immensely supportive to both professional carers and to the parents. People are hard pressed to define what it is that creates this comforting presence but it is sufficiently widely experienced to be more than an idiosyncratic quality found in a single individual, and clearly there are certain ministers who are exceptionally good at this task.

It is noteworthy that although almost all doctors and nurses esteem the chaplain and value his input, they do not see a place for him in the actual decision making. His role is rather to comfort and support and in a way put a seal of approval on what goes on in NICUs.

Ethics committees

There is scant support amongst staff in NICUs for the introduction of ethics committees to help them with these complex ethical dilemmas. Indeed many senior figures were vehemently opposed to such an idea and couched their objections in strong terms.

Since the Baby Doe regulations were passed in 1984, infant care review committees have been established in the States although their adoption on this side of the Atlantic has been slow and guarded. Many questions and concerns attend the use of such bodies.[187] The theoretical advantage of having an ethics committee scrutinise decisions is that multidisciplinary perspectives can be brought to the individual situation, although of course, simply having members of the different disciplines present does not guarantee that all points of view will actually be represented. The power structures and dynamics of the group, as well as the skills in articulation of each individual member will influence the relative strengths of different voices.

In general ethics committees have three main functions: a) education; b) policy formation; c) case consultation.[188] Certain paediatricians have supported the idea that such official groups have a useful role to play in all these areas:

> 'to educate, to set broad policies, to review experience, to act as a sounding board, to advise on special problems, to provide "ethical comfort" to the staff and even to protect paediatricians from pro-life activists, crusading lawyers or worst of all, crusading pro-life lawyers.'[34]

But these clinicians were quite sure that decision making should not be one of such a committee's functions. No matter how sincerely motivated, such a body of people cannot understand the complexity of these difficult choices in individual cases. An evaluative study of one neonatal ethics consultative group indicated that they did indeed form a useful sounding board for discussions of difficult cases and contributed an educative dimension, but it was emphasized that theirs was strictly an advisory role; they did not make treatment decisions.[189] There appears then, to be potential value in a forum for considered and balanced debate but no place for the intrusion of outside agents in what is essentially a highly specialized and inherently personal decision.

An alternative with certain advantages over a committee is the appointment of a clinical ethicist who makes his own assessment at the bedside and assists the health care team in working through the relevant ethical issues.[190,191] In this way they are not totally dependent on second-hand information from the doctors or nurses but meet and speak with the families concerned. They can then delineate the issues as they appear in the individual case and help health care professionals to develop their own frameworks for ethical reasoning in the clinical situation.

GPs and community staff

Considerable numbers of nurses do maintain contact with families and visit or meet outside the hospital setting. This is felt to be helpful for the nurses in their own grief resolution as well as for the parents in being able to share precious memories. But with the best of good intentions NICU staff may simply be unable to free up time to spend with parents whose babies are no longer the concern of a hard pressed team. They can rarely linger over one tragedy; there are always other sick babies requiring them to devote their energies to new problems. While it can be enormously supportive to keep contact with the staff who knew the baby best, there are, nevertheless, difficulties attending this prolonged tie. Returning to the scene of so much heartache can resurrect painful emotions which parents may wish to avoid; seeing their baby's space occupied by another child and their professional 'friends' deeply involved with other families can be painful; constantly reliving the past can at a certain point inhibit moving forward into the future.

In the support of such families some see a special role for the GP who has perhaps known the family for some time, meets them in their natural setting, has shared important life events with them, discussed their feelings on previous occasions, and who will see them at intervals for a long time to come.[192] He or she is in a position to keep a watchful but unobtrusive eye on their grief resolution. If there has been contact between hospital and community staff, there is an even better starting point for ongoing support and understanding. If the GP has also seen the baby in the Unit and shared something of his history he will be in a stronger position to pick up the ongoing care of the bereaved family.[168] Other community staff can also fulfil this important role. The exact identity of the support persons or the nature of their input will vary according to circumstances and need.

Conclusions

It is important to appreciate that the skills and insights of each group within the NICU are complementary. Together they make up a whole. Secrecy, fragmentation and inconsistencies dog the paths of some teams making a coherent and strong approach impossible. Genuine compassion, sensitivity to the feeling and beliefs of colleagues, an ability to articulate a considered view, attention to the pacing of discussion and events, and good and open communication are essential ingredients if the team is to work harmoniously.

Whilst there seems to be room for only a few people whose input is highly specialized in the actual decision making there is scope for many people to support and help both families and staff to work through this bitter experience. The contribution of each needs to be respected and valued if the maximum support is to be mobilized.

CHAPTER ELEVEN

Conflicts and Tensions

The sheer enormity of what is being decided is sometimes sanitized with euphemisms and half truths. Clinicians not infrequently refer to non-treatment as 'allowing nature to take its course', but as Kuhse and Singer have graphically shown,[30] seldom does such a representation of events bear close scrutiny. The underlying condition or illness, any medical omission, and what would have been standard treatment for an uncompromised infant, all come into the question. Although it is relatively easy to make the events more palatable and less personal by singling out any one of the conditions as *the* cause, it is the sum total of all of the factors both negative and positive which together contribute to the death. Doctors and nurses working with these babies and their families are forced to face human tragedy on a profound level. Deciding who lives and who dies is a weighty burden which affects people as individuals as well as in their capacity as team members.

As we have seen, deciding what is in the best interests of a neonate is a complex matter with few hard boundaries. It involves unravelling all the tangle of knowledge, historical precedents, perceptions, emotions, aspirations and beliefs. There is a considerable margin for individuals to draw their distinctions at differing points along the spectrum from aggressive treatment to palliative terminal care. Problems exist in trying to arrive at an agreed point and superimposed on these agonising processes is a pervasive feeling of helplessness and intense sorrow,[193] for the loss of infants is a painful experience for those who are trained to cure and to care.

Additional stressors are to be found both between groups and between individuals. Differences of training and roles, organizational matters or personality traits can affect team working and render individuals isolated or distressed. Conflict may result because of a range of factors: inadequate communication, differing ethical positions, divergent roles, ambiguous documentation, administrative barriers, an unstable workforce or inappropriate behaviours.[184,194–197] The combinations and permutations are legion.

The baby who fails to respond to treatment has a different 'social meaning' for the nurse who spends long shifts at the one cotside, compared to the doctor who flits in and out and sees other babies surviving and improving,[5] although of course, the consultant is the one whose reputation and medical skill are on the line. As Anspach has pointed out, the social origins of these different perspectives are radically different:

> 'One bases its conclusions on diagnostic technology, physical findings, and epidemiological studies; the other, the perspective of continuous contact, bases its inferences on social interaction.'[5]

These very differences represent a possible source of tension or conflict.

When all these factors are taken into account, it is hardly surprising that staff working in NICUs can at times become stressed, irritable and overly critical. These are troubling experiences. In order to explore the difficulties of each of the Units, respondents were asked to identify sources of tension, and to examine the ways in which efforts were made to resolve or reduce these additional pressures.

Tension in the Units

Since many respondents had worked in more than one Unit, strenuous efforts were made to ensure that only comments related to the study Units were included in the analysis. Eight respondents were too new to the Unit to offer comment on whether there was ever tension around when these decisions were being made. A further quarter (45, 26%) were unaware of any tensions. In general the doctors were less aware of undercurrents than the nurses with as many as a third of doctors (19, 33%) saying there was no tension in their experience compared with only 26 (22%) of nurses. However, when the consultants were singled out, far more of them (12, 57%) were conscious that there was tension in the team at these times: proportionately nearly twice as many. Even so, only just over half of the consultants were detecting tension themselves.

Sources of tension

Important similarities and differences emerged when respondents were asked to identify those things which caused tension or conflict (Figure 11.1). The exact numbers are not as important as an overall picture of the relative stresses staff experienced.

It was difficult to separate the sources of some of these tensions. For example, it was apparent that whilst the timing of events was a major problem for both disciplines, in the nurses' perceptions the tension between the disciplines was the most commonly cited source of conflict. Where the timing was not right in their judgement they saw it as doctors in conflict with them, so to some extent these categories overlapped for the nurses more than for the doctors. The nurses were markedly more stressed than the doctors by the actual management of cases as well as by the decision itself. Since the doctors were more in control of these aspects of care, this difference was to be expected.

When the different grades were separated, it became clear that the middle grades – the registrars and the staff midwives were the ones most troubled by doctor-nurse conflict. For the senior staff the timing of events was the most frequently cited stressor.

One group of doctors who appeared to be particularly sensitive to unrest in the ranks were the research staff. They were often in the Unit quietly attending to their study infants for long periods. They felt the nurses got used to them and almost did not notice them at times. As a result they heard the muttering and complaining which went on amongst the nurses and so became aware of undercurrents which were not necessarily overtly apparent on ward rounds.

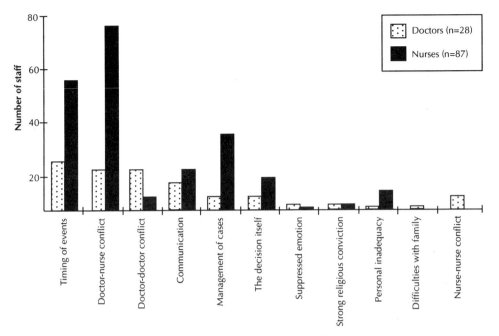

Fig. 11.1: Sources of tension or conflict identified by doctors and nurses

'Actually being a Research Fellow's quite an interesting position because you're almost considered not one of the doctors any more. My research is actually looking at [something which is seen to be of positive value to the comfort of babies] so I'm sort of seen as one of the goodies on the research side ... I think because of that, the nurses are on my side, whereas there's some research that could make you even less approachable to the nurses. It's partly my research and partly personality.' (Registrar, less than 5 years experience)

The nature of their research could indeed influence how they were received and many nurses spoke eloquently of their fierce protectiveness of the babies against too many invasive or disturbing procedures.

The timing of events

Overall a major source of conflict for both doctors and nurses related to the timing of events. It seems to be very difficult to time discussion, withdrawal of treatment and management of the dying in a way which meets with the approval of everyone involved. In general the nurses thought the doctors were too slow in arriving at a decision to stop treatment; the doctors thought the nurses were too hasty in their conclusion and did not fully understand all the factors which had to be considered. Junior doctors were irritated when nurses kept badgering them to get something done. Nurses were frustrated when the medical staff appeared indecisive. It was noteworthy that both groups tended to think the other did not appreciate the time it took for parents to be ready for such a major step; an important difference in perception which can only be illuminated by discussion with parents themselves. But whereas the consultants said their delay often related to needing to be sure the parents had fully grasped the situation and the consequences of this decision, the nurses considered that the parents had come to this point well before the doctors thought they had.

Interpersonal conflict

Interpersonal conflict came high on the list for all grades of staff except the SHOs. Consultants appeared to have more difficulty with other doctors than with nurses. Since in half of the Units there were major differences in approach and practices between the consultants, it is understandable that this should feature strongly. Furthermore the staff midwives reported that they did not share their anger or frustration with senior medical colleagues but with their peers or, where team relationships were good, with the sisters and/or junior doctors. Thus, unless someone relayed this unease to the consultant, it was difficult for him to appreciate it existed.

Doctors' behaviours and attitudes were considered as a distinct item but in reality they were linked to the problems of relationships too. Factors such as high handedness, poor communication, indecision, inconsistency and insensitivity all featured. Whether or not there was justification for such behaviours, they were sources of stress for those who experienced them. Team members felt vulnerable caught up in these delicate negotiations with parents, but not understanding or supporting what was happening. The way the doctors approached staff and parents, and the way they handled the decision making mattered enormously to colleagues. Their sensitivity could transform a difficult situation into an experience where the staff grieved but were left with a feeling of satisfaction about both the process and the way a family had been helped and supported. One consultant summed up his own softly-softly approach:

> 'It may take a week to get to that point [where the nursing staff realize this is the right decision]. But you're drip feeding them, not crashing them saying, "Look this is hopeless." It's a gentle approach. You feed them a piece of information. Then next time you start the conversation, they're already at the point you left them last time and so on.' (Consultant, more than 15 years experience)

There were two groups for whom the traumas of conflict between individuals took precedence over even the timing of events: registrars and staff midwives. This could well have been a feature of their being less responsible for the decision than for its implementation. They were left grappling with the consequences of delays, indecision and inconsistency.

Middle grade staff could be made to feel very uncomfortable with the treatment meted out by the nurses on occasions. Their very inexperience and availability made them a target for pent up anger or frustration.

> 'Frequent requests for me to go and see the baby or the parents, for no particular reason that you can see – being asked repeatedly to go and speak to them or to see them. And there've been a lot of comments: "Don't know why you're doing this," or "Do you have to do that?" Making you feel uncomfortable if you've got to go and say take blood or [site] another drip or something like that. Yes, you

get that, which makes you feel quite bad. Things like, "Do you not think we should call in the senior registrar?" Sometimes things that you've requested to be done, have not been done – or [are] taking an extremely long time to be done. It's very difficult ... Some people in here who're least experienced could become very defensive, probably – I wouldn't say aggressive, but I think maybe unpleasant. Or else you can just let it wash over you and ignore it. If there's any doubt in your mind, that's when it's hardest – it just becomes a conflict because you aren't sure whether you should be doing something and maybe if you're trying to get a drip [in], or you're doing something, you don't get it in first time, you think, "Oh, I must make sure I really am meant to be doing this." But it gets you very unsure of yourself.' (Registrar, less than 5 years experience)

There was clearly a tricky situation here with the nurses fiercely defending the comfort of the baby and the doctors trying to carry out instructions from their seniors. Both were made to feel worse by the actions of the other.

A variety of possible causes of interdisciplinary conflict were suggested.

Differing perceptions of death

Part of the tension appeared to stem from a different perception of events. Doctors sometimes referred to a sense of 'failure' when babies did not survive, whereas the nurses saw an opportunity to extend their nurturing role to provide a good experience of dying.

'I think nurses accept better that you can't cure everybody, whereas I think, having spoken to doctors as friends as well, it's more of a difficult thing to accept that you cannot save everybody, [if you're a doctor]. People do die. It's a natural part of life. So I think nursing-wise, perhaps we have it a bit easier. In fact we're helping people – you're nursing them to either health again or nursing them to a respectable death.' (Staff Midwife, more than 5 years experience)

That is not to say that nurses do not lament their inability to save babies. They do, but their regret reflects a general sense rather than a personal recrimination.

'There's a terrible sense of failure, because you think that with everything you've got in this Unit – all the equipment and all the drugs – you can't do anything for this baby. You expect to give these parents a normal healthy baby at the end of the day. You *want* to. You do your best and try to get to that stage – [but you can't].' (Staff Midwife, less than 5 years experience)

Responsibility

Another factor related to responsibility. It was one thing to have a definite idea of what should be done when the full responsibility rested with someone else. It was another matter entirely to be the final arbiter.

'I don't think the nursing staff, with the best will in the world, have any concept of consequences. They're not going to pick up the legal consequences. They're not going to pick up the hassle from parents afterwards if things go wrong. They're not going to have to sit and counsel them subsequently. So in some ways their advice is extremely valuable in that very narrow context of the environment where they live, where they work [the NICU], but in terms of the wider context then they are very restricted. They're not getting the experience of seeing children who are living with the problems and they don't have to live with the responsibility.' (Consultant, more than 15 years experience)

'Me, personally, I don't have any problems coming to the decision but then that's just me making the decision. But I'm not the one who has to go and tell the parents. I'm not the one who has actually physically to switch the baby off. But I think quite often we come to the decision before anybody else does – you think, "This baby's just not going to do it." I don't think we [have the same difficulty] because we don't have the same responsibility about making the decision.' (Staff Midwife, more than 5 years experience)

Perception of the baby

A third factor hinged on the way people perceived the baby. The nurses sometimes felt that their medical colleagues forgot that these were human beings.

'They're just doing another piece of research on them. But they don't always stop to think, "If that was my baby, how would I feel?" which I think, is what you must think. You know, they seem to divorce themselves from the fact sometimes, that that is actually a baby and *somebody's* – somebody's baby – in that incubator.' (Staff Midwife, more than 5 years experience)

Other respondents felt that junior doctors reacted more sensitively initially but had their finer feelings hardened over time.

'There was this comment made one day by a doctor about a baby and I think in some ways it summed up maybe how they felt. I don't think it was meant in any nasty way and it was said in a fairly jovial tone. But the round had got to this particular baby which was a particularly lovely baby and in fact it was the junior medical staff who'd said, "Oh, isn't this baby absolutely lovely," and "Isn't this baby nice." And the consultant said, "We're not here to be surrogate parents to these babies. We're not here to comment on how attractive they are. We're here to look after the clinical care." And it reminded you of those days of: "This is a paralytic ileus." And I thought that was quite a telling comment. Here are the juniors at the very bottom who still see babies as babies, and see them in terms of being attractive – or perhaps not so attractive. And this is the consultant who simply sees it as a condition to be made better and got out of the way.' (Staff Midwife, less than 5 years experience)

Communication skills

Some nurses felt that their training ill equipped them to 'fight' medical opinion. As has been said, they rarely confronted the consultant personally. Indeed some were aware that their methods of conveying disquiet were so backhanded that they suspected that the consultants neither noticed nor took them seriously.

> 'I don't think we're particularly good at confrontation. We channel it into a graceful confrontation – maybe again perhaps because our senior doctors are men and we're women, we feel as though it's the only way that they'll listen to us to an extent. But I think we have to learn. We have to really work at our communication skills and work out how we want to get ourselves across [so] that they will listen to us. If in some ways we have to dance in their waltz in order to make them listen to what we say, then that's what we have to do until they start to do that ... what happens is that it simmers under the surface and then eventually just dissolves until another situation arises. There's very little direct confrontation at all.' (Staff Midwife, less than 5 years experience)

It was interesting to find that even in those Units where the consultants were reported to listen to the views of all the team, nurses were emphatic that they would never go directly to the consultant if they felt worried about a decision. They acknowledged that the problems 'festered inside people' and were not resolved as a consequence.

Consultants' poor communication skills in relation to talking to parents generated a high level of tension in some instances. The nurses were seriously distressed when, in their view, parents were not adequately prepared for devastating news or were not well supported during the giving of such information. Not only was it disturbing to witness this kind of apparent insensitivity, but it made the nurses' own role extremely difficult. The staff with their specialised knowledge could appreciate that treatment was futile but the parents often could not. Knowing what to say and how much to sound a note of caution became a real problem.

Even harder to take was the kind of situation where the consultant's actions made it impossible to give what was considered to be good terminal care. One example was quoted of a consultant walking into the nursery, simply switching off the ventilator while the parents stood beside the incubator, and then walking straight out again without a word to anyone. The nurse looking after that infant had briefly left her post to collect some equipment so was not present when this act took place. Another nurse in the room was alerted to the baby's cyanosis by the slowing heart rate on the monitor. Both nurses were profoundly shocked and reported that the parents were bewildered. Such unilateral actions which inhibited the giving of good care denied the nurses their principal source of fulfilment where these traumatic cases were concerned: the opportunity to give high quality terminal care to the baby and supportive care to the family.

The management of cases

The way babies were treated and the way the dying was managed made a big impression on the nurses. Where they felt the doctors overlooked the humanness of the babies, treated them like specimens, or took too little account of their suffering or the exact manner of their dying, tensions mounted. As has already been suggested, a particularly difficult group were the severely birth asphyxiated babies who were breathing spontaneously but had no sucking reflex. These were cited by a considerable number of nurses as situations where things were not well handled.

The decision itself

It is interesting to note that the decision itself came relatively low down the list of stressors for all groups. This fact reinforced information given by the consultants earlier which indicated that the task of implementing the decision and dealing with all the people involved with all their different perspectives, was more stressful than actually deciding what was the right course of action. Nevertheless some of the consultants were not unmindful of the impact on inexperienced staff of these momentous events.

> 'The junior staff again – it's their first experience. It's going to mind blast them. They're going to end up having nightmares about it, whereas you and I will both go home and sleep and not worry about it. But there you're dealing with raw recruits who've not been through this process before.' (Consultant, more than 15 years experience)

Difficulties with families

Families who had problems coming to terms with developments or who appeared hostile or held entrenched beliefs which went against what in the staff's view were the best interests of the baby were an additional source of tension. Respondents recounted graphically situations where families had made their task extremely traumatic and stressful. It was evident that the staff in all six Units made enormous efforts to relate well to parents, but there were some parents who were particularly hard to get on with. Not only did this type of conflict engender personal feelings of discomfort but there could also be an underlying fear of recrimination or legal repercussions. Both consultants and the nurses giving the hands-on care cited this factor as a source of tension. In most Units these were the two groups most intimately involved in discussing the issues with parents so it is entirely understandable that they were the ones to identify this stressor.

A sense of personal inadequacy

Some staff felt their inexperience acutely, and tended to withdraw and get on with the other routine work of the Unit. Where they did meet the parents they were aware of the potential for difficulty and mostly referred family members to their senior colleagues. For others, particularly very experienced doctors, there was a sense of failure when a baby died.

People who had most difficulty with these decisions

Consultants mainly believed that nurses had the biggest difficulty in dealing with these difficult decisions. Not infrequently they were seen to be visibly upset and crying. Their emotional involvement was generally deeper and relationships with the family as well as the baby made them vulnerable.

'I suspect [it's] the nurses. We talk to the parents, and break bad news to them, and tell them their child's dying, we're going to withdraw care. And then we go away. And they go back to see the child, and they sit there, and the nurse is having to sit there with them. The nurse can't get out the room, can't run away like the rest of us do for a while, go and have a coffee and think, "That was awful! But at least I've got other things to do." The nurses build up a very close relationship often with the parents and with the child, and go through, often quite a grief process when the child actually dies. The nurses that we work with here appear to cope with that very well, and bounce back and get on with the job, otherwise I suppose they wouldn't be in the job, but they do have, I think, a lot of pressure on them at that time.' (Consultant, more than 10 years experience)

However, there were occasions where they felt their own role was the hardest position to cope with.

'It's variable. I think there are some situations where the consultant finds it most difficult because he or she is ultimately carrying the can, and wants to be completely sure there isn't a stone unturned. And that person can then be perceived as being indecisive or even avoiding the responsibility of taking the decision. But I emphasize that taking the decision is a corporate thing, and is not a unilateral thing, and mustn't be a unilateral thing. There are times, however, when I think the consultant may be the first to identify that a child's demise is inevitable. And then what his or her role is at that time is to inform everybody else and to say why. And that can often be extremely helpful to the team, to learn that this particular form of condition has got a zero outlook. So I think it's variable.' (Consultant, more than 15 years experience)

The sisters, staff midwives and registrars were more divided and ambivalent, understanding the special burdens both of those intimately involved in caring for the baby and the family, and of those who had to take the ultimate responsibility for the decision.

'I sometimes feel the doctors have a job to do and they do it and that's it. It's like them taking blood – it doesn't matter whether the baby's cyanosed or distressed, they take the blood and that's it. [But] when we're taking blood we feel every little stab in that heel, and we get upset when they're upset. And where they will just leave the baby crying, we're the ones that have to come in afterwards and soothe them. So possibly the nursing staff [have the hardest time with these difficult decisions] but I have seen doctors who've been quite upset.' (Staff Midwife, more than 5 years experience)

'I think the medical staff, yes. I think they [have the hardest time]. I suppose because they are the ones that are going to decide – after all this time caring for the babies, [trying to] cure the babies, and in the end they have to begin again. Makes it such a difficult decision.' (Staff Midwife, less than 1 year experience)

A considerable number thought it was the junior staff who struggled most.

'I probably could accept these decisions being made now more – a lot better than I could 20 years ago when I started obviously, because I've seen so many of them [where] the treatment hasn't been withdrawn and the parents have ended up with a [handicapped] baby for life. Again though, it's all very well saying to people, "This does get easier as you get on," but I don't think people believe that. I certainly wouldn't have believed it years ago.' (Senior Sister, more than 20 years experience)

Although this sister had found that the passage of time and accumulated experience had helped her there were many others for whom this did not apply – one just learned how to cope more effectively.

'It never makes it any easier. It doesn't matter whether you've been here 6 months or 6 years, it never makes it any easier. Some folk, I suppose, do handle it better than others. Some people are very, very sensitive – extremely sensitive and maybe go way over the top with their emotions. But you can't put them down for that. Everybody's different.' (Staff Midwife, more than 5 years experience)

Experience could, however, bring the stark reality of other options more clearly into focus, as the earlier quoted senior sister commented. This helped to make the present pain more understandable and thus endurable.

'Suppose in the situation where you had a term baby who's quite badly asphyxiated and brain-wise is very bad. And it's decided to withdraw care and just see how the baby sucks, rather than actually tube-feeding the baby ... You've got this term baby who's lying in a cot, who has been offered a bottle maybe every four hours. It is upsetting, but the alternative's going to be a tube for this baby if he survives, and you know mentally it has got a handicap. I think possibly, maybe, the rotating midwives [would have a problem with this] more so than your main [permanent Unit] girls. OK, it would be upsetting but you realize, well, the alternative is to tube-feed this baby and expect the parents to cope. I remember when I came first, the very first one I came across, I was thinking, "This is so unfair." But gradually as you gain experience you realize you're just looking at the short-term picture. The long-term picture is [bleak]. This particular family, they had other children. Money was very tight. They were really nice but they weren't exactly the brightest of parents and this baby would quite possibly end up maybe being a non-accidental injury – if he suddenly becomes too much for the mother and father ... So it's unfair, not just on the baby but also on the parents.' (Sister, more than 5 years experience)

Junior doctors could additionally be burdened with guilt about possible errors on their part. With experience came an acceptance that there were limits to modern medicine and that sometimes death was to be preferred to life.

'Your experienced people have been there before ... whereas if it's the first time, they can take it very personally, and they can go back and go over what they've done and what they've not done, when it's not been their fault.' (Registrar, more than 5 years experience)

Some very junior doctors admitted to being reluctant to ask for information or clarification in these difficult cases. It seemed somehow insensitive to address these delicate issues publicly. Not only did they recognize their own uncertainties but they perceived an inherent tension for everyone just because they are such sensitive matters.

> 'I think it's just because it's a very emotionally charged sort of topic and a difficult situation really. And nobody likes to discuss these sort of personal views at the best of times. And no one's really entirely sure of their own beliefs. It's bad enough having to confront them in yourself, without having to confront them publicly. I think everybody finds it all a bit tense.' (SHO, less than 1 year experience)

Manifestations of tension or conflict

It seemed important to explore those factors which alerted staff to the presence of tension in the team. Substantial differences were noted both between disciplines and between grades (Figure 11.2).

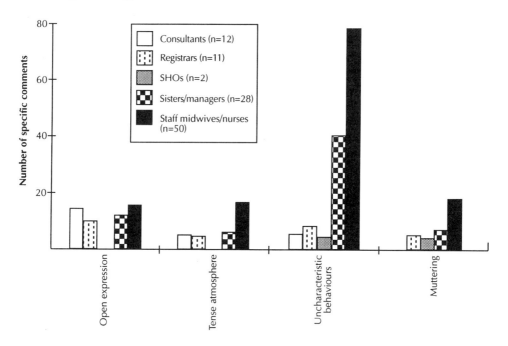

Fig. 11.2. Comparison of factors which alerted different grades of staff to tension

As has been pointed out, only just over half of the consultants were aware of tension in their teams at these times. The commonest way for them to detect it was by being directly told about staff disquiet. Some openly said that they relied on senior nursing colleagues or junior medical staff to alert them, since they were not in the Unit often enough to become aware of the tension for themselves and also they recognized the fact that team members did not confide their anxieties or fears to the consultant.

A generally tense atmosphere, with staff withdrawn or not chatting and smiling as they usually did, was however, noted by a fifth of the consultants. Uncharacteristic behaviour in colleagues with whom they had worked for years could also alert them to an incipient problem, although relationships in most cases permitted such colleagues to talk through their concerns more directly.

Registrars were more conscious of undercurrents of unrest. When nursing staff quibbled with their instructions or decisions, made seemingly inappropriate demands on them to do things for the parents or the baby, or made comments which criticised or questioned their actions, the registrars interpreted this as tension about the case. Clearly, on some occasions there was room for misinterpretation, and perceptions of tension have to be set against this backcloth. For example, one staff midwife reported an experience where she herself knew a baby was not for resuscitation but the SHOs were unaware of this order. When the infant collapsed she started to 'bag and mask' but when the junior doctors arrived she told them the baby was not for resuscitation. Asked by the interviewer why she had done so, she replied, 'I would always resuscitate. I couldn't take that responsibility. I'm a nurse, I'm not a doctor.' For the senior doctor who had originally informed her of the decision not to resuscitate, there could well have been a confusion about her position. It could have been interpreted as not supporting the decision. Registrars were more frequently in the nurseries than their senior colleagues and tended to hear and see more of the 'normal' behaviours of their nursing colleagues. They were thus aware of muttering and whispering, silences, irritability and a generally tense atmosphere.

Only two SHOs had experienced tension in relation to these cases. This had become apparent through staff weeping, or the whispering and muttering which went on amongst the nurses while they were in the nursery or coffee rooms. A considerable number of the SHOs were quite new to their posts and many expressed a sense of their own insecurity and inexperience which could well render them less sensitive to the emotional needs of others around them. Furthermore they did not know the staff well enough to know what kinds of behaviours constituted deviations from the norm.

If nurses were unhappy about a baby or a decision they tended to discuss it with their peers first. Having ascertained that others too were uneasy with what was happening, they would occasionally then take the matter to the sisters. Many sisters too were also delivering hands-on care themselves at least some of the time. As a result sisters were directly appraised of the feelings of their junior nursing colleagues. The sisters were also directly communicating with the consultants. This could well explain the fact that direct expression was commonly cited as a way that sisters had of knowing when staff were having a hard time with a decision.

However, they were also watching and listening to events in the nurseries and they listed many other cues which alerted them to potential problems: irritability, anger or aggression, silence, withdrawal of normal social exchange, whispering and muttering, excessive activity, nurses endlessly rehearsing the points which troubled them, and doctors procrastinating about decisions. Completely opposite behaviours could be indicators of stress. Thus excessive garrulousness in a normally quiet worker was as much a warning flag as silence in a normally outgoing happy colleague. A consultant slamming a door could demonstrate his tension but so could a consultant withdrawing to his office and not answering appeals to talk to parents. It was knowledge of colleagues as individuals which allowed these experienced sisters to detect uncharacteristic behaviours.

> 'Flying off the handle at the least little thing, [so] you just know that they're a bit [tense]. And they often look flustered as well. Or they say something that they wouldn't have said – out of normal. Or some people actually go away and have a cry – you *see* they've been crying. You know that they've been away in the toilet for 10 minutes and then you can see they've been crying. And things like that ... but you just also tend to go and talk about it afterwards. Go away for a cup of coffee, a wee break, if you've had a really hard time of it. Just a time away from the parents as well.' (Sister, more than 5 years experience)

The staff midwives and nurses tended to be a close-knit group who socialised as well as worked closely together. Mostly they knew one another well. As a result they could detect tension in their colleagues early on. Irritability and uncharacteristic behaviours gave them an indication that someone was struggling. This would lead others to ask the stressed colleague if she wanted to talk about what was troubling her, or seek out a colleague known to be a personal friend, and to provide a forum for a discussion of the difficulties. Whispering and muttering together about their feelings, as time and opportunity allowed, enabled them to work out a clearer assessment of the situation. Sometimes this sharing of their feelings, perhaps crying, was enough to relieve the tension. Where the consensus view was that things were not being managed well, they tended to go to senior nursing colleagues, looking to them to explain the rationale for the current position or to register disquiet to the consultants.

Part of the outward expression of their inner struggles was seen in the nurses who were giving the hands-on care, making comments to the junior doctors which questioned their actions, or in making snide or derogatory statements in their hearing. The SHOs and junior registrars found this kind of behaviour stressful. Sometimes they allied themselves with the nurses in their distress but reinforced the fact that they were only obeying instructions. Some kept quiet but inwardly resented these behaviours. Often when the nurses were uneasy, the junior doctors were too. It was hard to have the full battery of the nurses' anger and frustration directed at them, superimposing tension on an already high level of insecurity and uncertainty and sometimes a sense of failure or guilt.

Resolution of the tension

There was a remarkable consonance between the disciplines when it came to trying to resolve the difficulties. Top of the list for both doctors and nurses was discussion of the things which were causing tension in the team. Actions which helped people to feel supported and to defuse the tension were the second most commonly cited way of relieving the situation. These overall similarities held for each grade of staff separately too, but the staff midwives identified grumbling to colleagues as a major way of resolving tension. Although this could have the effect of providing an outlet for pent up emotion some other members of the team felt it was destructive.

'You just have to wade into it. Covert disagreement is very unsatisfactory and either you have to wade into it or else you have to overrule it. Now that sounds terribly authoritarian, but if in the end, a small coterie of people who are most involved in the care of the child have a particular view and they are confident that that particular view is as right as it can be under these circumstances, then sniping from outside is only destructive. And I would see my role as wading into that and saying, "Look, this is not acceptable. The team has taken a professional decision, with integrity, and I think now is the time to let that decision come forward. Please back off."' (Consultant, more than 15 years experience)

A considerable number of nurses (22/86) but only three of the 28 doctors who had experienced tension around decision making, volunteered that they thought their Unit was not very good at dealing with this kind of problem. It was interesting to find that the majority of these nurses came from the two Units where there were inherent tensions between the sisters and staff midwives, and the consultants did not enjoy good relationships with the nursing staff.

When respondents were asked whether these attempts were successful in reducing or resolving the tensions, there were essential differences between the disciplines. The majority of the doctors responding (22/28, 79%) felt that they were, whereas less than half of the nurses (39/86, 45%) thought so, although a further 20 nurses did concede that the tension was sometimes eased to some degree by these efforts. Both sisters and staff midwives shared these reservations about the efficacy of current attempts to minimize tension.

Continuing conflict

A question was then asked about what the team did where these initial attempts at resolution failed and there were ongoing differences of opinion producing tension in the Unit. Eleven of the 28 doctors and 18 of the 86 nurses who responded to this question had never experienced this type of ongoing conflict. A further 14 nurses said that the conflict was not resolved in their experience and six felt that the way things were handled was simply to ignore the problem.

For the remainder, the course of action was principally to concentrate on continuing discussion both with individuals and with groups of people working towards agreement or some form of compromise. Some doctors drew attention to the advantages of having dissension in the ranks to ensure that these decisions were always made carefully and could be justified to potential critics.

'Obviously if there was somebody who repeatedly disagreed, maybe for whatever strong religious beliefs, in what we were doing, then we would have to question whether in fact that person was suitable for work in the Unit. It's very difficult. I would not want us to have in the Unit, everybody who thinks exactly the same, or who are just "Yes-people" who, just the minute one of us says, "That's it, right, fine, pull the plug," they just say, "Yes, sir," and do it. No, we mustn't have that. But at the same time, of course, if there is somebody who is persistently and totally different to their peers – that's the thing you have to match them against. You've got this whole range but if you've got people on either extremes who will not move their position at all – I think that's the point. You can have very strong beliefs, but I think you have to – in the world today – be ready to actually move your position slightly. And if they won't move at all then I don't think they should be doing the job. But, yes, there have to be people who are outspoken and say, "I don't think this is right." And you have to convince them. You think it's right and you have to convince them. And it may be that *they* convince *you* that it isn't right.' (Consultant, more than 10 years experience)

In the perceptions of most of the nurses, it was either the most senior, the most assertive person, or the one who shouted loudest who 'won' at the end of the day, the implication being that this was the consultant. However, a few nurses felt that overall the decision went by consensus with strong dissenters simply being removed from the scene of these controversial activities. Some nurses saw it as a way forward to keep protesting. Only a very few respondents (4 doctors and 6 nurses) said they would appeal to a third party to arbitrate where there was this form of ongoing difference of opinion.

On occasion the delay meant that the baby 'made' the decision by dying anyway and a small number of people cited time as a way of resolving such dilemmas. To some extent in these situations there was nothing left for the nurses to do but accept the situation and get on with their work and this was the perception of two of the nurses and one doctor concerning how the controversy was dealt with.

It was interesting to hear some consultants explain the measures they took to avoid such situations. Some made it plain to the team that the consultant was the one who decided: other people's opinions, even if heard, would not really influence the final choices. Others selected colleagues who were known and trusted to be involved in these cases. They tended to be those who were experienced and perceived to be wise about these ethical issues, not the idealistic crusaders.

'I don't get myself into these positions of conflict with the staff. I've picked the people to be involved beforehand and I'll only talk in circumstances where I'm comfortable. That may not be organised. It may just [happen] because I've seen this spontaneous situation arise and I've capitalised on the moment. I wouldn't get myself into conflicts. I don't want a radical midwife. I've had enough problems elsewhere with people who are not really caring about these individual babies ... I only deal with people who are willing to talk about these things and I can look into their mind and say, "Now that's OK, I know where they're coming from."' (Consultant, more than 15 years experience)

By contrast, other consultants made the matter so open to scrutiny and debate that everyone had an opportunity to contribute their views; decisions to withdraw would not be made unless there was a strong consensus. In three Units, as already described, the decision was only ever taken very late on in the baby's life by which time everyone agreed that the prognosis was so awful as to make death undeniably preferable to life under these conditions.

The final responsibility

There was widespread agreement that the final responsibility rested with the consultant in all of the six Units. This was sometimes thought to be in conjunction with the parents. Three sisters and two staff midwives/nurses thought that senior nurses also shared the responsibility.

When respondents were asked if they thought this was the right place for such responsibility, 82% of the doctors (45/55) and 62% of the nurses (69/111) thought it was, with a further 3 doctors and 20 nurses thinking it was partially right but that the consultant should work closely with the rest of the team and the parents to be sure he was acting rightly. As one nurse put it, the consultant was the driver who picked up the trophy or carried the can for a crash, but the rest of the team were navigators who helped him to reach the finishing post.

> 'I think he's the right person to make the final decision, but I think he should always do it in conjunction with other folk, for instance ourselves. Because we have gut feelings about these babies as well, and we have experience, and we're with these babies – sometimes in intensive care maybe I would be on a 10 day stretch – 7 and a half hour day, every day for 10 days on the trot.' (Staff Midwife, more than 5 years experience)

A small number (3 doctors and 6 nurses) said they simply did not know if this was the right way to proceed.

However, 16 nurses were unhappy with the consultant taking such a role. Only four of these offered an explanation for their response. They thought there should be a consensus decision with the most senior person on the spot at the time taking the final responsibility. This reflected a degree of disquiet about registrars consulting consultants over the phone in relation to babies whom they had never seen. The nurses felt that the person who was with the child could best interpret all the signs and results, and make the appropriate choices. They were also concerned about the introduction of a complete or relative stranger at these highly charged moments.

> 'The parents have usually never seen this person [the consultant] before. Sometimes you think it should be somebody that they know – maybe a registrar who's dealt with them. And on occasion maybe the junior doctor, because maybe the baby's not been here very long, and the registrar's never been around or anything ... because it's a familiar face, instead of a strange face ... Even just the word, *consultant doctors,* can have [a sense of] "Stand back, he's God." And maybe the registrar who has maybe scanned the baby's head, or been there at the delivery, or been there when there's been a crisis – not even a known name, but even a known face – I feel it's nice if it's a face that they know.' (Staff Midwife, more than 10 years experience)

Nevertheless the more junior doctors themselves were not keen to accept this responsibility in general. They were only too well aware of their own lack of experience. It required maturity and a broad range of experiences and skills to do this job well.

'You can't learn [this kind of experience] out of a book. You can't. Experience, seeing it out [there] in experience, I think that puts them in the position of being the one who's most able to really weigh up things ... having the confidence to *know.* I think you can only get that with experience.' (Registrar, less than 5 years experience)

Discussion

The NICU is a micro-society with a unique culture combining two discrete but potentially incongruous aspects – the technological and the caring.[4] A degree of tension and conflict is probably inevitable when people are dealing with distressed parents and making decisions about life and death in an already highly charged environment. Indeed it could be said that a certain level of tension and disagreement is a necessary prerequisite to such decision making. The agonising which characterises these debates and the pain which their implementation generates, are feelings which emerge from the crucible of profound human tragedy. If staff members stop feeling that pain they could become blasé about the enormity of the choices. And if all staff agree with the decisions there would be no necessity for the team constantly to revisit the arguments and ensure that they can justify their decisions on the basis of science, of logic and of compassion.

Every individual perceives these situations slightly differently. To some extent people control how they perceive a situation by the interpretation they give to events. Thus, for example, endowing the child with the ability to decide, shifts the responsibility away from the health care team.[3] Many respondents in this present enquiry referred to the baby deciding in cases of delay caused by differing opinions, and this idea of the baby deciding is a common phenomenon in NICUs.[4] If the baby simply dies they speak of the infant having resolved the dilemma or conflict. Alternatively if the baby keeps fighting it can create a moral obligation on the staff to keep treating aggressively since it is interpreted as the child not wanting to die and having the stamina for the battle.

Given that the team is made up of members of different disciplines and of individuals with unique histories it would be remarkable if everyone agreed all the time. Even if they had no superimposed highly emotional situations to contend with, they would bring different opinions, beliefs and values to bear. The addition of these profoundly disturbing circumstances makes it the more understandable that feelings run high, people behave out of character and stress levels rocket.

Exacerbating factors

A number of underlying factors add to the complexity of this decision making and increase the likelihood of tension developing. Two of the main ones, already briefly referred to, are the uncertainties involved and the medical compulsion to treat.

UNCERTAINTY

Decisions are based on the best interests of the baby. But so much about the baby is unknown. Although in recent years attempts have been made to measure levels of stress through physiological and chemical changes, it is still extremely difficult even to be sure what a baby is presently suffering never mind how he would cope with probable future difficulties. There are no instruments for listening to his views and perceptions so staff are forced to rely on their own intuitive understanding. And '[h]umane care depends partly on these primordial skills.'[24] Since each person will form a uniquely based assessment there is already a potential for division.

The situation is further complicated by the fact that experience brings its own wisdom but also additional ambivalence. For on the one hand uncertainties can be the result of imperfect mastery of what is known, and with greater knowledge of the specialty staff can gain a confidence in their own judgement. But on the other hand, to some extent the more that is known the more senior people recognize how easy it is to be wrong. They have witnessed the disasters resulting from the application of imperfect understanding. They see how limited is the current state of medical knowledge. Their confidence is shaken by individual babies defying their predictions. Neurological compromise is a major factor indicating future quality of life when it comes to withdrawing treatment, and yet even where there is evidence of catastrophic brain damage there are still cases where babies go on to have a reasonable or even good quality of life. Increasingly then experienced clinicians accept the impossibility of talking in certainties. It is sobering to analyse the situation and conclude that decisions about whether a baby lives are predicated upon such shaky predictions of probable outcomes. This deep ambivalence has been exposed elsewhere[24,150] but is not the easier for being acknowledged.

THE COMPULSIVE DESIRE TO TREAT

We have earlier mentioned the fact that the desire to treat is strong. Other writers too have made reference to the sense of mission of doctors which motivates them to treat aggressively in cases where other members of the team feel the burden of suffering outweighs the benefits.[3] Sometimes doctors are satisfied with nothing less than hard measurable data to show beyond doubt that treatment is futile, and in such cases withdrawal cannot be undertaken until such evidence is to hand. Sometimes a fear of legal repercussions compels people to pursue an aggressive course to minimize the risk of a court action. The result of such compulsions is that overly burdensome treatment of dubious value is sometimes inflicted on babies.[3,4,6] It is salutary to find that staff themselves are more concerned with the practice of over-treatment than of too little treatment.[167]

But the harder staff work on a baby the harder it may be to give up. If they are unwilling to accept that their attempts have failed they may continue to 'throw good money after bad'. Time, energy, money and emotions are invested in these infants. Initial commitment may indeed be well intentioned, justifiable and morally right, but determining when the point has come to stop can subsequently be difficult.

The main sources of conflict

Within this general framework of tension, two main sources of potential conflict were identifiable in this study: the timing of events, and interpersonal conflict.

TIMING OF EVENTS

Again and again in various guises this bone of contention was seen. The fact that nurses are more ready than doctors to limit treatment has emerged from studies additional to this one.[198] Because of their relative goals and different orientations nurses have less to lose professionally by the death of a baby. We have already seen many of the factors which make the decision about when to raise the initial doubts, when to make the final decision and when to actually withdraw treatment, a source of tension and conflict. The manifestations of this inner unrest are many and varied as the data show. There appear to be few Units where the views of all team members are openly and respectfully attended to when these weighty decisions are being considered. Even where the questions are addressed in a fairly public way – on ward rounds for example – staff often feel that the opportunity to air their feelings is not appropriately orchestrated. Some feel their views are not really heard, or that it is a 'paper exercise.' Others feel inhibited in the face of a crowd of people. These are delicate and sensitive matters; articulating a defence of what one thinks is not easy. Furthermore sometimes feelings are a reflection of a gut intuition rather than a reasoned argument and nurses especially do not feel that their medical colleagues respect intuition, although nurses believe that these finely honed skills rarely let them down. They cannot bring hard evidence to support their belief that a baby wants to die, or that a baby is never going to win the battle against crippling damages, so they keep quiet, reserving their opinions for their colleagues who understand these 'sixth sense' assessments. Senior nurses are in a stronger position to voice an opinion since they deal more directly with the consultants in many ways but their contact with the baby and family is often less intense and on occasions junior staff resent their input because of this.

Doctors on the other hand are frustrated by the undercurrents which make their own position so much harder to bear. Consultants are carrying the heavy burden of the final responsibility; juniors are having to contend with delivering ongoing treatment which inflicts suffering on a baby in what may be his last hours or days. But their position is made more uncomfortable by the disapproval of their colleagues. Because although junior nurses rarely speak out about their beliefs, they make their feelings known in other ways. When they repeatedly make snide comments, challenge junior doctor's management, or present a frosty front they are sending signals which can potentially increase the discomfort of the medical staff without the benefit of an opportunity to deal openly with the differences in perceptions or with the developing hostile situation. Some doctors try to ignore the non-verbal onslaught. Others try to identify with the nurses and give them insight into their own reservations in an effort to ease the relationship at the bedside at least. But many appear insensitive to the cues which indicate that all is not well.

INTERPERSONAL CONFLICT

The main sources of interpersonal conflict arise from doctor-doctor conflict and doctor-nurse conflict.

DOCTOR–DOCTOR CONFLICT

This source of tension comes high up the list of doctors' stressors. But nurses too are aware of these conflicts. The sisters are a group who deal fairly directly with the consultants and are often party to their thinking and their doubts when others are not. Indeed a number of very experienced consultants said the senior nurses with whom they had worked for many years were their chief confidantes. More junior nurses see the direct consequences of medical conflict.

The main components of tension between doctors are inconsistency and opposing practices. Given the fluctuating circumstances and the uncertainties around these situations it is not surprising that doctors change their minds about whether and when to withdraw treatment. The least hint of an improvement in a deteriorating baby can give them pause for thought. The enormity of what they are deciding remains a constant brake on too precipitate action. But doctors often discuss possible measures casually walking along the corridor or over coffee. A colleague might suggest, 'Have you tried such and such a treatment?' If there is nothing to lose the doctor might decide it is worth one last ditch effort to be sure no stone has been left unturned. But the origin of the idea, and the rationale for this eventuality, are not always conveyed to the nurse looking after the baby or even to the other doctors in the team. As far as they are concerned this morning's dictum that there was nothing more to be done, this evening has been overruled in favour of yet another treatment plan. Many and disturbing were the descriptions of such apparently inconsistent decisions.

As has been shown in a number of Units the different consultants are themselves working in opposition. This situation has serious repercussions for the team. Not only are they left personally insecure and bewildered, but more importantly their care of infants and parents is compromised. A totally unacceptable position develops if one consultant tells staff and parents that treatment for a given baby is futile but subsequently another orders aggressive and invasive therapy. It is not unknown for consultants to be so much at odds that one waits until another has left the Unit or is on annual leave before moving in and countermanding a decision which he considers is not in the best interests of that baby. Irrespective of where the rights and wrongs lie in relation to the decision itself, such discord needs to be worked out in private and away from the serious business of saving lives or allowing death.

DOCTOR–NURSE CONFLICT

Doctors and nurses have different and complementary orientations and access to different kinds of information. It is almost inevitable that they will sometimes see the patients' best interests differently. But it is sobering to uncover the extent of the problem. For nurses this inter-disciplinary conflict is easily the most commonly reported stressor.

Watts and his colleagues identified five main sources of conflict between nurses and doctors: inadequate communication; differing ethical positions; divergent professional roles; ambiguous documentation and administrative barriers.[196] All of these factors were identifiable in the present study as sources of tension. The *inadequacy of communication* has already been explored.

The effect of *differing ethical positions* relates principally to the perceived duties of the two disciplines. While a doctor might feel it is ethically acceptable to withdraw a life sustaining treatment, a nurse continues to have an obligation to care for that patient. Sometimes the withdrawal of a treatment can have serious consequences for the overall comfort and wellbeing of the patient which compromise the nurse's caregiving. This is seen dramatically in those cases where a consultant orders a regime of oral feeds for a severely birth asphyxiated baby who cannot suck.

The very fact that doctors and nurses espouse *divergent professional roles* creates a potential divide. Nurses provide physically intimate and continuous care; doctors make brief clinical visits. Discussion with distraught parents is usually a short experience in a varied professional day for a doctor; close involvement with those same parents may occupy up to 12 hours of a nurse's more repetitive working day.

Ambiguous documentation, the fourth factor, is an area of great complexity. Doctors sometimes deliberately veil their reports, at other times the limitations are a feature of slovenly practice or poor training. But whatever the cause it is difficult to sustain a concerted team effort if everyone concerned is not fully in the picture. A guarded 'Parents agree to withdrawal of treatment over time,' can mean that at the next emergency, resuscitation will not be attempted; or that existing support will be gradually withdrawn; or that all efforts will be maintained until the parents say they are ready for everything to be withdrawn. The interpretation will materially affect the way the rest of the team will proceed both in their own discussion with the parents and their management of this baby.

In all Units there are *administrative barriers*. Sometimes these are matters of etiquette and protocol. In some they have arisen by force of habit. In others they are features of individual perception. But however they have arisen, the end result is that there are no readily identifiable avenues through which to arbitrate in cases of dispute. This situation is particularly acute in those Units where junior doctors are inhibited from discussing their concerns with their consultants, and the junior nurses with their seniors. If the system of line management within a specific discipline breaks down, even the commonly accepted way to relay unrest is removed. Staff are caught in a spiral of frustration and moral unease if they are disturbed by what is being done but cannot attempt to rectify the perceived wrong because of the fear of breaches of confidence or ridicule, or because of damaging career implications.

Because nurses tend to show that they are upset when things are going badly for a baby, there is overt evidence that they are emotionally involved. Some doctors clearly view these shows of emotion with some disdain, others are grateful that the nurses care so deeply. But nurses themselves sometimes interpret doctors' more stoical approach as indicating that they do not get personally involved. Clearly doctors vary in this regard as indeed do nurses. But an absence of visible signs of unrest should not be interpreted as a coldness. As one consultant in Alderson's study said:

> 'we cannot possibly attend to everything fully and we have to decide what are the priorities. We are already overstretched. It is not that we do not care, or that we are not aware, or are not trying hard enough. You have to care to go on

working here. But the doctors who stay have to be, not tough because we do get distressed, but emotionally resilient. It is very wearing, physically, emotionally, and socially to go on working here. We need the government to fund far more supporting services for the patients and the staff.'[24]

Whether the doctors are given to displays of emotion or not, more important to the nurses is a demonstration of sensitivity to the baby's needs. It is a widely accepted fact that nurses are concerned about the potential exploitation of their patients.[199] Subjecting a baby to painful or insensitive treatment when their outlook is poor, is a source of grave disquiet amongst nurses. Relentlessly to pursue a syringe-full of blood or a successfully sited IV in spite of evident distress in the baby, is to appear to have ignored the humanness of a baby prone to suffering, and to be regarding him as a mere collection of veins. Some nurses commented that they would rather have an advanced nurse practitioner do these tasks than a doctor because she would be more likely to look at the baby and pace procedures alongside his tolerances. But there are junior doctors who themselves agonise over the need to inflict pain on a baby for whom continued existence is highly questionable. Contributing to the suffering of babies can be a hard act to perform and it is not surprising that many doctors feel the need to detach themselves to some extent in order to carry out the necessary tasks.[4] Overly identifying with either the baby or his parents can be paralysing but detachment can potentially lead to insensitivity in time. A balance has to be struck. Perhaps the extent of junior doctors' unease is inadequately represented since a sense of loyalty to their seniors, and their own insecurity often prevent them from sharing their reservations. But failures to express their distress coupled with efforts to hide their emotions create a situation which breeds further misunderstandings.

There are, however, problems amongst the nurses too, attributable at least in part to a failure to communicate their feelings. By their own admission they rarely convey their disquiet beyond the confines of close friends and their peer group. Studies have shown that women and nurses try to avoid conflict, and turn the problem inwards resulting in stress, low morale or depression.[200] Valuing caring and attachment, they tend not to face conflict head on but to make compromises in order to preserve relationships. There is a sense in which characteristics such as assertiveness or confrontation are seen as antithetical to caring and nurturing, the traditional roles of nurses. But adopting these distinctions can handicap nurses from exercising their autonomy and dealing healthily with differences of opinion in clinical situations.

> 'Passivity by caregivers who spend the greatest amount of time in direct patient contact is both wasteful and potentially dangerous.'[197]

Another factor in this interprofessional conflict relates to the tasks of each group. Although the doctor makes the decision it is very often the nurse who must deal with the effects of decision making at the point of impact.[201] Yet the nurses may be divided in their loyalties – to the patient and his family and to their medical colleagues. This conflict can be a source of moral anguish superimposing stress onto an already emotionally overloaded situation. Sometimes nurses have felt forced to take extreme measures. On one end of the spectrum they may behave surreptitiously: there is ample anecdotal evidence that over the years nurses have slipped unrecorded feeds to infants scheduled to be starved to death. At the other end they may blow the whole matter out of the water in a dramatic way – 'blowing the whistle' on their colleagues and so bringing activities which they find morally reprehensible to public attention. Either way discord and damage will be the result.

Sensitivity to tension

Individuals are variously sensitive to tension within the team. In general consultants rely on overt expression of unease. Sometimes this comes from discussion with their junior medical colleagues, sometimes from senior sisters representing the nursing staff and very occasionally from nurses providing the hands-on care. The more involved the consultant is in the daily care of the child, the more likely he is to pick up dissension if it exists. Being a remote figure calling in for official ward rounds and only reappearing if called to attend a crisis, tends to isolate him in terms of respect as well as from a practical point of view. There is an increasing unlikelihood of anyone confiding their doubts to him. For those consultants who are working closely with their colleagues there is opportunity to get to know them as individuals and to find out in the process how they think and feel. Some have indeed developed relationships which have withstood the years, and they are grateful for the support and friendship offered. In return they gain insights into the beliefs of other team members and hear their intuitive hunches.

Registrars occupy a different place in the team and tend to mix more with the nurses. Spending more time actually beside the babies they pick up opinions from shared discussion with these colleagues as well as by overhearing whispers or muttered conversations between the nurses themselves. Sometimes they are the uncomfortable butt of repeated quibbles which betray the nurses' disquiet. If they get to know the nurses well, they are also able to detect uncharacteristic behaviours which indicate raised stress levels or sadness.

SHOs are new to this area and have much to learn about the practice of neonatology. Although they are the doctors who most frequently appear at the cotside, they appear to be sensitive only to the overt expressions of upset such as tears or muttered conversations overheard. It seems likely that their attention is concentrated on getting their own contribution right and they have little space for the tensions of others who appear to be more competent and experienced in this high powered environment.

When it comes to the nurses there are grade differences to be seen. The staff nurses and midwives are numerically the largest group and they are the ones who rely heavily on sharing their disquiet with colleagues. Close friendships and common tasks and beliefs make sharing feelings an acceptable and accepted practice. In this way they are party to the opinions of a range of individuals. Additionally because of their close associations geographically in the Unit and in terms of acquaintance, they are in a position to detect uncharacteristic behaviours which indicate when someone is having a hard time with a situation.

Sisters, where they work closely with the babies pick up cues in the same way. Where their role is more managerial but they enjoy close relationships with the other nurses they are privy to information because the nurses confide in them when they are seriously concerned about developments. They are also the people who hear what the doctors are thinking on ward rounds and in meetings about babies. They are then in a key position to bring together opposing viewpoints and work towards an acceptable resolution of difficulties. But if they are remote figures resented by nursing colleagues because they do not appear to pull their weight, or not respected by their medical colleagues for whatever reason, they can remain unaware of opinions and so are unable to effect any sharing of different ideas and working towards compromise or settlement.

The way forward

It is widely accepted that consultants are the people with whom responsibility for the final decision lies. But very few believe it should be a unilateral decision. The consultant is part of a team and as such, relies on others to work alongside him in the provision of a total package of care. True consultation and collaboration offer a much more productive way forward. But success presupposes open and honest communication, mutual respect, and on occasions even a degree of compromise.

Nurses and junior doctors in all Units express genuine anxieties about the suffering of babies and families when treatment is prolonged but the prognosis is bleak. Real conflict exists where they are required to act within narrowly defined roles which limit their capacity to do what in their judgement is in the best interests of the child and his family. Where there is a clear hierarchical structure and little real communication between the ranks, frustration and distress build as they carry out instructions against their better judgement. This further adds to the barriers between groups and a vicious circle is perpetuated. In those Units where caring is openly acknowledged as a legitimate approach and where team members are encouraged both to express their reservations and to share their grief, open clear lines of communication are facilitated and supportive environments are fostered. If they have shared in the decision making they are more likely to be committed to implementing the agreed programme of care.

Everything appears to hinge on effective communication. Without the knowledge of different opinions and attitudes there can be no effective resolution of conflicts. Although the existence of a communication gap between the two disciplines has been acknowledged elsewhere,[198] there is evidence that consultants and cooperative teams can overcome inherent problems. Careful and sensitive team management based on genuine respect and open communication can produce an environment where decisions are made with the maximum amount of team participation but the minimum of unhealthy tension and conflict.

The General Medical Council[202] has recognized the central role of communication in a doctor's practice. It points out that 'Deficiencies in this area are responsible for a high proportion of complaints and misunderstandings.' Such deficiencies are certainly seen as key factors in bringing about both complaints and misunderstandings in NICUs. The ability and willingness to listen well and to offer explanations which are comprehensible and at once compassionate and logical, is essential in any honest and open sharing of information with others, either fellow health care professionals or patients and their relatives.

Conclusions

Tension is high in the busy and specialized environment of modern NICUs. Making these momentous decisions about which babies will be treated superimposes further stress. Keeping conflict to a minimum depends on staff communicating effectively and being consistent in their approach. Serious consequences to the baby and family as well as to the team members may accrue if the timing of events or relationships between people are not attended to wisely and sensitively.

CHAPTER TWELVE

Parental Involvement in Decision Making

It has often been suggested that the survival of a handicapped infant results in the creation of a handicapped family. There are, of course, many examples of families finding amazing reserves of selfless devotion and strength in such circumstances. But, even though stress is not of necessity dysfunctional in these families,[93] there are also countless examples of lives sorely tried or even broken by the chronic sorrow and daily toil.[203–205] Nor should it be forgotten that considerable numbers of such parents support the idea of euthanasia for handicapped children.[206] Parents then, differ: 'Some can find virtue in what is, for others, a bleak necessity.'[30] Opinions too may well differ over time as situations change and the child does or does not develop.

Knowing how far to involve parents in decision making requires judgements to be made. To date there has been no reputable, empirical work carried out to identify the issues from the parents' point of view, although a companion study to the present one is scheduled to commence this year (1996) to explore parents' perceptions about involvement in decisions regarding the withdrawal of treatment from their babies. Many factors relating to expectations, ambitions, values and knowledge will impinge on parents' reactions, but to some extent is seems likely that the outcome for that child will influence how parents remember the circumstances. Success may well lend a rosy glow to memory; problems and tragic outcomes may cast a black shadow of criticism. Although anecdotal evidence abounds of bereaved parents writing appreciative letters or energetically fund raising for the NICU, nevertheless it is not unknown for parents who initially appear grateful and cooperative, to become militant and confrontational later in their search for some form of legal or public redress when things went wrong.

When a decision has to be made about possibly stopping treatment, three options are available. The doctors can decide that this is a medical matter and accept full responsibility for this momentous choice just as they do for other major decisions on behalf of their infant patient. Alternatively they can judge that this is a decision which has profound consequences for the family and only they are in a position to make such a choice: it is part of parental responsibility. The third option is to have the parents and doctors together making a joint decision. There are persuasive arguments both for involving the parents and for protecting them from the burden such choices may carry, and exponents of all three courses are to be found in the vast anecdotal literature on this subject.

Arguments against involving parents

There are six main reasons offered against asking parents to decide.

They are too emotionally stressed to make such a decision

Delivery of a severely impaired infant or an extremely premature baby, is a shock to parents. Having to make vital decisions while they are still reeling from the impact of these events, might lead to subsequent doubt and remorse. Opinion is indeed divided on this point, although paediatricians themselves have argued persuasively over the years that given the right support and help parents can deal with even these momentous events. After conducting a lengthy study exploring parental consent to major surgery on behalf of their children, Alderson concluded that parental emotions might well have been misinterpreted:

> 'Parents' distress tends to be seen as a disadvantage, crippling their thinking and understanding. I think this is a mistaken view. Lauren's parents were "shattered" *because* they understood the danger she was in. Moral feelings, such as anxiety and compassion, need to be seen as a vital part of proxy informed consent. They deepen understanding.'[24]

The burden of responsibility is too onerous

Some people believe that deciding for their own baby that death is to be preferred to life, is too weighty a decision for parents to make. They will have to live out the rest of their lives with the knowledge of their own involvement. This may engender powerful feelings of guilt at a later date. Doctors, on the other hand, are well used to making crucial decisions and their involvement with this child is a more detached one, making it less likely that they will be unduly stressed by the thought of what they have done. However, whilst any effort to protect parents from a burden of guilt may be a laudable motive, questions have to be asked about such a paternalistic assumption of what is best for the parents. One study found that 'members of the nursery staff systematically underestimate parents' competency to participate in life-and-death decisions, whilst overestimating the negative consequences of incorporating parents in these decisions.'[5] It has been suggested that, ironically, attempts to protect parents from guilt may well produce the very effect they are designed to minimize, since regret after the decision is more likely to ensue when parents are given neither sufficient information nor sufficient time to weigh up the alternatives for themselves.[5]

Parents' own interests might conflict with those of the baby

It is sometimes thought that parents might decide to allow the child to die, because they are more concerned about the burden they will shoulder, not because it is better for the child. Clearly this risk does exist but it can also be argued that parents make decisions all the time on behalf of their children. As has been suggested:

'there is nothing improper in the parents' giving weight to their own interests; impropriety would arise only if the interests of the person who the infant may become were not properly considered because they clashed with the interests of the parents or of the family as a whole.'[30]

Parents lack medical knowledge and experience, and therefore might make inappropriate decisions

Of course, there will be circumstances where the parents' decision is unacceptable to medical staff. But just because parents perceive a level of impairment in a certain way, or decide that they cannot personally cope with the burden of a damaged child, it does not mean that doctors must simply comply with their wishes without discrimination. They are under no legal or professional obligation either to abandon the care of a treatable child, or to continue to offer futile treatment.

Decision making may be prolonged at the expense of the baby's wellbeing

If parents are to have their awareness awakened they have to bear 'the pain of thinking' which is much more than an intellectual problem.[24] It is not a comfortable experience to be forced to face the reality of having a damaged baby, or of the suffering their child may have to endure. For the majority this will be a new experience and it may take them days or even weeks to fully grasp the meaning of risk. They may well initially feel an overwhelming desire to have the child survive at all costs, and it may take a considerable time for them to begin to feel that the cost of survival for their particular child is too high. Warnings may pass them by, unrecognized and unassimilated until a particular reality is witnessed or impinges on their understanding in a way they can grasp. Sometimes they may need to go through a phase of everything being attempted before they can contemplate the possibility that treatment is futile or at least not in the best interests of their baby. These processes take time. Delays may seriously add to the burden of suffering for the baby, and there are considerable stresses on the staff waiting for the parents to arrive at a decision, which their greater experience of these matters told them a long time ago was the best course of action for this baby. There are those who consider that the interests of the baby take precedence over the parents' comfort and that doctors are in a stronger position to make the decision to stop treatment earlier to minimize the suffering the baby must endure.

Parents are ill prepared for such a momentous decision

There are organizational matters which further complicate this issue. Ample evidence exists that parents are not always involved in decisions about the day to day affairs of their infant's management[168] – what he will wear, who will visit him, how and when he will be fed. If parents are not consulted about small matters, they are not encouraged to take responsibility for the infant's welfare. Falling into such a vacuum, the profound decision about whether their baby lives or dies, may be quite overwhelming. There has been no preparation for such a task.

Arguments for involving parents
Parents have themselves argued eloquently for their own right to decide
Doctors can walk out of the lives of these families and carry on a normal existence. Parents are left with burdens which few professionals would wish to bear.

> 'We believe there is a moral and ethical problem of the most fundamental sort involved in a system which allows complicated decisions of this nature to be made unilaterally by people who do not have to live with the consequences of their decisions.'[7]

Only parents can know their own tolerances
The point is often made that pain and burden are matters of individual perception. As Tolstoy put it, happy families are 'all more or less like one another' whereas each unhappy family is 'unhappy in its own particular way'.[207] What is within the bounds of the tolerable for one family is not for another. As a consequence, only parents can decide for themselves what is right for their baby, since only they can really appreciate their history, their aspirations, expectations and breaking points.

Because of this very fact, clinicians as well as parents have advocated involving the family in spite of the problems and consequences inherent in doing so. In 1988, Campbell and his colleagues wrote plainly that in their view parents and the responsible doctors should have the primary power of decision making.[34] As practising neonatologists they were very aware of the complex interplay of clinical judgement, the interests of the baby and the family concerns. Fine balances have to be considered between the doctors' autonomy, leadership and advocacy of the baby's interests; and parental wishes and autonomy. But, with their shared commitments in examining the issues, making the choices and living with the consequences, doctors and parents together form a sort of 'moral community'. (It is noteworthy that in a later paper[137] whose authors included one of the above neonatologists, the medical contribution was extended to include taking account of the views of the nurses and other members of the health care team.)

Parents have very different perspectives
The very different perceptions and yardsticks of doctors and parents, in relation to the baby himself, represent another reason why parents' voices should be heard. Families' main concerns are often relatively minor, visible symptoms and how to cope with them. Doctors, on the other hand, tend to concentrate on major, invisible problems and how to manage them. If the medical staff make a unilateral decision, matters which are very important to the parents may not be adequately addressed, and they in their turn may disregard or imperfectly assess the interests of the rest of the family. They cannot know intimately all that needs to be known in order to make such a judgement. Only the family can.

People respond better to a burden they choose to carry

In general, experience shows that people respond less well to a burden which is thrust upon them than to one they have elected to carry. If other people say they must accept a total disruption of their normal lives, both day and night, and accept it for the rest of their lives, such a decision is likely to engender a feeling of resentment. Tensions will mount as time makes the prospect a reality. Families not infrequently break down under the pressures.

It was against this background of divided opinions that respondents considered the involvement of parents.

Information giving in the NICU

A context is needed in order to understand parents' involvement in decision making about withdrawing treatment. Respondents were, therefore, first asked who provided information for parents on a range of matters. It has to be appreciated that each respondent speaks from his or her own perspective and it was clear that perceptions could differ markedly within the teams. For instance, in one Unit the nurses reported that a senior consultant was just not available enough for parents. He himself said that he believed the nurses liked to be the ones to impart information. In his opinion they made him seem unavailable in order to keep the communication within their own domain.

The provision of information

There was overall agreement that as far as the everyday clinical care of the baby went, both nurses and doctors supplied information. The contributions of each varied according to the setting, opportunity and condition of the baby. Thus for example, when a father visited his baby newly admitted to the nursery, it usually fell to the nurse looking after the child to explain the equipment and the basics of current treatment. But if parents were present when the ward round was in progress or a doctor was carrying out a research procedure on the child, the medical staff might well discuss things with them.

The giving of information about medical progress was also shared to some extent but the general feeling was that nurses would rarely impart new information, only reinforce what doctors had already said. In some Units however, certain experienced nurses were trusted to use their judgement and inform parents as they felt appropriate. Consultants who supported this situation commented that senior nurses had many years of experience and knew where to draw the line and when to call in their medical colleagues. In other Units, the doctors made it clear that medical facts remained in the doctors' remit and both the nursing and medical respondents reported this clear demarcation.

Universally it appeared that the more grave the information, the more likely it was that it would only be given by senior doctors. Diagnoses were also usually conveyed by medical staff although as some respondents pointed out nurses could well inform parents about a simple non-life-threatening diagnosis such as hyperbilirubinaemia. Frequently respondents referred to the practice obtaining in all Units, of nurses re-interpreting the information for the parents at all levels of gravity.

> 'Obviously if they've got [something quite serious like] a pneumothorax, the doctor would go and tell them, and try and explain. But what I find is that you can explain until you go blue, they don't understand. And they come and talk with the nurse who'll explain it to them right. So you actually have an interpreting system. At first I thought it was my accent – it's the way I say it!' (Senior Registrar, more than 10 years experience)

> 'I've seen the parents not understanding maybe what the doctor's said to them, or you just have to help to clarify. He's maybe used terminology they're not familiar with, and you've just got to bring it down to laymen's terms a bit for them.' (Staff Midwife, more than 5 years experience)

Nevertheless the nurses were aware that information coming from a doctor had a different weight from that of their own messages. It was a source of frustration for some that parents on occasion needed to hear things from a doctor, no matter what his or her seniority, before they would believe them. The facts conveyed could be identical but they were perceived differently by the recipients. Things were even more frustrating when the nurses felt the doctor was not good at this task. Examples were given of doctors who always smiled broadly when delivering bad news, or who remained remote and cold, or who wrapped everything up in unintelligible or ambiguous language.

The doctors appeared less aware of the practice of nurses re-interpreting information but the picture given by the nurses was the same everywhere. The parents were overwhelmed by events, shocked by the situation and the environment, ignorant of medical matters, and felt overawed by the knowledge and power of the consultant. Not infrequently, the nurses reported, the parents came out of a session with the consultant and, when asked whether they had understood what they had been told, volunteered that they had taken in nothing. The language was unfamiliar, the concepts alien, and the parents too emotionally shocked to absorb the facts. If they had been present at the interview themselves, the nurses undertook to rephrase the information, explaining it in simple terms and phasing it so that the parents had time to absorb it in stages. Where they were not included in the original exchange, they had much more difficulty in knowing how far to go and how much of the parents' understanding was correct. It was then that misunderstandings and conflicting information could complicate the picture.

From the consultant's point of view certain situations presented major obstacles. For example, there were particular problems if there had been no opportunity to establish a relationship with the parents.

'If this is an acute event – the first time [the consultant has] met the parents, then I would alter my way of management. I wouldn't expect them to believe me. I wouldn't expect them to trust me. If it's an immediate decision then I am quite open with them. I say, "I'm sorry, this is the first time I've met you. We're very quickly going to have to understand each other over what's happening here. We haven't got time to build up an understanding of each other, but believe you me, I will try to do my best for your baby" … in the first five minutes I have with the parents, I'm desperately trying to think of what they want me to say. Do they want me to say, "What do you think about this situation?" Or do they want me to say, "This is the situation". Or do they want me to explain things in great detail. Or do they just want to know she's been delivered. So the first 5, 10 minutes of the interview with a parent, I'm desperately looking for signs and signals – vocal, bodywise, everything – just to see how I can get these parents on my side. How can I get them to trust me … If they are aggressive, that makes it difficult. If you are aggressive in turn back to them, you've lost it – but sometimes it's difficult! If they are polarised, if they are as polarised as you are, it doesn't matter which end, you've lost it.' (Consultant, more than 10 years experience)

Almost all respondents put the prognosis squarely in the doctors' court. Once again nurses had a role in helping parents to understand the facts and assimilate the implications, but only a tiny minority of very experienced sisters said that they might themselves offer such information if the parents asked them outright. In this context the point was made that it could sometimes be more damaging to parents to have their questions evaded than to have a straight answer from the person they asked. Some believed that the parents would only ask those staff whom they had grown to respect and trust, but others felt that parents shopped around for the most hopeful prognosis and great harm could accrue from a practice which allowed several people to convey uncoordinated facts. Most nurses said they would simply refer the parents to the consultant. For their part, the consultants were conscious of the risks of others muddying the waters before they themselves deemed it was the right moment, with sufficient concrete evidence to put the case to parents.

Referring parents to a later appointment with another person was an inadequate response to immediate need, but few apart from consultants were prepared to be the ones to impart devastating information. Some nurses felt that their own relationship of trust with the parents could be compromised if they had themselves known about a poor diagnosis or prognosis but had not imparted anything of this to the parents.

'Sometimes I have quite a problem with that … we're sitting with the parents, with their babies, maybe many hours of the day. The doctors are popping in and out. Very often you will be aware of the diagnosis and you're perhaps sitting with this mother and father for half a day before they're spoken to by a member of the medical staff. And they ask – they're looking in your eyes, – "Why couldn't you have told me that?" And I often feel very compromised. And I feel I've failed the parents because I've not been totally honest with them … to be honest, I feel if a diagnosis has been made, I wouldn't have a problem, I would quite like to discuss it with the parents. But in this Unit it isn't the prerogative of midwives and nurses to do that.' (Sister, more than 10 years experience)

Nurses recognized that consultants were not always instantly available to come and talk to the parents, so they particularly valued those doctors who not only responded courteously to such a request but also made these tasks a high priority. It was traumatic for a nurse to say she would call the doctor and then have to stall for time or keep comforting or calming parents during a long wait until he appeared. On the other hand, senior doctors sometimes resented the nurses apparently forcing their hand when it came to imparting bad news. If they were not yet ready to present the full picture to the parents they did not like to be put on the spot, having to convey uncertainty or disquiet prematurely. In their judgement this gave the parents anxieties which they might not need to know about if they could be kept in ignorance of certain developments for a while longer.

'I sometimes think parents are told things a bit soon now – I've found this more in nursing staff than medical staff. They don't like knowing something that hasn't been shared. And I found that particularly with Down's. They're *desperate* that the parents should be told about this, and they'll drag – I mean I have known this happen – they'll actually drag the only doctor round, who may be the SHO there, to see this baby, to say it's a Down's, to say something to the parents. And of course the parents get in a terrible tizz. Whereas if you say, "OK, it looks like a Down's, but it's all right, there's no immediate medical problem," we can take it a bit more leisurely and get the parents to know the baby. Often the parents themselves will actually begin to realize that maybe all is not well, which makes it easier then when you go to say to them, "Have you got any worries?" I myself would prefer not to have to tell parents that diagnosis until I'd got the chromosome result. But nowadays it often isn't possible to do that. They have been given an indication that there's something wrong with their baby beforehand and so they're wanting to know.' (Consultant, more than 25 years experience)

When all these matters hinged around stressed parents and tense staff, it was small wonder that resentments and conflicts sometimes arose. It was all too easy to blame the nurse or junior doctor for an incautious word to a parent, or to blame the doctor for not responding instantly to a call to attend the nursery. Nurses not infrequently criticized the doctors' use of language which was 'incomprehensible' or 'confusing'. Doctors felt the nurses could be too involved, too emotional and too gullible at times. The researcher herself witnessed more than one exchange between consultants and nurses which implied or explicitly stated that parents were upset because they had not been told what was going on. The consultants were understandably annoyed when they had spent hours talking to those parents – they felt they could hardly be blamed for the parents' failure to take the information in. Here again it was apparent that it was vitally important for nurses to accompany doctors, and for staff to share information carefully about exactly what had been conveyed.

When it came to imparting information about life and death matters, such as withdrawing treatment, almost all respondents considered that this was the exclusive province of the consultants. Four doctors and six nurses felt that senior nurses were also involved at times in their Unit (they represented five of the six study Units) but only in conjunction with the consultants. Many more had already made reference to the necessity for nurses to be involved in order to rehearse the facts with the parents subsequently and to support and help them through these difficult experiences.

Satisfaction with communication with parents

Respondents were asked whether in their judgement the current system of imparting information to parents in their Unit was satisfactory. Overall 25 of the doctors (44%) thought it was, with a further 18 (32%) believing it usually worked satisfactorily if everyone did as they were expected to do: clearly, occasionally staff made errors of judgement. More than half of the nurses (73, 61%) were satisfied that communication with parents was effective, a further 11 (9%) reporting that it usually was, and 17 (14%) that it was some of the time. This means that as many as a quarter of doctors and a sixth of the nurses were unhappy with the existing service.

When each of the Units was examined in turn, it became apparent that the least satisfactory communication systems were to be found in two of the Units. In one of these, there were poor relationships between the consultants and the nurses, and between the sisters and the staff midwives. In the other, there was great hostility between the consultants who practised very differently, communicated with each other and with nursing staff poorly, and frequently did not involve nurses in discussions about the babies. In the three Units which were rated the most satisfactory in this respect, there were certain consultants whom the nurses singled out who responded well to requests to talk to parents, who listened to nursing opinion, and who were seen to make appropriate and timely decisions.

Areas for improvements in communication with parents

The table given below (Table 12.1) shows the areas identified where things could be better. The items are presented in descending order of frequency with which they were cited.

Doctors	Nurses
Better communication between staff	Better communication between staff
More continuity/consistency	More team involvement
More consultant involvement	More continuity/consistency
More team involvement	More consultant involvement
Better documentation	Better documentation
More staff	

Table 12.1: Areas where improvements might be made in communication with parents

Overall there were four main areas where things could be improved in order to enhance communication with parents.

Communication skills

General communication skills and practices gave the most problems. Both doctors and nurses singled out medical communication as a particular area of concern. This was something more than simply the way doctors spoke to parents:

> 'I've heard a couple of consultants wanting to get across the reasons for why treatment should be discontinued. One of them, she certainly got across what she wanted to say, but she spoke in words of one syllable and very simply and very rationally. Whereas somebody else, perhaps using a lot of long medical terms and talking medical-legal language and stuff like that, I didn't think, listening to him, came across as easily for parents to understand. I think it's perhaps silly little things that concern parents, things that maybe doctors don't think about, or nurses even ... I remember one lady, it was her other child's birthday and she didn't want this to be the day that she was going to remember that the ventilator was switched off. And other things like – everybody told them what'll happen after the baby dies, you have to go and register the death, you have to do this [and that], but they were unsure what was going to happen for the 5, 10 minutes exactly after the ventilator was switched off.' (Sister, more than 10 years experience)

Good communication included a fine degree of sensitivity. In conveying these difficult messages to parents, it was crucial to be in tune with parents' thinking and acceptance of the situation. Unless the doctor could appreciate their concerns and level of understanding, he had no yardstick by which to pitch information.

When it came to inter-professional communication, a number of doctors volunteered that medicine could learn a lot from nursing in this respect: from the way they handed over from shift to shift, kept detailed records and reported happenings to seniors on a regular basis. A picture was built up of how parents were reacting and coping which enabled staff to be responsive to their needs. Because medical involvement tended to be spasmodic and fragmented, and there was less obvious attention paid to communicating sensitively, it was harder for doctors to assess parents' level of understanding. One doctor even recommended that this matter should be given policy status to encourage doctors to be more conscious of the issues and more precise in their practice.

Once again the matter of nurses being in the dark was raised. It was extremely difficult to function effectively with parents if they did not know what was happening or what parents had been told. In some ways good reporting by the nurses helped to ameliorate the situation but nurses intimately involved with particular families resented finding things out secondhand. Furthermore, where the primary nurse was given all the information but did not necessarily convey it to others, a situation could result where another nurse subsequently looking after that baby felt disadvantaged. Communication had to go in all directions if the team was to work cohesively.

Continuity and consistency

Another issue raised was that of consistency of approach. Not only was good communication essential for parents but there needed to be continuity: either the same people seeing them or the messages being consistent. They were confused enough by events and new information without being bewildered by conflicting messages.

It was not just consistency of information which was needed. Respondents considered that there should be an element of continuity about the handling of the baby and the parents too. There were large numbers of staff working in most of these Units. Parents were perplexed by the changeovers. It helped to anchor them if they could identify key people with whom to relate, who could keep them informed. These individuals would grow to know the different family members, appreciating something of their background and circumstances. It could be wearisome and frustrating for parents repeatedly to establish new relationships and go over old ground.

A particular problem was seen in the adequacy of medical cover. This was acute where the consultants were part time in the Unit or where they were people who worked more in research labs or offices and were not seen regularly during unsocial hours in the nurseries. Night time could present especial difficulties if it was not possible to have known individuals communicating with the parents. Stressful situations arose at night just as during the daytime, and at weekends as well as Monday to Friday. Fragmentation of care added to the parents' burden.

Consultant involvement

In three of the six Units a small number of staff looked for more involvement on the part of the consultants. One of these Units had only part time consultants and the nurses played a major role in communicating with parents, often having to wait some time for doctors to answer calls for assistance. In the other two Units, the issue was more about the timing and nature of their interventions rather than their physical presence. The approach of the consultant was a crucial factor in the quality of communication at these sensitive times.

> 'I think it's knowing that somebody's available and approachable – if somebody's aloof and we hardly see them, then it's extremely difficult to get to communicate. It depends who your consultant is as to how good the communication is down the line. And the personality of that consultant – approachability, availability, giving a sense of being trustworthy, it may be that, and giving a sense that they are so enthusiastic about their job, and about what they do, and about the people that they care for. And I think that has the back effect that people aren't backwards in coming forward, wanting to communicate with them, and they themselves want to communicate with other people.' (SHO, less than 1 year experience)

Colleagues wanted them to take an early and ongoing interest in families, to get acquainted with the parents from early on rather than appearing for the first time when things deteriorated. It was hard for parents to have to meet a new and 'important' senior doctor when a crisis presented. Building up trust and getting acquainted over whatever time was available helped them to assimilate information at a more reasonable pace and to build on it gradually. It also helped parents to believe what they were hearing if earlier explanations were understood and seen to be accurate. As one consultant pointed out, parents noticed if the consultant was around a great deal and were inclined to interpret his involvement favourably.

> 'I think if you explain things simply to them, you put it into context – not only their baby's illness, but based on nearly a quarter of a century's experience now. They do feel that they can trust you. And I think that's what it is – it's trust. Also I think this is quite important too – if they see that you work hard and are around the Unit a lot. They'll find it easier too. If they notice that you are an individual – [not one] who comes to work at 9 disappears at 5 and they don't see you again until the following day, I think – [but] even when you're not supposedly on call, you're always around, they realize, well, it means this person does care.' (Consultant, more than 20 years experience)

Team involvement

A real rather than 'paper' team effort was seen to be an important part of effective communication with parents. Everyone involved needed to be in possession of the facts, presenting a coherent picture to the parents and discussing things openly together. If nurses were in the dark about intentions, or doctors held private sessions with parents, or different consultants gave conflicting instructions, the team approach was lost. Competing interests and uncertain behaviour led to tension and misunderstandings.

Whilst many nurses felt that they tended to be left out of deliberations, some medical respondents felt that lapses in team effort were unintentional. They tended to have sudden ideas for alternative courses of action at odd moments or in response to test results which were not always conveyed to their colleagues.

> 'You sort of whizz round on the ward rounds and I don't know whether we always think of the nurses. Decisions in medicine are often suddenly made walking along the corridors – "Let's try and do this" and "Maybe it could be that". But then that's often not passed back to the nurses. On the ward round they may catch up with what we're thinking, but so many decisions actually often don't happen on the ward round. It happens – sometimes we get a result back and, "Oh, it might be this" and "Let's try that," and it's not that we mean to but ... the nurses only find out maybe hours later.' (Registrar, less than 5 years experience)

Personal preference in relation to parental involvement

Having established the pattern for communication with parents, the researcher then explored just how parents were involved in decision making about treatment withdrawal. As has been outlined earlier, three general approaches to parental involvement were identified:

a)   parents making the decision themselves;
b)   doctors taking full responsibility for the decision;
c)   parents and doctors sharing the decision making.

In order to try to present each as a viable option and not to prejudice responses, a brief rationale for each was given. Respondents were then asked which approach they personally favoured before moving on to the problems which might be encountered in following any one of these practices. The results are presented by discipline in Figure 12.1 and by grade in Figure 12.2.

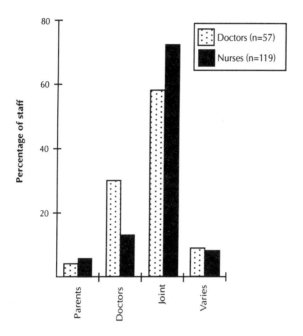

Fig. 12.1: Comparison of the preferences of doctors and nurses in relation to who should decide about withdrawal or withholding of treatment

As can be seen from these figures, overall the majority of staff preferred a joint approach (33, 58% of doctors and 87, 73% of nurses). It is important to record that even some of those who declared another preference added a rider to the effect that where parents accepted the final responsibility they should be guided by doctors; and where it fell to doctors to decide, they should take the parents along with them.

A joint approach

As many as 33 doctors (58%) and 87 nurses (73%) favoured a joint approach. There was a strong sense conveyed that if the task was properly handled parents felt that the doctors had actually decided, even though they were asked their parental opinion. The parents were then able to say that the doctors had recommended withdrawal of treatment as the best thing for their baby. In this way they were not left with a burden of guilt.

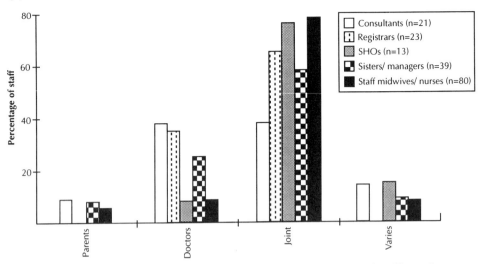

Figure 12.2: Comparison of the preferences of different grades of staff in relation to who should decide about withdrawal or withholding of treatment

> 'I think if we're doing the job correctly, then we are telling them what we expect them to say and so they don't feel they've made the decision ... I think if we do it well, and make it as easy as possible for them, they are actually – we are making the decision but they are kind of rubber stamping it and saying, "Yes"... Obviously the parents will want to ask questions and the final responsibility is the doctors' because they're the ones with the facts ... and they're quoted in such a way that the [parents] actually agree with us without actually feeling they have killed the baby.' (Staff nurse, more than 20 years experience)

However, even with a shared responsibility, some consultants wondered about the welfare of families. It was difficult to know how they reacted later on and whether in time they came to terms with events in the nursery.

> 'I wonder how people are doing *now*. It's not the actual decision and so on that bothers me because I can rationalize that. But it's – did these people heal afterwards? Are they OK? That's the bit I often don't get fed back and I'm very interested in meeting those parents again, just to see how they go on.' (Consultant, more than 15 years experience)

Nor was it always easy for consultants to share the decision with parents who varied and could be so unpredictable. Doing so required them repeatedly to adapt to all shades of opinion and degrees of wisdom.

> 'I can tolerate a lot of greyness – because that's what medicine's all about. You can't dictate what kinds of patients you'll get or how they view their problems. As long as it's within our remit and my values and my professional values, then I'm happy to go along with [what parents want]. I can divorce myself from them and not value judge them.' (Consultant, more than 15 years experience)

A parental responsibility

A very few respondents (2 doctors and 7 nurses) thought that it should always be the parents who bore the burden of the final choice. For them this was part of the responsibility that went with parenthood. As one consultant put it:

> 'They accepted the responsibility when they conceived the child. They didn't come to me and say, "Dr X, we're thinking of having a child." They came to me with a problem. I give them the facts. This nannying idea that you can't load parents with decisions [is a nonsense]. Does that mean you can't load them with the decision to take out a mortgage, or to have an operation for a hysterectomy? The decision has been made. They decided for whatever reason to have a baby. It went wrong. They should be supported because it went wrong ... I am not going to carry this can because it's too emotionally damaging to carry that [responsibility].' (Consultant, more than 10 years experience)

This consultant was adamant that the doctor's task was to give the facts, it was the parents' task to make the decision. Another respondent was of the view that parents' capacity to cope was seriously underestimated:

> 'The human spirit has got far more resilience than we give them credit for. And I think people can tolerate huge stresses and responsibilities as long as they are given some guidance and support. I think we underestimate parents' tolerance.' (Consultant, more than 15 years experience)

But people who thought in this way were in a decided minority. Other respondents felt that parents lacked the requisite knowledge and understanding of medical matters to shoulder this responsibility.

> 'The parents are helpless ... the doctors are the people who know ... if they need the input of a paediatrician and they're at this critical stage, these people know that the expert for their baby is that doctor, and his decision ... is probably accepted more than it would be at any other time in anybody's life. I think a lot of parents abdicate their role to the paediatricians – to the experts ... It take us years to get to this stage – how can parents know in a matter of days?' (Staff Midwife, less than 5 years experience)

Some pointed out that handing responsibility to the parents could result in real abuses.

> 'What worries me is that if you have consultants with no power at all to go against the parents' wishes, you could have babies with lovely prognoses at 32 weeks gestation, with no sign of damage to the central nervous system, and the parents so stressed and saying, "Look, I don't want you to do anything." And in those circumstances – you can't actually deprive a child of a chance of life like that.' (Consultant, more than 15 years experience)

The majority considered the final decision far too heavy a burden, likely to engender subsequent guilt. However, a small number (5 doctors and 8 nurses) felt that circumstances could sometimes make this an appropriate option. Much depended on the coping capacity and knowledge of the parents. Indeed there were parents who insisted that this was their baby and they would decide. Given such circumstances, however, some consultants volunteered that the strong opinions of such parents would make them question motives even more rigorously than usual. Furthermore, they felt they would probably be even more cautious about withdrawing treatment and would institute delaying tactics to prevent an inappropriate choice being made against the baby's best interests.

A medical responsibility

Proportionately more doctors than nurses would make doctors the prime deciders (30% as against 14%). The reasons given varied. Relieving the parents of the burden was adequate defence for some.

> 'I don't think we're doing anyone a service by giving them [the parents] an extra sort of piece of emotional baggage to carry around for the rest of their life, when usually that decision is inevitable anyway. And in that respect I think that we are the advisors of these parents. We are the people they've entrusted to do the right thing for their child, and we've got to take that responsibility on our shoulders ... I think they should be left feeling that their doctor's told them that the future was hopeless for their child and that the kindest thing to do would be to make their child comfortable and end [his] suffering ... and that they understood that and believed that it was right.' (Senior Registrar, more than years experience)

Others considered that this was simply a task they accepted with seniority. Since they were the ones with the knowledge and experience only they were the ones who were equipped to make the necessary judgements.

Some consultants however, considered they had to take a lead role since parents were in no position to make such a momentous decision.

> 'I would actually say to many parents, "I'm not giving you that responsibility." And I certainly said that to Baby N's parents. "I've decided myself that medically her outlook is bleak and I can tell you why I feel that. I can tell you what her future would be. But I want to make it quite clear that *I'm* taking the responsibility." It's a question of how you say it in some ways. I would then try very hard to take the parents with me. If you're very cynical you can say you're actually twisting parents' arms and you're pushing parents into one way of thinking. And I freely admit that. I think at a very emotional time nobody can make clear rational decisions.' (Consultant, less than 10 years experience)

Only one consultant went so far as to say that the decision was an entirely medical matter, he simply informed the parents of his decision. Most added that they did their best to take the parents along with their thinking and to gauge their reactions and wishes in an ongoing way.

It appeared to be fairly common practice to tailor the amount of information and the speed of giving it in line with the consultant's perception of the parents' abilities and expectations. In this way some doctors accepted a larger responsibility than others and a few nurses described cases where, in their judgement, parents had been railroaded and did not appear to understand why treatment was being withdrawn. Nurses were disturbed by such paternalistic behaviour, particularly where the decision appeared to be made on grounds other than a recognizably bleak prognosis. They were particularly incensed by decisions which appeared to them to be based on social factors which discriminated against the less articulate and affluent.

Important differences emerged when the different grades of staff were separated. No registrars or SHOs believed that parents should ever accept this awesome responsibility. In addition, much larger proportions of junior doctors and junior nurses considered the decision should be a joint one rather than their senior counterparts. Consultants and senior nurses were more inclined to think that doctors should actually bear the bulk of the responsibility.

Potential difficulties

Trying to arrive at a decision which both parents and doctors feel is right, is sometimes a hazardous task. A number of difficulties have been identified. Only five doctors and five nurses said there were no problems, it was simply a matter of building up trust. There was remarkable concordance between the two disciplines about the commonest stumbling blocks. In descending order of frequency with which the different factors were cited, the problem areas were:

- parents' lack of experience and understanding;
- emotional readiness/timing of events;
- communication;
- different perceptions or values;
- doctor-parent relationships;
- rigid attitudes or beliefs;
- factors related to the doctor;
- reluctance to accept responsibility for the decision;
- inter-family conflict.

Exact numbers of staff citing any given factor contribute little but it is important to underline the overwhelming number of staff who cited the influence of parents' lack of understanding of these matters and delays in their emotional readiness for decisions to be made. It was clear that such parental factors dominated in staff's perception of areas of difficulty.

The top four factors were the top four in all six Units and were easily the most commonly encountered difficulties. Since the consultants were the people most intimately involved with the parents in making the decision, their comments were studied separately. For them the parents' apparent lack of understanding or emotional readiness, and factors related to the timing of events, were those most commonly cited, with less than a quarter of the group citing any other factor as a cause of difficulty. Clearly in their perceptions the problems stemmed almost exclusively from the parents.

Parental factors

Parental factors represented the commonest stumbling blocks in the experience of all groups of respondents. It was recognized that these were momentous affairs for parents who were undergoing a profoundly stressful experience. They were almost always unfamiliar with the world of sick babies, and even where they had some knowledge or experience of medical matters, they were usually not well acquainted with the highly specialized field of neonatology, or could not take a detached professional view now they were so intimately involved.

> 'You have got parents who may have no medical knowledge at all. Even if they are medically trained, for instance doctors or nurses, they know nothing about this sphere of neonatology, and it's difficult to be objective when it's your own children that are involved. So I think you need someone else to take a degree of responsibility for the decision that's been made, who can think objectively, who is up to date and knows as much as possible about a baby in that situation from experience, from literature, from common sense and intelligence, to say "Look, these are the facts. This is what I think. I have discussed it with X number of colleagues, and we believe this. But in the end we can't tell you what to do. We'd like to know your views too."' (Registrar, less than 5 years experience)

Intense emotions could make parents appear irrational and lead to extremely difficult situations developing.

> 'At one point it was felt, "This baby's going to be grossly handicapped, going to be blind – horrendous problems." And the parents insisted they wanted everything done, didn't matter to them what happened, they wanted this. And the baby did survive and is quite poorly, and is blind, and has horrendous problems today. Now that Mum said to me many times later – although I personally knew, I'd *heard* her being told of the implications – "Nobody ever told me." So you really [wonder], did she understand? ... And she's not proven that she's a particularly capable mother. Now the last I heard she's insisting that the Health Board pay for residential care etc. etc. because the full implications of this weren't put to her. But they *were*. Where would you stand legally if [you didn't go along with her initially]? I think you'd have to, because I think really the medical staff today, in both obstetrics and I suppose in neonates, are so vulnerable. Everyone is jumping on the bandwagon for the compensation and you really are open to so much abuse of what you've said – being turned round or whatever. And this is why I think documentation is absolutely essential.' (Staff Midwife, more than 10 years experience)

There was clearly a potential to misconstrue parents' behaviour. Everyone was labouring under great strain and this could produce uncharacteristic aggression or unpleasantness which should be interpreted with compassion.

> 'Really pushy parents are the ones that we all go, "Ttch, what's right for *them?*" – the ones that actually cause us a lot of anxiety – the ones who tend to get the best deal. And the parents we tend to see as, "Oh they're a lovely couple.

They're so nice."– it's often because they're not hassling me or pushing me and asking me difficult questions. [But] it doesn't mean they don't want to know the answers. I've become really aware of this. Sometimes we get very defensive with the parents who are truly just anxiously wanting [information]. They are basically expressing their dissatisfaction with the level of communication they're getting. Yes, some of them are difficult people but most of them [are not] – it must be the most awful thing ... Sometimes the most aggressive parents you sit down and you start talking to them and they just break down. They're not aggressive at all – just terrified.' (SHO, less than 1 year experience)

In the perceptions of the staff, almost all parents lacked experience and understanding of the circumstances and conditions they were now being asked to think about. Some observed that parents were seriously disadvantaged in not knowing the extent of their own ignorance. Indeed it was common for the nurses and doctors spontaneously to say they would not want a baby of theirs treated under certain circumstances, even though they were themselves party to such treatment being given to other people's babies. Specialized knowledge brought its own reservations.

Parents' expectations of medicine often appeared unrealistic, not infrequently fuelled by extravagant media claims. Many respondents bemoaned the tendency for newspapers and magazines to run articles on tiny infants and dwell exclusively on the good outcomes. They felt that the public needed a more realistic understanding of the limits of medical achievements.

Sometimes parents were seen to have serious doubts about their own capacity to cope with the outcomes predicted for their baby. Hearing about the assessed risk of their child's having serious impairments required them both intellectually and emotionally to grapple with unknown facts: the relative risks, the medical, physical and psychological ramifications, the whole family's stability and ability to deal with the consequences. Contemplation of the death of their baby, on the other hand, was painful and again so much was unknown. They were seen to be fearful about what the dying would be like and how they would themselves behave and respond during that time. Dealing with these profound issues in the here and now, it was difficult for them to project themselves into the future and logically consider the consequences of the various choices available to them, and difficult to be rational about much that was happening when they were so deeply affected emotionally. Their own attitudes, and backgrounds, the family's coping strategies and support networks, could all influence parents' perceptions and ability to grasp the enormity of this decision. It sometimes happened that parents themselves were not in agreement, or that grandparents exercised an unhealthy influence, or that the stress exacerbated incipient problems within the family and major conflicts broke out. These family troubles added additional layers of stress to this traumatic time for parents.

In a few instances, parents were either unable or unwilling to be present with the baby in the nursery, during his dying or death or funeral. Where significant relatives were travelling to see the baby while he was still alive, staff sometimes went to enormous lengths to keep the infant breathing until they arrived. It was a source of profound stress to them when these efforts failed. But sometimes parents could not be present because of illness, or stayed away for religious reasons or because they were denying the reality of events in the nursery. Their absence made it extremely difficult to make the necessary decisions.

There was a general sense that parents were ill prepared to make these momentous choices. Other people decided even what the baby drank or wore, where and when he slept, and who saw him; things much more basic than how much oxygen or medication he was given, or which investigations or tests he underwent. Into this vacuum fell a request to make the biggest decision of all: whether he lived or died. Already disempowered parents could easily be overwhelmed by the enormity of the responsibility.

The timing of events

As has already been recorded, the timing of events caused major problems. In relation to parents this had to do with their perceived emotional readiness for the decision and death. Respondents recognized the necessity to be sensitive to their needs but when parents kept delaying the decision, it was sometimes at the expense of the baby and this caused great distress to staff. Juggling support for the parents with the comfort of the baby was difficult for those closely involved in the decision. One case was reported where it took three months for parents finally to accept that it was futile to continue treatment. During this time the condition of the baby and the circumstances of the case created a high level of stress for all the staff in the Unit. The consultants were unable to overrule the parents who categorically denied permission to stop treatment. Respondents described it as 'three months of pure hell.'

It was apparent that consultants' assessment of parents' readiness was rather different from the perceptions of the sisters and staff midwives giving the hands-on care. The nursing staff tended to feel the parents were ready to have treatment stopped a considerable time before the consultants felt they were. This further added to the problems of both groups: the doctors feeling under pressure and misunderstood; the nurses distressed by 'unnecessary' delays. The consultants were, however, acutely aware of the difference between having an opinion about the right decision and actually taking responsibility for it. It was imperative for their own peace of mind that they waited until they were absolutely sure that the parents had understood and accepted the position. It was they, the consultants, who would follow up the parents in the bereavement period and they were all too conscious of the risk of parents changing their minds or apportioning blame in their hurt and bewilderment.

Communication

In any social exchange between individuals there are inherent communication issues. Where the participants come from totally different backgrounds and knowledge bases, these are likely to pose real problems. In the NICU, consultants have a detailed and highly specialized knowledge of neonatal issues and a wide range of experiences to draw on. On the other hand parents usually have little understanding of the problems.

Problems in communication include a range of issues. The way information is conveyed can materially affect the way decisions are made. Nurses frequently made reference to the inability of parents to understand what the consultant said. In their judgement this related to the use of complicated terms with which parents were unfamiliar, a basic lack of understanding of the parents' ignorance of anatomy and physiology, the state of shock parents were in, and the awe in which many parents hold senior doctors. This was sometimes further confounded by the lack of time or opportunity for the consultant to build up a relationship of trust over time with the parents.

Communication difficulties were not all in one direction. Parents too could give complicated and confusing messages. They might well tell the consultant they had understood what he had said, even repeating the main points if asked to do so. But where the significance of these facts was lost to them, they could not readily translate the facts into meaningful reality for their own personal circumstances. Respondents were aware that it was on occasions important to the parents that they, the parents, appear knowledgeable, calm and rational. They lost face if they admitted that they had no idea what the heart looked like or where the intestine or liver was.

Disadvantage was added to disadvantage if they became upset and confessed to bewilderment or socially unacceptable emotions. It was often easier to reserve these revelations for the staff they met on a different level and whom they had got to know more intimately. The nursing respondents, as well as a considerable number of the doctors, reported that parents perceived the nurses as speaking their language and feeling the same kind of emotions. They grew closer to them, spending long hours together beside the baby and seeing the affection the nurses developed for the babies in their care. They were thus more likely to tell the nurses that they had not understood medical information. If they were totally in the picture themselves, the nurses could re-interpret the information, pacing it in line with parental understanding and levels of stress or distress.

Some consultants however, were seen to be particularly good at establishing relationships with the parents, synthesizing information appropriately, and being sensitive to the needs of different individuals. Where they demonstrated this kind of skill, respondents felt parents had the best possible service because the information was consistent, and from the most knowledgeable source. The rest of the team could then support both consultant and parents free from the doubts and confusions which attended less effective communication.

The parent/doctor relationship

Inevitably personalities influenced communication. It is noteworthy that more nurses than doctors perceived problems in the relationships between parents and doctors. No respondents were asked how they rated their own ability at this part of their work, but a small number of consultants specifically volunteered that they considered themselves particularly good at communicating with relatives, with a few adding that they had letters of appreciation from parents to demonstrate the truth of this statement. But only one of these people was actually rated as a good communicator by their nursing or medical colleagues. The consultants the nurses singled out as good at relating to parents did not themselves say they were. It could be that they knew their colleagues would supply such information, or it could have been that they were unaware that theirs were exceptional qualities, or perhaps it was natural modesty.

Some consultants were perceived by colleagues as particularly likable people who inspired confidence and trust. Others were seen as less assured and sensitive. Similarly parents could be more or less easy to get on with. As might well be expected, staff reported that parents who persistently challenged decisions, or who were aggressive or critical, were harder to deal with. Doctors sometimes admitted that they exercised particular caution which such families, aware of the potential for litigation if they were unguarded in a comment or did not fully inform the parent of treatment decisions. Even though they intellectually accepted that it was often the stress they were suffering that made the parents appear belligerent or volatile, it was still a tense time, very draining on staff morale and emotional resources. 'Difficult parents' were present in more than one Unit while the researcher was carrying out fieldwork in those Units. It was interesting to trace the emergence of an understanding of why parents were behaving in this way as information was unravelled. But sometimes along the way relationships between the team members could become strained. And it sometimes happened that even when enlightenment came, junior staff were not told why parents had behaved so 'objectionably'.

Respondents described certain circumstances as causing particular difficulties. For some babies, the time between their birth and withdrawal of treatment is quite short. Traumas follow one upon another for the parents. In such circumstances parents can feel the doctors are synonymous with bad news. Doctors can feel they have no opportunity really to get to know the parents and their needs and wishes. Communication is often less than optimal in these cases.

Another circumstance is where deterioration is less rapid, and doctors and nurses have time to build up comfortable relationships with parents gradually. Perhaps the professional realization that the infant's prognosis is poor emerges slowly and following various tests. The parents may be unaware of the turn of events or may be clinging hopefully to the good indicators even where hints are given that all is not well. It can become a difficult matter to broach the delicate question of the prognosis or withdrawal of treatment in these circumstances, particularly where emotional ties have developed between staff and families. If parents have openly expressed their trust in the team to pull their baby through, failure to do so can leave staff feeling guilty and upset.

All parents have certain expectations and hopes for their children. It takes time and effort on the part of staff to understand what these expectations are for different families. Good communication depends on a sensitivity to the cues participants offer, and clearly doctors and nurses possess the necessary skills to varying degrees. It can be difficult for professional staff to appreciate where parents are coming from or to sympathize with their point of view if they adhere strongly to entrenched and rigid ideas or beliefs: where they reject a child because of a relatively minor defect; or refuse treatments which are commonplace because of religious scruples; or insist futile treatment is continued because of a belief in miracles or divine pre-ordination. If the parents' preferred choice of treatment is seen to be detrimental to the best interests of the baby, there are serious conflicts for those caring for the child as well as those faced with deciding how to proceed. Inability to comprehend or support such parental views can lead to major problems in communication which sometimes require outside arbitration.

A major problem for consultants is one of medical uncertainty. There are few certainties in neonatology and yet grave decisions have to be made. It appears to be easier for nurses to feel certain that the right thing to do is to withdraw treatment, than it is for senior medical staff. Their reputation is not on the line. Many doctors and some nurses described the problems of having to say things like, 'There is a strong probability that ...,' or 'In our experience these babies do not do well ...,' or 'We think your child will never walk or talk or know you ...,' all the time only too well aware that some infants defy such predictions. It is usually impossible to be categorical about conditions. However, a very few consultants were perceived to be too inclined to present facts as black and white issues in their dealings with parents. Nurses especially were troubled by such behaviour, considering it a flaw in communication and a form of medical arrogance.

One doctor commented that a major problem in communication related to the time of day and the level of fatigue the doctor was experiencing.

> 'If it was now, I'm fairly awake, I've had a good night's sleep, I feel ready to discuss it. If it's 4 o'clock in the morning and I've been up the previous night and I've worked the full day and I've been in bed for 2 hours, then they're going to get short shrift. My decision making ability is not terribly accurate, and I'm going to fall asleep. And that is a barrier which is real. And all I want to do is get home to my kip, because I know I've got a clinic at 9 o'clock in the morning and I'm going to face parents who are – compared to the disastrous [circumstances we're talking about] – are complaining about trivial bedwetting, constipation – trivial to me – till it happens to me! All these trivia, and I just think how much longer am I going to have to go on. So tiredness [is a factor].'
> (Consultant, more than 10 years experience)

It was not as easy to be patient, logical and sensitive at such times. But drafting in substitute communicators ran the risk of fragmenting care and increased the probability of misinformation or conflicting messages.

Conflicts and dilemmas

It is apparent that a potential exists for opposing points of view between parents and staff. The two ends of the spectrum illustrate such dilemmas. The parents might wish treatment to be discontinued when staff believe there is still hope of a reasonably good outcome for the baby. On the other hand, parents might wish aggressive treatment to be continued when staff believe such measures to be futile and counter to the best interests of the baby. Respondents were asked to consider both scenarios independently and state what they believed their Unit would do in such circumstances. Sometimes respondents were basing their answer on actual examples of conflict. Others were surmising on the basis of known opinions and practices within their Unit. Having already offered a personal preference about the extent of parental responsibility and involvement, respondents were brought to consider their own view in relation to difficult conditions: first, situations where parents wish treatment to be withdrawn but staff are opposed to the idea; and second, situations where parents wish treatment to continue which staff believe to be medically futile. In focusing their thinking in this way, some subsequently recognized that they had contradicted themselves and acknowledged the dilemmas of real life practice. Others re-thought the issues and where they corrected earlier responses, their amended or qualified answers were accepted as their considered view.

More than one consultant commented that it tended to be the articulate middle class parents who took up polarized positions. They often have certain expectations of their children which are infringed by circumstances such as very premature delivery, intracranial bleeds or birth asphyxia. They can recognize the distinct possibility that their life style is likely to be substantially altered if they take home a severely damaged child. Other senior doctors remarked that it was the parents who adopted inflexible positions based on entrenched religious convictions who posed the most intractable problem. In most cases, other reasons for disagreement could be addressed by persuasion and logic and an appeal to their desire to make the baby's best interests the paramount concern. It was then often only a question of time before they came to see things more clearly. But deeply held religious beliefs were not amenable to these tactics.

Situations where parents wish treatment to be withdrawn but staff are opposed to the idea

Such situations occurred less frequently than the reverse scenario but occasioned less controversy so will be dealt with first. Eight doctors and 27 nurses volunteered that such a situation had never arisen in their experience. For a small number of doctors there was no dilemma here: babies had to be treated if treatment could be beneficial.

> 'I think if the baby is recoverable, it's nothing to do with the parents.' (Consultant, more than 25 years experience)

The consensus across all Units was that every effort would be made to discuss things with the parents to understand why they held these views. Energy would be devoted to getting them to understand the true nature of the circumstances: by repeated rehearsal of the facts, by giving them concrete indicators of progress, by involving them in the baby's care to demonstrate more forcibly that he was responding to treatment even if in a limited way. It could also have been argued that involving the parents in the baby's hands-on care was likely to increase their emotional attachment to him and make it harder for them to contemplate deciding he should die. But this possibility was not put forward by these respondents.

Most staff believed that given accurate facts and time to assimilate them, parents would usually come round to the doctors' point of view. Cases were reported where parents had initially reacted with horror to a situation and demanded that treatment be stopped. To some inexperienced members of staff, or those with strong opinions, parents' apparent rejection of their child, or a desire to get the event behind them and get on with grieving, was hard to tolerate. But most appreciated that it was a feature of the parents' insecurity and ignorance. Staff had to explain gently that they could not simply stop treating an infant for no good reason. Parents usually saw reason as time and a better understanding gave them a more balanced view of this novel experience. Sometimes it was a question of their needing reassurance about the comfort of the baby or about the burden of current treatment. A tiny minority suggested that parents could be manipulated by devious means, by giving information in certain loaded ways or selecting facts to convey to them, but most preferred a gentle and sensitive pacing of information to allow parents sequentially to assimilate the reality of what was happening.

Very few respondents (13, 10% of doctors and 10, 4% of nurses) felt that the appropriate thing to do in these circumstances would be to draft in a third party. Mostly this meant other neonatologists or neurologists or other specialists who could offer a second expert opinion. This might be in order to reassure the parents about the outcome for this child, but some consultants said it helped them to be sure of their own assessment, giving them the confidence to override parental wishes. One senior consultant elaborated on this point drawing out some of the issues relating to appealing to colleagues elsewhere. In his judgement, parents could well interpret a second opinion as merely a rubber stamping exercise because in their perception the first consultant would hardly call in someone who did not share his or her own way of looking at these issues. But there were senior people in reputable establishments who were held up as the experts in neonatology, and they were useful people to approach in difficult cases. One consultant appreciated their role but felt they carried a heavy burden:

> 'There are exceptional people in the world who will actually do it for the sake of pushing out the boundaries of what can and cannot be. And they may at the end of the time be crucified for it. And there *are* some martyrs around – bless them! – who have to be crucified to get the message over. But there are others like poor old Leonard Arthur who didn't turn out to be a martyr, he turned out to be a criminal. And I think you don't know as a martyr whether you're really right or going to be a martyr and be pilloried for it, but at the end of the day, you'll be the one with the halo and wings, or whether you'll be the guy who ends up in the stocks. And I think that's where there's a moral fibre required which is beyond what I would have been willing to take on in my professional career. I always find a little burrow! But it's not fair to some people, because if I'm the one who starts to throw the really awful situation in their face then that could be very hard for them. Having said that, there's a great deal of kudos comes out of being perceived as the last man in the line to make the decision. Now if you're in that position and you're willing to take that responsibility that can be a very satisfying thing to be able to do. It could also be an extremely tiresome thing, that somebody hasn't got the gumption to make the decision.' (Consultant, more than 20 years experience)

There was some reluctance expressed about going along the route of appealing to an outside agent if it meant that legal powers overtook medical responsibility, since so much emphasis was placed on trust and continuing negotiation. To call in legal advice and have parents overruled by someone else ran the risk of breaking down this special relationship irretrievably.

'I hope I'm never in the situation [of going to the courts for arbitration] because I think if the courts agree that we should withdraw care, the parents then go away with the feeling that, "Yes, the hospital has killed our child." And I don't think you would ever win them round at all.' (Consultant, more than 10 years experience)

Some respondents went to considerable pains to emphasize that calling in an outside expert commonly did not transfer responsibility from the shoulders of the consultant in charge of the baby. Such people were simply advising. The parents and the doctor had the choice of accepting the advice or not.

A third party did not necessarily have to be medical. A few of the nurses suggested that an opportunity to talk with other parents who had been in similar circumstances, or with a chaplain, social worker or counsellor, could help to persuade parents to change their minds.

Following such concerted efforts at communication and explanation, however, differences might still persist. Not all respondents volunteered what they would do in such circumstances. Some relied on ongoing negotiation to effect an acceptable decision. Others used a variety of means to reach a compromise. Yet others adopted a short term approach, bargaining with the parents at intervals for a little more time to see how the baby responded and to establish which course of action or which treatment would be best in the longer term. However, a considerable number did have a definite response as to which group would take ultimate responsibility.

Four junior doctors and two nurses thought they would simply tell the parents that it would be illegal for them to stop treatment which they believed to be in the baby's best interests. Interestingly no consultants who had had to make such a decision, offered this as a way of dealing with such a situation. Over half of the doctors (33, 58%) and just under half of the nurses (57, 48%) said that if they were sure they were right, they would override the parents and continue to treat the baby. As many as half of the consultants (11, 52%) would take this line. However, seven doctors (12%) (but only one consultant) and 15 nurses (13%) were reluctant to do so believing that parents had a right to decide this way. As long as they were aware of the facts and understood the consequences of their decision, parents should be allowed to exercise their parental responsibility in this regard. It was pointed out that they could have sound reasons for deciding against continuing. Only they really knew their own tolerances and breaking points. An intolerable situation could be created if doctors pursued treatment and then handed a severely damaged child to his parents for a life-time of pain and suffering.

These essential differences held true across all Units. In summary then, in all six Units far more staff believed they would override the parents on this matter than believed that they would give in to their wishes to withdraw treatment. Concerted efforts were made to reach compromises with other experts being consulted as necessary.

Situations where parents wish treatment to be continued which staff believe to be medically futile

Seven doctors and ten nurses volunteered that they had never encountered a situation where parents wanted futile treatment to continue. As in the reverse scenario, the majority of respondents placed a heavy emphasis on continuing discussion and negotiation. Finding out why parents held such definite views helped staff to assist them in coming to a more realistic understanding of the situation. Fears about the mechanics of the dying, or about the baby's suffering could be allayed. Events could often be orchestrated so that uncertainty was reduced and parents' own needs and wishes were taken into account in the timing and management of affairs.

Sometimes, where parents had falsely high expectations, or were clinging to vain hopes of miracle cures, it was a matter of explaining the limitations of modern medicine. In presenting the probability of certain impairments or of death, it is always possible to offer different pictures each giving the same facts but with varying emphases. 'A 20 per cent chance your baby will survive this treatment,' feels different from 'An 80 per cent chance that your baby will not come through this experience.' Indeed, as one consultant said, 'Consultants have enormous power because of the way they describe things.' Respondents suggested that it was on occasion necessary to spell the facts out in different ways or even to be brutally honest in order to bring parents to a realization that treatment was no longer effective. It was crucial for parents to grasp the implications fully of the course of action they were advocating. If for example, continuing treatment would result in their being saddled with a grossly impaired child who needed 24 hour care for the rest of his life, parents needed to know that the burden would be excessive.

It was sometimes the case that parents held out for treating the baby even when they recognized the implications for the family. In these circumstances, many respondents worried about just how much the parents did appreciate of the burden involved: unless they actually had first hand experience of similar circumstances, it was debatable whether they could ever truly foresee what life would be like with a seriously damaged child. Nevertheless staff considered that parents had a right to take on such a task for themselves in some situations.

> 'There's one case that we counselled four years ago that we really ought to withdraw care. And the parents said, "No." And that child's now still alive, with a number of handicaps, but not [nearly] as bad as the medical profession would have feared. The baby had bilateral IVHs – bad IVHs – necrotising enterocolitis, jaundice, and all sorts of things, and was 700 grams. And that child was in the Unit for over a year, and is very significantly damaged, but has enough intellect and enough physical capacity to have an independent life in the future – not a very good one – but ... So I think you do have to go along with the parents if the parents are very forceful and wanting everything continued. I don't think it's my position to go against the parents. If you believe that the parents are making the decision with the best information that you can give them, and with the knowledge that they're going to have to look after a damaged child, then it's not my business to say, "Time to Stop".' (Consultant, more than 25 years experience)

Short-term indicators could help to reinforce verbal messages: 'Let's see if your baby responds to such and such a treatment. If not I think it means that his brain is very severely damaged indeed;' or 'We are going to try this new course of treatment. As I've said, it's a new treatment. It hasn't been tried on many babies and we really don't know much about it. But nothing we've tried so far has been effective in stopping your baby's condition deteriorating. This is our last hope.' It not infrequently happened that while negotiations continued the baby 'decided' for them and just died. Some staff commented that this was often the kindest way out of a difficult dilemma.

When parents were taking a long time to come to terms with the medical facts, doctors sometimes limited the extent of the treatment. Not initiating resuscitation or antibiotics could allow death to occur without parents feeling that their views had been overridden. Suffering for the baby was one circumstance which gave staff enormous doubts about the wisdom of waiting for parental approval for withdrawing treatment. Some respondents volunteered that in these difficult circumstances where parents were withholding consent for withdrawal they would give additional analgesics which might have the effect of hastening death anyway. Parents too were reported to find the idea of the baby being in pain intolerable, and this fact alone could sometimes persuade them to alter their view and allow the child to die peacefully.

In rare circumstances however, parents' views which conflict with medical opinion stem from immovable religious convictions. Staff reported that it was extremely difficult to counter such preconceived ideas and these situations were the hardest to resolve satisfactorily.

Where continuing discussion did not resolve the differences, 9 doctors (16%) and 10 nurses (8%) advocated bringing in a third party to try to help the two sides to reach a decision. As can be seen, rather more doctors would resort to this strategy when the conflict was in this direction than when the parents were wanting beneficial treatment stopped. Hearing from a specialist from quite outside the Unit could bring an air of authority to a prognosis. It could also help to reinforce the consultant's own sense of the right way to go.

There was overwhelming agreement that it was not an appropriate course of action to override parental views and withdraw treatment in these circumstances. Only 5 doctors (9%) (just 2 of whom were consultants) and 7 nurses (6%) suggested this. By contrast 44 doctors (77%) (14, 67% of the consultants) and 76 nurses (64%) specifically said they would go along with the parents, keeping the baby alive while they continued negotiating, doing whatever they could to bring parents to a realization of the futility of further treatment. Aside from these specific comments, almost all respondents emphasized the need to keep negotiating. There was nothing to negotiate if the baby was dead.

Again these differences held true across the six Units. It was clear that in all Units there was a great reluctance to override parents in this circumstance. Some people suggested that to do so would be morally wrong. Others added that it would be inviting litigation. Nevertheless, it was this kind of dilemma which posed the greater problems. It was harrowing to keep babies alive who were suffering or visibly deteriorating. Respondents described skin sloughing off, bodies discolouring, infants 'smelling of death', babies writhing in agony every time they were touched, miserable days or weeks where everyone concerned was profoundly distressed by the inability to implement what they firmly believed to be the right decision.

The final decision makers

When respondents had considered both these scenarios they were asked who then did actually take responsibility for the final decision. A breakdown by discipline is presented by numbers in Table 12.2 and graphically in Figure 12.3. One doctor and five nurses had never experienced such conflict. A further four nurses declined to comment either because they were undecided or because they were too newly in post to have formulated an opinion on this matter.

Staff perceptions		
Final decider	*Doctors*	*Nurses*
Whoever wants treatment to continue	27 (47%)	66 (55%)
Doctors	12 (21%)	15 (13%)
Parents as far as possible	10 (18%)	23 (19%)
Varies with circumstances and time	3 (5%)	1 (0.8%)
Third party	2 (4%)	3 (3%)
Whoever wants treatment to be withdrawn	2 (4%)	2 (2%)

Table 12.2: The perceptions of doctors and nurses about who should make the final decision where staff and parents do not agree

When these results were further broken down by grade, it was apparent that the various grades perceived things rather differently (Figure 12.4).

As can been seen from these comparative tables and figures, most people in all groups favoured going along with the side who wanted treatment to continue, at least until circumstances dictated otherwise. Sometimes the baby's condition changed, sometimes he died in spite of efforts to keep him alive, sometimes one or other party changed their minds and both sides came to agree that withdrawal of treatment or the opposite was the appropriate choice. Staff recognized a peculiar poignancy in overriding parents. It was their baby and they were the ones who had to live with the consequences most closely and for the rest of their lives.

'Where you get conflict between what the nurses looking after the baby say, and [a sense of] "What the heck are we doing this for?"; and the parents are saying, "Look, we want you to go on," I would probably side with the parents, but then talk to the nurses about it, rather than simply overruling. I think I'd say, "Look, the reason we're doing this is because of this, that and that. I understand your feelings, but I think we've got to show that we've done everything for this baby. You and I know this baby's going to die – but in a year's time the parents can sit back and say what we did was right. And for the extra two or three days that this baby might be in intensive care, I think that's worth it." ... On the whole at the end of everything, I'd like the parents to remember the good things about the baby rather than the possible antagonisms that might have occurred with the management [of the case].' (Consultant, more than 15 years experience)

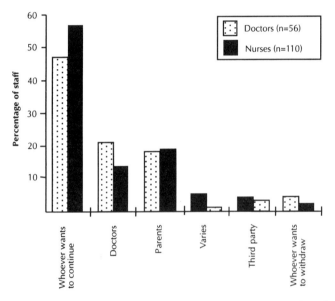

Fig. 12.3: The perceptions of doctors and nurses about who should make the final decision where staff and parents do not agree

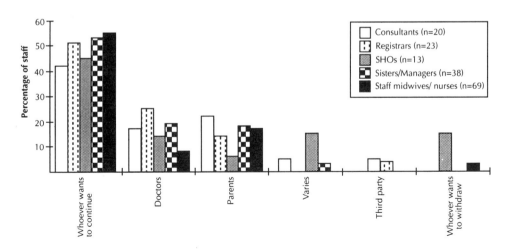

Fig. 12.4: The perceptions of different grades of staff about who should make the final decision where staff and parents do not agree

Very few doctors or nurses advocated a third party decision although they frequently sought outside opinion. This was a matter best kept within the close confines of the nursery and decided by those who knew intimately the exact circumstances of the case. However, some differences can be observed in the responses of the different groups. Senior doctors and nurses were more inclined than their junior counterparts to make the doctors the final arbiters.

When respondents were asked if they felt the right people were actually taking the responsibility when both sides could not agree, most felt they were. About three quarters (42, 74%) of the doctors but only just over half (65, 55%) of the nurses gave an unequivocal yes. One doctor and six nurses said the wrong person was deciding. The remainder qualified their responses. Some felt that there was no viable alternative, this was the way it had to be. Others felt that it was only partially right: it was right legally but not ethically; or other members of the team should also be involved. It was pointed out that in reality medical opinion usually carried more weight and parents gave in to pressure of facts and greater knowledge. However, where parents' views prevailed, a real anxiety was expressed that the decision could well be right for the parents but wrong for the baby: if parental preference meant that the baby suffered there was something far wrong. Some parents should not be permitted to accept too much responsibility.

There were no easy answers about how these criticisms could be answered. In general, staff felt that while doctors could usually bring the greater knowledge and wisdom about the medical condition, likely outcome and future consequences for the baby, they could not know the tolerances of each family nor decide what was right for them. The parents were the ones who had to bear the physical, psychological and social consequences of these momentous decisions for the rest of their lives. Their wishes and decisions should not readily be over-ridden. It was vital that earnest and continuing efforts should be made to arrive at an acceptable compromise which did not jeopardise the wellbeing of the baby.

Discussion

When a parent of a sick baby enters the nursery he or she generally adopts a certain role. Gone are the usual freedoms, autonomy and self direction assumed by parents of newly born infants. In their place are various controls. But, alongside those controls comes a degree of protection from responsibility. However, in recent years there has been increasing emphasis on partnership between the health care professionals and the parents, giving parents the task of juggling the competing messages they are receiving in these unknown and uncharted waters, and both parties the task of negotiating roles and degrees of involvement.

For years it has been argued that doctors should approach parents as allies, not adversaries, in the task of finding the least tragic solution to extremely difficult situations.[208] But the expectations of staff vary and the exact nature of the parental role appears to be open to interpretation. What one clinician expects and encourages is to another beyond the scope of parents. However, some illumination of this complex issue emerged from this study.

The majority of staff in NICUs do favour a joint approach. But they believe that, while parents have a role in the deciding, it is important to ensure that they are as free from guilt as possible. Most recommend that doctors make it clear that this decision is the one they think is right for this baby. Indeed the experienced senior clinicians in both disciplines more than their junior colleagues are inclined to move the burden closer to the doctors' end of the continuum.

Differences of perception

There appear to be important differences in the perceptions of parents and staff, and parental concerns are different from medical ones.[168,209,210] It is perhaps not surprising then that when it comes to ethical decision making these differences persist. It can be hard for those familiar with the sights and sounds and smells of neonatal units to appreciate the shock and bewilderment of parents. And to doctors and nurses it can seem incongruous to be worrying about a small blister or a bruised leg, when an infant's lungs are deteriorating and his vital systems failing. But parents often are more concerned about visible minor problems and staff with invisible major concerns. In addition, while staff can readily accept that sometimes continued existence is a fate worse than death, facts and figures mean different things to parents and they interpret information using common expressions of probability differently from medical staff.[211] For the parents intimately involved in the life of their infant, it is difficult to 'let go' and this phenomenon is well understood and recognized.[212] Emotions, while central to their involvement, can be complicated and sometimes conflicting.

> 'Parents' love and anxiety for their child can impede thought but also enable it, confuse yet enrich their thinking. Without emotions real understanding is impossible. Far from being irrelevant, emotions are a central part of the consent process.'[24]

When it comes to ethical choices then, it is perhaps small wonder that parents are not always aware even of having actively participated in the decision making, although it is important to recognize the fact that they are not necessarily upset by their own passivity in these matters.[210]

Parents' needs and wishes

By careful observation and real listening, staff can learn where parents are in their understanding and emotional acceptance of a seemingly intolerable situation. Their focus on a trivial happening may be disguising a deep seated anxiety about what the actual dying will be like. Such an unspoken fear may indeed prevent them making a decision to have treatment withdrawn. But it is unlikely that just one staff member will hold all the pieces of this jigsaw. Each in their own particular dealings with the family will glean a little information. They need to share these glimpses behind the masks parents wear and together build up a more accurate and comprehensive profile of the parents.

Of course, parents cannot be totally shielded from the harsh reality of these tragic circumstances. But they can be helped. For example, it is clear that they value honesty and full information as long as it is imparted with sympathetic understanding by someone they can trust.[209] [213] [214] There is a general consensus in the literature that imagining the worst is worse than knowing the truth about a poor prognosis.

But just by virtue of their own ambivalent feelings, there is a potential for problems. For instance they want to have faith in superior medical knowledge, and this is sometimes accompanied by a degree of remoteness and awe. On the other hand they also want the security of shared understanding and this may discourage honesty if the parents are fearful of disrupting a close relationship by being critical. The two may be incompatible.[24]

Staff however, can only take the parents so far. Warning of an eighty per cent risk of death or severe damage is very different from the 'inner labour of imagining'[24] what that really means. That is a task only the parents can do for themselves.

These are awesome issues. Profound emotions are involved. Sometimes parents can be 'difficult' to manage. Staff in this present study found the parents who appeared aggressive, domineering or entrenched in rigid beliefs, added to the stress of an already emotionally overloaded situation. Indeed domineering parents make staff even more cautious about their decisions and actions. But it is all too easy to misinterpret the outward signs. Some respondents were perceptive enough to realize that powerful negative manifestations could well be a cover for great sadness, insecurity and fear. Easily the most intractable group are the parents who hold extreme religious convictions about the sanctity of life. Most other ideas which may appear misplaced to staff, are amenable to persuasion or the appeal of logic, but such entrenched scruples are usually not.

Special relationship

For the most part staff take their duties to parents very seriously. They build up very special relationships, sometimes engaging in intensive and time consuming counselling sessions over prolonged periods of time. Where they are able to endure expressions of powerful emotion without taking it personally the relationship which develops can be a strong one based on trust and respect.[170,213] Both the doctors and the nurses are keen to preserve this shared intimacy and almost all are resistant to the involvement of outsiders who, they feel, cannot truly appreciate the fine nuances of each set of circumstances. Outside arbitration is reserved for those rare cases where all other avenues have been exhausted.

It seems that a degree of sharing of the peculiar pain of this particular baby's predicament is part of the service to which parents are receptive.

> 'Personal trust looks for a particular doctor with a personal concern for the child to guide the family through the impersonal and threatening world of intensive medicine.'[24]

They value warmth and personal concern at least as highly as technical efficiency in the people they entrust with their child's life. They are looking not only for 'the heroism of cure', but also for 'the vulnerability of care' from the people who have the task of helping them to cope practically and psychologically with this moving experience.[24]

Practicalities

Actually dealing with the parents is not always easy however, even where such good relationships exist. Organizational barriers between parents and staff may arise from things as diverse as the atmosphere of high technology, staff rotas, hierarchical systems, an imbalance of knowledge and power, regionalization of services. It is important for staff repeatedly to re-evaluate these issues and assess how the parents will perceive them. They all have a potential to complicate decision making as a joint enterprise.

Two key factors which bear repeated scrutiny are communication and consistency.

COMMUNICATION

Simply to say that parents should be involved in decision making does not take into account the 'highly complex and delicate negotiation *process*'[5] required. Inevitably clinicians make assessments about the parents they are dealing with. They vary their language and style of communicating in response to their perception of the level of medical and moral sophistication of the parents. To some extent, however, stereotypical judgements about parents' background can influence the staff's assessments of parental ability to understand the detail of the baby's condition and prognosis, and in consequence they may overly inform or withhold information which may in turn persuade parents in one direction or another.

Furthermore both the pace and manner of communications are important matters to parents and not just what is said.[24] The way in which parents are given the news that all is not well with their baby is crucial to their subsequent coping.[215]

In theory it is easy to see how all these factors impinge on the way parents perceive events and work towards their decision. The reality is far more complex. Parents themselves perceive the roles of different staff to be distinct. For example, they tend to rely on doctors to give them highly specialized detail about the baby's medical condition but the nurses to keep them abreast of daily developments.[216] Staff too have different perspectives. For example, doctors do not like being rushed into early communication, before they have evidence to present. But nurses feel compromised if they are obliged to withhold crucial information and to appear not to be telling the whole truth. It is an extremely difficult matter for junior members of the team to be asked for information which they do not feel empowered to disclose.[178]

These potential and real difficulties make it imperative that the team works together. If the timing and pacing of communication is to be maximally effective, it is not just the consultant or just the nurse at the cotside who needs to understand where parents are in their acceptance. But here again the consultant's role is crucial. If he is a good communicator and approachable, responsive and sensitive, not only will his messages and information giving be clear and appropriately paced, but staff will be more inclined to want to talk to him. In this way they keep him informed of developments. This two way exchange can have a knock-on effect in as much as he can then be even more sensitive to parents' needs and wishes. There will consequently be no talk about heaven-going with parents who do not believe in this phenomenon; no suggestion of withdrawing treatment on a date which marks a special family anniversary.

CONSISTENCY

Consistency is the second major requirement of staff dealing with parents during these delicate negotiations. Some teams indeed emphasized the importance of discussing the issues thoroughly together before presenting them to parents in order to present a coherent and consistent picture. But this united front approach has a down side. For example, there was a sense conveyed that if the staff were not prepared to go through with different options there was no point in offering them as options to the parents. Although one of the purposes was to avoid confusing the parents, this approach could be seen as operating against the parents. Where the decision is to continue treating, the parents will probably not be asked for their opinion; in general their consent is only really sought for discontinuation. Additionally the parents are not then exposed to the full range of opinions amongst the staff. As Anspach concluded: '"Presenting a united front"' obscures controversy in favour of consensus and narrows the options presented to parents.'[5]

However in general parents will prefer a consistent approach. To hear mixed messages and conflicting advice adds to their burden. As we have seen, they already frequently shop around for the most hopeful prognosis, so any ambivalence will compound their doubts and insecurities.

But a real problem exists by virtue of the organization of care. Services are fragmented. This becomes a major issue when we consider the divide between hospital and community. For most NICU staff an infant's story begins when he enters the Unit and ends on his death or discharge unless there are occasional visits at special times. But for parents of infants with severe ongoing problems, it is at the point of discharge that the story really takes on a new momentum, and for parents of those who die it is later in the community that the full impact of what has happened becomes a reality. However, it is then that the staff who have built up this special relationship, who have shared this emotional start, are absent. Even where a new support team out in the community is available, parents may not know of its existence or may be unwilling to tap into a resource which they consider inappropriate.

When they take time to contemplate these matters staff in the Units are fearful for the welfare of such parents. Deep emotional scars may exist which no one truly appreciates since care is so fragmented. Even paediatricians attached to the Unit follow them only so far. GPs and health visitors commonly know little about what has actually happened during the short life of a particular baby.[168 209] Who is there to make the relevant connections and trace grief resolution as a long-term process?

Cases of conflict

It is inevitable that on occasion parents and doctors will disagree about the decision which ought to be made. But it is a tribute to the skill and caring of the professionals concerned that these circumstances appear to be rare. For the most part the pattern adopted where differences exist is first to try the effect of time. Sometimes parents cannot accept the reality of what has happened and are in denial. If they are given a few more days to accept the dashing of their dreams, or to see for themselves that the infant is not responding to treatment or is in pain, they may of their own volition change their view. If not, the art of gentle persuasion is the next step. Persuasion may be accompanied by negotiating tactics. Saying, 'We will give your baby until Friday on this treatment but if he is still showing no improvement then I'm afraid we will have to conclude that continuing to treat him is futile and not in his best interests,' may be the next move. Such a tactic gives parents the opportunity to recognize for themselves the fact of their infant's condition, as well as the time and space to accept the likelihood of his death. These negotiations may themselves take time and it not infrequently happens that in the meantime the child dies anyway. Some staff believe this is the kindest option. Others suspect that parents sometimes avoid the necessity of deciding by being unavailable for the task of discussing what their choices are.

It has been suggested that staff allow more latitude for parental discretion in those cases which they perceive to be morally ambiguous.[5] This fact would appear to be borne out by this present study. If the outcome for the infant is thought to be certain death there is less room for discussion than where his probable future quality of life is the major issue. It is after all the parents who will bear the brunt of the consequences of the decision if the prospect is of severe impairment. All children try parents to breaking point on occasions; severely impaired ones may try their parents 'every hour of every day.'[217] And it requires a special generosity of spirit to withstand these demands. If the parents judge themselves able to deal with such a burden and elect to shoulder it, it is difficult for staff to overrule their decision. But sometimes there are conflicts for the staff if they believe that the parents are not understanding the weight of suffering which the baby must also endure. Where there is considerable uncertainty about the decision, more weight may also be given to the opinions of the other team members as well as of the parents. Indeed team effort has been identified as one way in which inappropriate behaviours such as paternalism, may well be controlled or exposed.[218]

Rarely a situation arises where the medical team and the parents cannot arrive at either an agreed decision or an acceptable compromise. A clear majority view emerges: whoever is in favour of the baby's life continuing holds the stronger hand. If it is the parents who want treatment to stop, staff have much less difficulty with the notion of overruling them than they have if the conflict goes the other way. Even where they are seriously concerned with the present suffering of the child, they have found themselves forced to continue treatment at least for a time. The fear of possible legal repercussions as well as a natural reluctance to end a life against parental wishes, seem stronger than the knowledge that doctors are not obliged to give medically futile care. When it comes to infants, emotions run high. The staff as well as the parents can be seriously overburdened by such conflicts and tensions.

Conclusions

It is widely accepted that the decision about whether or not to treat an infant should be a joint approach between the parents and those most intimately involved in the care of the baby. By involving a number of people all with slightly different perspectives and insights, a composite picture can be built up of the parents' understanding and tolerances. But these negotiations require enormous sensitivity and good communication. Sometimes conflicts persist. When parents request withdrawal of potentially beneficial treatment, far more staff would override the parents than would give in to their wishes. When the parents request continuation of medically futile treatment, staff are more reluctant to override them, although the delays can sometimes mean a baby's suffering is prolonged as a result. They rely on time and continuing negotiation to help resolve the situation. There is currently too much fragmentation of services which results in a lack of continuity and inadequate follow-up care, both of which potentially add to the weight carried by these already heavily burdened parents.

CHAPTER THIRTEEN

Support

NICUs are high powered environments with a degree of tension existing much of the time. Being involved in critical decisions about whether a baby lives or dies is a stressful experience superimposed on this inherent tension.

The burden

Since the doctors are the ones who accept responsibility for these decisions, they were expressly asked whether they found the task burdensome. Eleven of the doctors admitted that they did, while others recognized that they had developed mechanisms for dealing with the stress which cushioned them from some of the effects of these difficult tasks. A few commented that they did not enjoy this part of neonatal medicine but accepted that it was an inevitable part of the job. However, one consultant with over 25 years experience in neonatology confessed that, although it was not a happy time, he did find it stimulating: 'quite an exciting part of the job, because it's highly emotionally charged. I mean, it makes the adrenaline run, and makes you think about lots of things.'

To some extent doctors learn to deal with the burden and keep stress to a minimum, but inevitably some have developed their defences more strongly than others. The point was made that there is merit in feeling the distress of these experiences keenly since it helps to keep doctors sensitive to the emotions of the parents and nurses. Additionally personal pain ensures that deliberations are careful and are agonized over. Concern was expressed by one respondent who felt that changes in medical career structures eliminated the apprenticeship element which helped doctors to develop adequate coping strategies.

> 'The modern practice is going to get rid of the senior registrar. Big mistake. Big, big mistake. As a senior registrar you make the decisions but don't carry the responsibility. It allows you to build the [protective] wall, brick by brick. Now with the modern training, you're going to be a consultant in four or five years. Quite frankly, bollocks! You know, you're going to end up with a whole lot of burnt out shells five years on from that.' (Consultant, more than 10 years experience)

A few qualified their response by saying that it was not the decision itself which was burdensome since they only made it when the prognosis was hopeless, but it was the process – the carrying out of the decision – which troubled them: dealing with parents, watching the baby die, coping with the distress of staff as well as their own sense of failure or grief. It was not so much burdensome as emotionally draining. One consultant confessed to feeling very depressed after such events, needing time to recover before returning to the general work of the Unit, but most doctors actively immersed themselves in their other duties seeing this as the way to keep these difficult cases in perspective.

> 'When you are working, you are sort of on auto-pilot … there's a job to be done and you do it. But it bothers you afterwards.' (Senior Registrar, more than 10 years experience)

A number of consultants pointed out that their role in relation to treatment withdrawal was actually not as stressful as some other tasks.

> 'I've had more self-criticisms on occasions where I've actually had to go and tell parents that the baby has died, and it's been something unexpected, and it's been because of their condition, not because of this other process when I think you always feel you never did it right, than I've had with this process where obviously there is time and there has been discussion and there's more control.' (Consultant, more than 25 years experience)

Furthermore there was a sense of satisfaction afterwards if things had gone well which brought its own reward. But 'if it doesn't go well, it can be very disturbing,' as one consultant with more than 20 years experience commented.

Coping strategies

There are various ways of dealing with stress in the workplace and each is variously effective at different times and in different circumstances. It is important to take account of the effects of individual strategies as well as of the whole approach within the Unit towards support of the team.

Tactics adopted to protect the individual are not necessarily in the best interests of the team, and vice versa. For example, cool detachment might well be a defence against pain but hurt may then be buried on a deeper level.[24] Protecting oneself may be at the expense of instinctive compassion. Simply not acknowledging hurt or conflict may protect colleagues from damaging revelations but can add substantially to the burden carried by the person internalizing these powerful emotions. If colleagues are unaware that one of their team members is struggling, they are not likely to mobilize assistance. And they in their turn may not recognize that someone else shares their own disquiet which leaves them isolated and unsupported.

What appears to be needed is a general ethos of rational concern, based on knowledge and sensitive awareness, which permits the expression of feelings, and offers support to the individual as well as to the team, without impairing the ability to make decisions. But how may this approach be fostered in the busy and competitive environs of NICUs? In order to address the whole area of staff's ability to cope with these momentous decisions and to support families effectively, this enquiry explored the level and sources of support staff received in each of the Units.

Existing systems of support

The majority of the respondents (38, 67% of the doctors; 79, 67% of the nurses) answered immediately that there was no support system in their Unit. Only 3 doctors (5%) and 15 nurses (13%) responded with an unqualified yes. But a further 8 doctors (14%) and 19 nurses (16%) said a type of support system did operate in their Unit.

Identified support systems varied in form:

Trained counsellors

In one Unit staff could go to a counsellor in a nearby hospital. No Unit had a trained counsellor on their premises, although one Unit had had previous experience of employing such a person. The experiment did not work, however, and was abandoned in favour of an informal vigilance within the health care team itself.

Specific departments

The Department of Occupational Health was the source of formal support if requested in another Unit. Staff who felt the need for additional help could apply directly to this Department for access to someone to supplement internal Unit support.

Chaplains

Two doctors and seven nurses identified the chaplain as a source of support for their teams. It was noteworthy that the nursing staff who cited the chaplain were those who were giving the hands-on care. They said he just came around and chatted informally, sometimes just reassuring them by his acknowledgement of the pressures and tensions they were experiencing, sometimes giving them an opportunity to express their anxieties without the threat of repercussions.

Senior staff

A very small number nominated senior staff in the Unit as their mentors and support people, but one doctor pointed out that even though the consultant was the person to whom they could go officially, there were barriers to confiding in someone in his or her position. To betray uncertainty and distress might be to jeopardize future appointments. And if the junior doctor was troubled by the decision being made or the way things were being managed, going to the consultant could appear to be a personal criticism of the senior's practice. The problems attending senior staff acting as mentors were mentioned by a number of nurses too. In more than one Unit staff were allocated mentors but the juniors volunteered that they did not use them because there was too little confidentiality and their comments were used against them.

Specific meetings

One sister identified occasional debriefing meetings set up by staff in the team as the way difficult situations were dealt with and staff supported.

In planning

Two of the Units had recently sounded out their staff to see whether there was support for a formal system being implemented. In both, the general consensus was that the team did not want any formal set up. However, in a third Unit a support system was in planning (according to six nurses) but no details were supplied.

Personal coping strategies

Given that a recognizable formal system did not exist, respondents were then asked to identify and explore their own sources of support. As many as 13 doctors (23%)and eight nurses (7%) replied that they did not need support, they could work things out for themselves. One senior registrar pointed out that it was natural to be upset for a while, but it was not necessary to take any active steps to deal with this kind of distress. Proportionately more male doctors (9/34, 26%) than female ones (4/23, 17%) adopted this position. One consultant said he had early recognized the potential for stress in neonatology and had quite deliberately built a protective wall to defend himself. However, most respondents acknowledged a personal need for coping mechanisms and identified their resources.

Colleagues' sensitivity

A widespread sense was conveyed that people did obtain support at work. Easily the most commonly reported source of support for both disciplines was that obtained from colleagues. Knowing themselves the intense emotions involved, staff were vigilant on behalf of those around them.

> 'I work with girls that I've known for years. There's a lot of us have been here around the 20 year mark. We've worked together for a long time and we're friends, so we do pick up the vibes if there's any single one of us [struggling] ... We are aware of it.' (Sister, more than 20 years experience)

For all grades of staff except the SHOs, this was the most frequently cited source: the SHOs identified friends and family slightly more often than colleagues. The majority were referring to an informal arrangement which relies on the sensitivity of the staff. Individuals notice stress or distress and offer support in whatever way seems appropriate. Some mentioned just asking the colleague if they wanted to talk about whatever was troubling them. Nurses tried to relieve their peers of their duties for a time so that they could go away from the nursery for a break, to have a coffee, to cry or just be alone for a time.

There were certain people who gave rise to particular anxieties. Colleagues who never talked about their feelings in these traumatic situations were one such group. Staff who went home to an empty flat apparently with nothing and no one to help them to restore a measure of balance, were another. Brooding on these painful experiences could potentially convert a normal grief reaction into pathological stress.

But talking about these cases appeared to have different connotations for doctors compared with nurses. Doctors appeared to learn to cope without sharing their uncertainties and tensions verbally. They looked more for confirmation that they were right in their judgements. Indeed, some senior doctors voiced the opinion that if they got to the stage of needing outside help to cope they would feel it was time they got out of neonatology. Junior doctors admitted they had got caught up in this general stoical philosophy and it was only sitting down and listening to others' uncertainties and pains that helped them to see that they were not alone in their struggling. But they perceived it as hazardous to let seniors know about their vulnerabilities since the older generation might see such 'weaknesses' as indicators of an unsuitability for medicine or at least for this specialty: a consultant hardly wants as his registrar a person who is not coping with babies dying. And in this way the myth that doctors are tough and unmoved by profound human tragedy is perpetuated. Nor was it a phenomenon exclusively reserved for medicine: a number of doctors spoke rather slightingly of nurses' excessively emotional behaviour.

Nurses, on the other hand, considered that it was proper and healthy to be upset when babies deteriorated and died, their very tears showed that they had cared deeply. They spoke warmly of the sensitivity and compassion of their peers. Sharing stresses with understanding colleagues was to them a normal healthy reaction which helped to keep things in perspective. But they were selective. They too were alive to the possibly damaging consequences of confiding their struggles to people outside their immediate colleagues. In some Units staff midwives said they certainly would not tell the sisters if they were having a hard time since they feared such information would be used against them. With job prospects uncertain they could ill afford to jeopardize their positions in the hospital.

It was not just outward obvious expression of inner turmoil, however, which betrayed a need for support. Some senior nursing staff felt that sickness rates told their own story: staff would keep going during a crisis and while the Unit was busy, but subsequently they tended to be off work for various reasons. It was quite conceivable that these absences could be related to unresolved stress. However, in one Unit where sickness rates were exceptionally high, the junior nurses attributed this more to lack of support from senior colleagues than to the stresses related to the care of dying babies and their families.

Support from senior staff

A particularly valued form of support was seen to be that offered by sensitive seniors who acknowledged difficulty but gave the junior staff the opportunity to deal with it in whatever way they themselves deemed best.

'You shouldn't *have* to rely on your friends and colleagues in here. You should be able to rely on the nurse in charge to realize you *are* in a stressful situation. In situations like that where a baby is dying – often you need to come through to the quiet room to speak to parents. You can't always be with that baby. But you want to be with the baby all the time – you don't want to leave that baby on its own. So you need someone there supporting you to let you out when you need to. You're torn.' (Staff Midwife, less than 5 years experience)

Sometimes senior staff frustrated nurses' efforts to adopt coping strategies which they knew were appropriate for them in dealing with the loss of babies.

> 'There's been a bit of frustration ... about going to funerals, about staff being on duty. Some feel they *need* to go to the funeral, just like the parents need to go. And a lot of the staff feel it's appropriate that they go because they've been involved in the baby's care. A lot of the time they've been the main person looking after the baby – closer even than the grandparents and other relatives. And I think it's very important that staff are allowed to go for the parents too.' (Staff Midwife, less than 5 years experience)

Staff recognized that administrative and financial constraints inevitably imposed certain restrictions but simply having others sensitive to their troubled feelings was supportive in itself. This support could be seen in a number of diverse ways such as arranging a social event, providing an opportunity to talk, or giving a hug at the right time.

> 'The senior doctor and the senior nurses – they're the ones that have to pick up the pieces, and they have to share with each other those pieces. And they have to be sensitive to the needs of their staff and each other ... If there's a low phase and you've lost a number of babies that have been long-stay patients on the ward, then it's an evening out bowling that brings the Unit together and supports them, not someone wandering in in an arbitrary fashion discussing one's own personal and private feelings. It's an arm round the shoulder at the time and, "Are you all right? Can I get you a cup of tea?". That's the way to deal with it, I believe.' (Consultant, more than 25 years experience)

A few respondents drew attention to the difficulty some male doctors found in expressing support by touch. Although they might instinctively feel that a quick hug or a pat would convey more than words, they were conscious that physical contact could be misconstrued. One doctor from a foreign country said he hugged male and female colleagues alike since in his culture this was a recognized and effective mechanism which he believed worked. But he was aware that this was an alien practice to his British colleagues. Listening to the staff on the receiving end of gestures such as these, it seemed to be the case that the touch itself could not be isolated from the overall demeanour of the person. If he showed in other ways that he was sensitive to distress and supportive, then the touch was accepted as merely symbolic of the whole tenor of care and valued as such.

Actual needs appeared to be quite basic. Stories were recounted where senior colleagues had shown no sensitivity to the morale of the team when there had been deaths in the Unit. On the other hand appreciation was expressed for times when experienced colleagues – especially consultants – had simply voiced a comment which showed they understood why everyone was subdued. All that was wanted was some acknowledgement that they had been through a traumatic time: this in itself lifted moods.

Discussion with colleagues

Another form of informal support was that provided by confirmation of one's ideas and assessment. This was a support identified principally by senior doctors. For them the stress was of a different kind. Discussing the issues with other knowledgeable colleagues enabled them to sort out the facts and deal with the uncertainties. Support and reassurance came in having these other doctors agreeing with their decision.

There is a degree of isolation at the top and some consultants recognized the need to be cautious about what they divulged. Inherent dangers lurked in sharing too much of one's thinking.

> 'I think the problem arises where you really do not know people you're working with. You know them very superficially and usually not in the depth that you know certain other people in your group of friends. Maybe I'm a private individual. I have a lot of bizarre thoughts – not bizarre, different – and I say, "Well, I don't really want to throw this one out in case people pick it up wrongly." And there's a sense in which I want to control how much of myself I want people to know. Oh yes, there's no doubt about that. Unless you know me well, some of the things I say would sound extreme probably. But they're not how I *am*, but it's the way I *think*. You've got to be able to think radical new thoughts – to get over the hurdles. What excites me are ideas. And you've got to chuck out an idea and you maybe chuck it out to somebody who then says, "This guy is two standard deviations beyond the mean!" Which may be true and they may be very astute – but I don't think so! You need to be as close to them as they are to you. If you're going to throw out these ideas then they've got to be of similar mind to you – people you're comfortable with.' (Consultant, more than 15 years experience)

Talking to senior staff could also be helpful to more junior staff and nurses. If the consultant's decision was causing unrest, it was clearly most effective to discuss it with him or her in person rather than through third parties, but many felt uncomfortable in taking this path. Nevertheless there were consultants who volunteered that they actually found it useful to be challenged by junior colleagues who tended to come to these things with fresh eyes. In a number of the Units there appeared not to be a mechanism for direct discussion with the consultants and the frustration this engendered was seen in the amount of muttering and complaining engaged in within peer groups.

Family and friends

After informal support from colleagues, the most commonly identified source of support was family and friends. Spouses were singled out for mention by seven doctors and 11 nurses, although some of the nurses qualified their statement by saying they used their husband as a sounding board, just someone to let off steam in front of, who would comfort them even though he did not understand the issues. Other family and friends also supported by providing a listening ear, comfort and recognition of the worth of the individual.

Religion

Personal religious conviction was cited as a source of support more by doctors than by nurses. This was something other than the reassurance provided by the chaplain. Prayer and meditation formed part of it. There was too a sense that a basic religious belief influenced the whole of a person's life, offering them solace when times were difficult as well as a frame of reference in decision making.

Other work

The doctors had opportunities to move away from the most difficult scenarios. Attending to other babies or children who were making good progress was comforting and helped to keep things in perspective. For the nurses there was no escape during the long hours of each shift, but a few said that a form of support was provided where they were permitted to go to less intensive areas on subsequent shifts to give them a break from the tension. Some did point out however, that these troubling cases, where treatment was being withdrawn, were usually allocated to the more experienced staff, so these people often had quite long periods without reprieve.

Outside interests

It was generally agreed that having a balanced outside life helped to keep things in perspective. For some, vigorous exercise helped, for others, quiet reflective hobbies enabled them to regain a measure of tranquillity. Leaving the problems at work appeared to be difficult to achieve when the issues were so profound and staff so burdened, but some staff volunteered that that was what they tried to do. Having many demands on their time and energies at home made it imperative that some did adopt this practice. Considerable numbers of the respondents were also running homes and bringing up small children. This did not always offer relief from the dilemmas since they reported that going home to their own robust children was in stark contrast to the homecomings of the parents whom they had been dealing with at work. Comparing their lots brought sadness and a burden of responsibility as well as a renewed appreciation of their own family life.

Giving vent to emotion

Small numbers confessed to the healing power of a good cry, or vigorous swearing and raging.

On-going contact with families

A considerable number of the nurses said that actually attending the baby's funeral helped them. It rounded off the experience and was a final gesture of support to the parents indicating that they too had cared deeply. Some extended their support into the ensuing period maintaining contact sometimes over several years. Not only did this offer them the comfort of feeling they were helping the parents with their on-going friendship but it also provided a legitimate opportunity to go over the experience and analyse emotions and events until meaning or acceptance softened the hurt.

Other avenues

A stiff drink, or black humour could also offer temporary relief from the stress to a few staff. Most people relied on a mixture of strategies by which they managed to cope with the pressures and tensions produced by these difficult decisions and their implementation.

The need for a formal support system

For years debate has continued over the value of formal support systems. Questionnaires had been circulated in two of the Units to ascertain staff views on the subject. Several of the Units in the present study had considered various options in the past and, as has been mentioned, one Unit was currently planning to implement a new system. By contrast, however, another Unit had abandoned a formal system because it had not worked. Respondents were asked for their own opinions as to whether a formal system should be available.

Considerable numbers of both doctors (24, 42%) and nurses (76, 64%) thought that some recognized system of support should be available, although many qualified their statement with an observation that they would not themselves use it; rather it needed to be available for those people who otherwise had inadequate sources of support – those who lived alone or who were very young and inexperienced. A structured system might simply be formalizing the informal arrangements already existing, or it might be introducing an alternative form of support. Either way there was merit in having something which was known about and which reflected the ethos of the Unit: namely that it was normal and acceptable to need support in this stressful environment. In a sense adopting a formal stated approach to support put a seal of approval on individuals seeking it.

A further 18 doctors (32%) and 19 nurses (16%) were ambivalent about the need for a formal service since they would not themselves wish to use it, but they recognized that others might feel a need for something more than the present informal arrangements. One doctor wondered if there was not merit in retaining the status quo since a form of 'survival of the fittest' screened the unsuitable out of the specialty.

There were potential dangers in implementing a formal system. Some people felt that doing so ran the risk of exaggerating difficulties, making transient tensions into major issues.

> 'What might be a transient problem for us could be gelled into a definite problem, if we had a formal [system]. Whereas if you can resolve it in your own way and in your own time, I think you work through the emotions and you get over it. You don't forget the experience and it doesn't make you feel any happier afterwards, but you can more or less get back to normal. [Formalizing it] sometimes makes a mountain out of a [molehill] – not that I'm saying this *is* a molehill. But it makes things out of proportion, and things that you could deal with amongst yourselves, are taken out of your hands and dealt with differently and possibly not appropriately for the person.' (Staff Midwife, more than 10 years experience)

There was a perceived danger that the experience of going for specialized counselling might turn out to be more damaging than beneficial. An element of stigma attached to people who sought professional help and this too could militate against an individual. Some respondents believed that even were such a system to be formalized, staff would not use it.

Formal support could include a number of different sources and forms of help. One such example was to employ a trained counsellor. But an additional hazard was identified here. One experienced consultant had reservations since he felt that introducing a psychologist as a counsellor could escalate into their becoming involved in more than the support of staff: he did not want such a person to start interfering in the decision making itself.

Confidentiality was a thorny issue and a considerable number pointed out the difficulty in confiding in people outside the rarefied world they inhabited. Some volunteered that they did talk to other people but it was on certain specific grounds. Names were not mentioned, only the general issues were discussed. Confidants were hand-picked because of their empathy or known integrity. A few nurses who had tried to talk to others had discovered that these people were either not interested in the problems or stresses, dismissed them as just part of their job, or were too upset themselves at the mention of dying babies to be of use to anyone else. The nurses had therefore abandoned the effort to seek help outside in order to balance the support they received from within the Unit or to relieve their colleagues of a burden. There was a general feeling that people who had never experienced these traumas could not really understand the issues.

In the perceptions of NICU staff, the possession of a counselling qualification puts people outside the Unit into a different league. Such individuals are offering a specific kind of support. Their skills can turn the encounter into a specific professional service which is of value in itself, irrespective of whether or not they understand the fine nuances of neonatal care. Indeed some respondents suggested that such people could be usefully dispassionate and slightly removed from the intensity of the emotions generated. A few felt that skilled counsellors definitely had a place: where staff encountered a run of deaths, or were involved in particularly traumatic situations, or were simultaneously grappling with profound personal experiences, then their needs tended to lie outside the scope of peers, and professional counselling could be beneficial. However, even then there were potential problems for some. Going to anyone else and confiding one's vulnerability could seem like a dangerous expression of inadequacy.

> 'I wouldn't want to let anybody outside know that I'm inadequate. I don't mind my colleagues knowing that I am inadequate in coping but I don't want to go and tell somebody [else]. I mean if the counsellor was somebody like [our chaplain] I could go and talk to him, but if it was somebody in some bereavement council of the [Local Health Authority] council, there's no way I'd go and let myself down.' (Sister, more than 20 years experience)

Introducing specialist counsellors as part of the formal support system presented problems to a considerable number of respondents. Perhaps the biggest drawback was that outside agents were usually not available when they were primarily needed. Staff often felt an urgent need to discuss troubling matters. Being required to set up an appointment at a later date or to wait until the following Thursday afternoon for the visiting counsellor, was entirely unsatisfactory. Similarly when the counsellor *did* appear there was a need to find staff for her to speak to; a number of respondents described such circumstances encountered in other Units where 'sacrificial' staff had to be found to justify the counsellor's regular visits. One person suggested that research was urgently needed to explore the efficacy of trained counsellors in NICUs.

A few nurses in the study Units had undertaken counselling courses. They had the capacity to offer special opportunities for their colleagues to unburden themselves of painful emotions, although none of them appeared to be being utilized in any structured way. Since they were all involved in the normal hands-on care of the babies, scope for exercising their counselling skills appeared to be limited. A specialist colleague, in-house but slightly removed from the clinical care, it was suggested, might provide a viable alternative but confidences were not always respected in the experience of many respondents and they were understandably wary of promoting a system which forced them into untenable positions. It was noteworthy that very many medical and nursing staff spontaneously said that participating in the interview for this current study had been a useful and therapeutic experience. Some even extrapolated from that feeling a sense that such exchanges would be a valuable source of support for the team in an ongoing way.

Senior doctors could obtain little help from outside sources since they were looking principally for confirmation that they were right in their assessment. Such reassurance could only come from those who were experts in the field. An interesting difference was observed between medical grades. Proportionately more consultants than junior doctors wanted to see a formal system implemented (38% as against 26%). This could have been an indication that the juniors were content with the current provision, or it could have reflected an unwillingness to acknowledge need. A sense was certainly conveyed that requiring support cast doubts on an individual's suitability for medicine. Amongst the nurses there was a high level of support for a formal provision at both senior and junior levels.

Discussion

NICUs are hotbeds of tension and stress. However, doctors and nurses tend to be stressed by different things.[219,220] Nurses are overburdened by shortage of staff, relentless tension, failures of equipment, parental demands, the grief of infants not getting better, the tension of organizational pressures. Doctors carry a relentless burden of responsibility which often cannot be shared, they face the anxiety of making crucial decisions with uncertain facts, imparting bad news to parents who are ill prepared for tragedy at the beginning of a life, they are confronted by the evidence of earlier decisions when survivors visit follow-up clinics, and sleep deprivation is common. All have to cope with frequent change-overs of colleagues and the influx of new and raw recruits to a field of medicine demanding specialized skills. Most Units in the United Kingdom are working at below the recommended basic levels of staffing,[158] in spite of a long series of reports outlining minimum standards concerning the structure, staffing and equipment required for NICUs.[221–225] Furthermore 'success' and 'failure' in the neonatal world are often held up to public scrutiny – in perinatal figures as well as through cases which hit the headlines – further adding to the pressures of a high powered existence.

> 'The stresses and psychological wear and tear that come from the nature of the job itself are, in many units it seems, exacerbated by organizational factors and staffing problems. Effective team-work and support are difficult to maintain in these circumstances, but are essential if nurses are to want to stay in this specialty.'[131]

Into this taut scene drop the immensely stressful experiences of deciding whether or not to treat very sick infants.

Although the stressors vary between disciplines, the relapse or death of an infant is universally stressful for both groups. But in the face of their own profound sense of helplessness and intense sorrow, they are required to fulfil a multiplicity of roles. After sometimes a few brief hours or days, the parents will be left with only a birth certificate, pictures, the memories the staff have helped to create and a death certificate. The staff must be counsellor, advisor, friend and substitute relative, sometimes chaplain or psychologist. There is only one opportunity to get it right. These are burdensome responsibilities and tensions run high.

For the doctors and nurses themselves, of course, there are repeated losses as babies they are struggling to save do not get better or deteriorate and die. It is right that they should have opportunity to grieve for those babies with whom they have developed a relationship, and they need compassionate support from other people in order to effect a healing process. But the endless demands of a busy environment make it difficult for colleagues to provide such opportunities or to offer on-going support for very long after the death.[193]

An individual's ability to function competently and adapt to the range of stresses which characterise life in a NICU, depends on the adoption of effective coping strategies. To some extent a degree of personal hardiness can be a buffer against the deleterious effect of these stresses.[226] A strong social support network can also positively influence outcome.[226] But the main source of support comes from within the Unit. Colleagues are uniquely qualified to provide this support since they alone know all the circumstances of this particular case and understand the issues. Often too they share the same emotions. The strength which comes from this source has been identified elsewhere too.[193]

The NICU has been likened to a war zone and as with any intense, separate and dangerous context, survival and individual as well as collective wellbeing depend on teamwork.[4] Each needs to be sensitive to the needs of others if the whole team is to function effectively. As discussed before, the consultant occupies a special place in this regard. He is the person leading the team in discussions around this decision; he is the one who must finally decide on the best course of action. His unique need for support should not be underestimated although it is often unrecognized. But his support comes mainly from two sources: in having his decision confirmed as the right one, and in the reassurance of a team united behind him.

For the rest of the team, needs are at a different level. They need to be comfortable with the decision itself and supported in the working through of its consequences. As far as the decision itself is concerned, there is a real sense in which most people benefit from talking directly with the consultant where there is any ambiguity or uncertainty about which option is to be preferred. But currently few have this opportunity. By understanding the rationale for what is decided they can have a better appreciation of why this course has been chosen. It is then easier to implement the management of the baby and his family. Coincidentally such open communication can be helpful to the consultant since being repeatedly challenged to think through the arguments around a decision and justify actions can be confirming. A few very experienced neonatologists acknowledged the value of young fresh minds addressing these issues, seeing them in a different way. Their challenging can help everyone to proceed with more confidence in the end. And this two way benefit is also instrumental in encouraging more open discussion. Different members of the team get to know one another better and feel less inhibited in sharing their feelings and doubts. This circular effect facilitates a deeper level of support all round.

As far as the support in caring for the family goes, the senior staff (including the consultant) can offer much if they acknowledge the special place of those who are helping the parents to have a meaningful and optimally satisfactory experience through the dying and subsequent period.

> 'It is important for the senior staff to communicate that the skilful provision of terminal care to ensure a baby "dies well" in the loving arms of his parents may be as much a successful outcome of neonatal intensive care as ensuring the survival of an extremely sick preterm infant.'[155]

Nurses spending long hours with distraught parents and deteriorating babies, can feel much less stressed if senior colleagues acknowledge both the burden of their task and the value of what they are doing.

Whilst the nurses tend mostly to rely on sharing their stresses with their peers, doctors seem to adopt a wider range of supportive strategies, perhaps because they are not openly showing tensions and talking to their peers. The whole working structure for the two disciplines is different and the more fragmented tasks of doctors for the most part do not permit the close working arrangements which nurses experience and gain from. But it is salutary to realize that junior doctors enter the nursery feeling the grief and helplessness and yet soon feel that they must learn to suppress their emotions if they are to live up to the example set by their seniors. Those consultants who have the courage to share their own distress and uncertainties to some degree are providing what would appear to be a healthier template both for the individual and for team wellbeing.

Managers have an important role to play when it comes to support. It is decidedly unsupportive to staff busy Units inadequately. Nurses are frustrated when the calibre of staff sent to relieve pressure in an emergency is wholly unsuited to the tasks at hand. Certainly staff ratios for these patients are high but the skilled tasks involved demand expert hands.

Setting up a structure which says to staff that stress and tension are inevitable parts of the work acknowledges that individuals are not deficient if they experience stress.[227] Simply having a system in place can be supportive in itself and may well lead to less demand for counselling services. There should be no sense that to seek help is to lose face or that in doing so individuals betray unsuitability for the job. Indeed it could be argued that a person who has so inured him- or herself to the emotions of these momentous affairs is the more unsuitable. As one experienced sister commented: 'I think when you don't feel, that's when you've got to start worrying.'

Although the bulk of the needed support comes from within the Unit, other sources supplement it and are valuable. Family and friends can provide loving support which is usually unconditional, and there is no loss of face in showing human emotion to those bound by social or familial ties who have known one intimately over prolonged periods of time. Simply talking through the events can help people to grow through the total experience and is supportive. Talking to the chaplain offers a form of such 'talk therapy.' Going to the funeral is seen as a supportive gesture for the family but it may also be an important element in the nurse's own grief resolution. Vigorous exercise or quiet contemplation alike can offer solace. All these and many other activities as we have seen, can be used as outlets for tension which reduce the burden of stress for staff. The permutations are legion.

The need for greater emphasis on support for staff is not a new phenomenon. A group of organizations concerned with promoting good support practices for staff in health care recognized that people who care are a 'most important resource' and that the need for support is both 'legitimate and acceptable.'[228] They identified six ways of preventing the damage caused as a consequence of occupational stress:

> **Recognizing** that stress exists
> **Acknowledging** the need for support
> **Educating** staff in prevention and management of stress
> **Providing** adequate support services
> **Creating** a caring culture in the workplace
> **Promoting** good staff support practices throughout the system.'

As they concluded, staff who are cared for provide the best kind of service. Our data reinforce the need for more rigorous application of these principles.

Conclusions

Every NICU needs to embrace an ethos which regards support as essential for all members of the team. The structure needs to be known so that it is available to those in need but neither intrusive nor imposed. Individuals must have the autonomy to seek out those supportive strategies which are most appropriate for them. In feeling personally valued and cared for, each person will be the stronger to carry on performing this demanding role. These are not new concepts but they clearly need reiteration.

Open communication, particularly as far as the consultant is concerned, and sensitive awareness of the strengths and weaknesses of colleagues, go a long way towards cultivating a harmonious team approach, thus minimizing unnecessary tension and conflict. Each member of the team has a part to play in providing such an environment, but managers have a special responsibility both to ensure staffing levels are adequate for the tasks in hand, and to foster an appropriate and available structure which makes support a standard part of practice.

CHAPTER FOURTEEN

Education

In recent years there has been a growing emphasis on teaching ethics to both doctors and nurses. Exploration of the morality of what is done is as important as learning technical skills. Research has identified the need for health care professionals to be aware of their own opinions, beliefs, prejudices and feelings in order to minimize the risk of such factors impeding the giving of good quality care.[227] Furthermore official bodies endorse this need. The General Medical Council has recently published a document recommending a swing away from the acquisition of factual information and towards a process of self awareness and self learning which gives attention to the cultivation of appropriate attitudes and the development of communication skills.[202] Gaining an understanding of ethical issues is a stated part of this deeper awareness.

In the current study, efforts were made to find out how adequately respondents felt they had been prepared for dealing with the sensitive issues around withdrawing treatment from babies.

The adequacy of training of doctors and nurses

The point was made that there is so much teaching to cram into training (particularly for doctors) that it is impossible to cover everything. Competition for teaching slots is great and one successful bid is often at the expense of some other important topic. Nevertheless, even given this understanding, the vast majority (43, 75% of the doctors and 99, 83% of the nurses) felt that their training had been inadequate. A small minority (1 doctor and 5 nurses) however, had limited expectations: for them these were not issues which *could* be taught outside of the actual experience, so they did not look for classroom input on such matters.

> 'I think you can give them guidelines like that but *how* to do it only comes from watching and seeing and doing. The only way they can do it is by getting in amongst it, I think. It's a practical training process.' (Consultant, more than 15 years experience)

> 'You can tell somebody as much as you like, and yes, it's all there on paper. But until you experience it it doesn't mean very much.' (Sister, more than 10 years experience)

To some extent, respondents felt that undergraduate students were too young and inexperienced in life itself to be receptive to these issues. It takes understanding of deep realities to be able to comprehend the enormity of these decisions. A considerable number of nurses remembered with feeling their own early experiences of dying patients and the uncertainties and powerful emotions they had often suppressed. Indelible memories were created by particularly traumatic experiences; feelings of remorse attached to early indiscretions brought about through a general unpreparedness.

'My friend who trained at Hospital X did her first ward duty with a single auxiliary. And [when the first patient died] my friend went to open the window. And the auxiliary says, "What you doing that for?" And my friend said, "I was told I had to open a window to let the spirit out." And she said, "There's enough f... cracks in this building, the spirit'll find it's ain way out!" And that was her dealings with her first death. All she had been told was she was supposed to open a window and let the spirit out. From then, she went to look after other people, deal with a dead body with more sensitive people. But to send a first year student with an auxiliary who had an attitude problem like that is horrendous. We can laugh about it when we've got a bit older, but I couldn't believe it – that she even swore in front of this person, this dead person.' (Staff Nurse, less than 5 years experience)

'They could maybe have had a priest – some kind of spiritual input to say that death isn't the end for lots of us. Its not the end for any of us, but eternity can be a whole different place. And I just feel that it would have been nice to have had something like that. And also to have had people who were going to be more understanding. I called my sister tutors – I was absolutely terrified of them! They were really dictatorial and they were away apart from us – we were just minions. And yet as a very young nurse ... I think back and I think, "We had no preparation for [dealing with death]." But because you were young, you just went on and you did it, and I can't remember feeling particularly emotional or anything. It was just a kind of non-event. And I could remember even at times, you know, *laughing*! And it's a very serious thing. I think it would be good to demonstrate to young girls the kind of reverence that we should have in a situation like that – there's a certain amount of reverence – seems a daft word – [solemnity?] yes – what on earth would relatives think if they thought you were there attending to this body and [larking around] just like life was going on [the same] because that's their nearest and dearest. But even then we had no support.' (Staff Midwife, more than 10 years experience)

Doctors recounted their horror initially when they lost patients in spite of their best efforts. Some respondents spoke eloquently of facing death in their own families for the first time and being suddenly much more acutely aware of the importance of what people said or how they reacted to the bereaved. One senior doctor with a wealth of community experience observed that as a new graduate it had never occurred to him that some people might actually choose to have an impaired child or might feel able to care for incontinent relatives for years and years; his own ethical position had been very black and white then. As a result of meeting many such families over the years, he had changed his ideas and opinions about what was morally permissible or desirable.

Satisfaction with preparation

It is commonly suggested that things are improving and it seemed likely that younger, more recently qualified staff would report more satisfaction with their education in these matters. This did not appear to be the case in reality: all, except one of the SHOs who had completed a more recent training, were not persuaded that current provision met needs. They all gave an unqualified 'No' in response to a direct question about whether their training had prepared them. And only three staff midwives were satisfied with their preparation out of the total population of 119 nurses.

Only three doctors of any grade and three nurses said that their own exposure to these issues had been good. These respondents praised a medical/nursing school which was enlightened enough to prepare students for the human side of caring.

> 'I was lucky, I went to Medical School X. And we had a medical ethics course and nobody wanted to go to a medical ethics class because they were on a Friday afternoon. If you *didn't* go to the medical ethics lectures you didn't get to sit your exams! So everybody *had* to go. Otherwise you got hauled in front of the Dean. And they were probably the most entertaining two or three hours that we had. Because it was this debate – like this [interview] – and it was great. Small rooms and it was great. And you may not [speak], [all the issues] may not be addressed, but they give you a forum to express your views and listen to other people's views, which is what you need.' (Registrar, less than 5 years experience)

In some ways other respondents recognized that the clinical environment was now more conducive to openness and team work: staff were more friendly, parents felt freer to talk to both nurses and doctors about their feelings, the nurses at least felt able to show their own emotions in a way that was unacceptable in the past, and some Units even had on the premises equipment such as videos and reading material specifically on these issues. But overall, this newer approach had not been reflected in adequate preparation for the rigours of difficult decision making.

> 'A thing people don't like to talk about is death. They scurry across it and you get factual things like grief – these are the things you go through. But you're not prepared for what you're going to see [or experience].' (Staff Midwife, less than 5 years experience)

Sources of learning

When the respondents were asked how they had learned about these sensitive issues, interesting differences emerged between the two disciplines. Overall, however, the main way staff learned was through clinical experience. As many as 88 of the nurses (74%) and 27 of the doctors (47%) cited this as the way they had acquired understanding of these issues. A further 20 nurses and 7 doctors had received some formal input in addition to what they picked up in clinical practice.

But for doctors there were additional sources of learning. A type of apprenticeship system enabled them to learn from their seniors and mentors and some very experienced doctors reflected with gratitude and affection on the insights they had acquired through affiliation to wise and innovative practitioners during their formative years in medicine. Others identified specific opportunities they had had which had opened their eyes to deeper realities. These included being sent to a hospice for a short time; having the chance to talk to parents and child patients; taking part in lively discussion groups which explored difficult topics either with medical groups or lay people; and being influenced by a philosophy in medical school which encouraged students to think rather than to assimilate facts passively.

Nurses on the other hand did not in general identify such sources of learning in their system of training. They rarely singled out particular individuals as role models, although a very few did observe that older experienced nurses had shown them an excellent example.

> 'I learned a lot by just listening to what older [people say] – especially people with kids of their own – they are very, very good, I don't know why. Just saying the right thing at the right times. ... there's one person, I've learned a lot from her. Because she's a Mum, she's been through having kids, she knows how it feels to have a baby – she knows the emotional side. I think the older people, they are experienced. They are the ones who've got a lot of life under their belt and I find the [parents] get a lot of comfort from the older ones because you can trust them. You do tend to watch what they do.' (Staff Midwife, less than 5 years experience)

Some nurses did mention having had experiences in other specialties which gave them insight into life and death issues, but they considered this to be learning on the job and adding to the sum total of their nursing experience, rather than as specific opportunities to be educated in the ethics around prolonging life. This could have been a feature of a number of differences in the training and experience of the two disciplines. Roles and expectations are quite different. Student nurses are intimately involved, over long shifts, in the hands-on care of patients, tend not to be engaging to the same extent in discussions either with senior nurses away from the patient or around stopping treatment, and concentrate on gaining experience of different diseases and nursing different clinical groups.

> 'I suppose in basic nursing training you were faced with a fact of having to care for people in their last hours. But we were never given any instruction about the moral or ethical side of it. It was assumed that whatever decision was made would be right and we would support it.' (Sister, more than 15 years experience)

On the other hand, student doctors initially flit in and out of different fields of practice, detached to a large extent from the intimate lives of their patients, attend to fairly mechanical tasks, and rely on extracting the essential issues from their various clinical placements rapidly and selectively. There is so much to be learned that they have to concentrate on the important factors in each specialty and try not to worry about the bits they are missing.

'Where I come from, you've got lectures in medical ethics and stuff like that, but you're not dealing with it at the moment so you don't worry about it. You don't even want to go to the lectures because it's so boring. But once you're there – when you see your first person dying, it's [different]. I was very shocked. So it's quite difficult then. And you need them to talk about it. I think they must when you're a house officer. It's then that lectures must be given, rather than when you're a student, when you don't worry about it.' (Registrar, less than 5 years experience)

Naturally, understanding could come from sources not immediately identifiable as training for health care professionals. Reading, informal discussions with many people and a variety of life's experiences were all ways in which some respondents had explored these delicate issues for themselves.

Postgraduate opportunities

Sometimes opportunities to explore a subject in depth only come later, once a basic level of knowledge is acquired and some clinical experience gained. For some it is not until they have specialized in neonatal care that they really face these difficult questions. Respondents were therefore asked to reflect on postgraduate/post-qualification experiences to see whether preparation had been more effective in subsequent years.

Identifiable postgraduate opportunities appeared to be more available for nurses than for doctors. As many as 49 of the nurses (41%) had had some opportunities to address these issues after qualification. Some admitted the openings were very limited but nevertheless had helped them to think more deeply. Study days, specific courses on topics like bereavement or euthanasia, and degree courses they had undertaken, had all offered new insights. A few cited studying for their neonatal qualification as a time when they had been brought face to face with the complexities of loss and decision making in relation to babies. Eight other nurses said that they were aware that courses were available but they had not had the chance to enrol on any of them. Only five doctors had availed themselves of specific training opportunities although a further five acknowledged that the openings were there but for a variety of reasons had not been taken up.

For the doctors, the learning was still predominantly in clinical practice. Tagging along with a consultant or experience in general practice had shown them what these decisions entailed. In some hospitals, specific training goals for junior doctors helped them to identify the issues, and enabled seniors to ensure that the less experienced continued to develop in understanding as well as exposure to new situations.

It was not just the availability of teaching which left room for improvement. The majority of the respondents, both medical and nursing, felt that what they were taught was largely irrelevant. Once they knew at first hand what these difficult decisions entailed they looked back on their training and saw it as deficient. Several qualifying statements gave insight into how staff felt about this. To some extent these things cannot be taught cold. A basic framework can be supplied but it is repeated exposure with ongoing discussion which helps doctors and nurses to formulate their ideas and inform their practice. Some accepted that when they were very young and inexperienced, they had problems knowing what to say in sensitive situations anyway. They also felt their immaturity and naiveté probably rendered them unreceptive to ideas centred on deep experiences which they had never encountered and which seemed peripheral to the factual information they had to assimilate. However, more senior people remarked that these young people sometimes thought they had all the answers and the most helpful and instructive thing to do was to challenge them to really think about the specifics of a case and justify their strong beliefs.

Suggestions for education

Having established that the present system of educating both doctors and nurses about ethical dilemmas in neonatology appears to be largely inadequate, it seemed useful to explore respondents' ideas for what would have helped them to be better prepared for these complex and often traumatic situations. A large number of suggestions were offered (80 different ideas). These have been assembled into categories for ease of reference. No attempt to quantify these citations has been made since excellent ideas were provided by single individuals and deserve equal recognition alongside the more obvious suggestions.

Reserve specific educational efforts on these issues for postgraduates
Youth, inexperience and other demands made it difficult for students to take on board the real issues underlying decision making in life or death situations. Such matters were best reserved for those who were facing the practicalities of these dilemmas.

> 'Learning medicine as an undergraduate and clinical practice are very, very different. Training people – I'm still in training and I'll be in training till I'm 60, I think! And I think that's the point. We can't expect everybody to be perfect after five years training. I think our primary goal has to be that they know how to – they know about the mechanisms of disease; they know about diseases and the treatment of diseases; they know how to elicit the signs of those and investigate them and sort them out; and they are *aware* of some of the emotional and ethical and moral issues. But we learn so much every day and every week and every year that to talk about training only in an undergraduate sense to me is pointless because most of our training is postgraduate. And I think that we should really worry about these issues in the training of people who are actually having to do it because they are going to be able to approach the learning situation with a lot more maturity and understanding than a second year medical student who's so detached from it that it's largely pointless. And if you take someone who's actually looked after this patient, who's tried to keep them alive and is now facing the fact that they couldn't keep them alive, and intervene in *that* situation, there's a hugely greater benefit than there is in trying to get some 20-year-old to imagine this situation. I think there's a serious deficiency in the training of postgraduates in these issues.' (Senior Registrar, more than 5 years experience)

When junior staff were confronted by the reality of their patients dying, doctors felt these issues had so much more meaning. The consequences of their own decisions and their own practices were so much more apparent then. They could appreciate that thinking about the ethics of what they did and looking at the arguments around various choices was an important element of their work and could influence the quality of their practice.

> 'Further training and continuing education as a routine part of your junior house officer year would be most beneficial, because it's there that you confront death for the first time as your responsibility. And a lot of the deaths that occur when you're a junior house officer – you may feel that your inexperience has contributed to these deaths, where it probably hasn't but you don't know. You're insecure enough in yourself, and I think that's a biggie that should be targeted.' (Registrar, less than 5 years experience)

Formal sessions

Large numbers of respondents recommended specific sessions providing a framework of the relevant areas: law, moral philosophy, ethics, outcome statistics, psychology, psychiatry. It was important, they said, to have the facts as a basis from which to work. For example, staff needed to know what the law allowed them to do. They needed to have a grasp of fundamental ethical principles. It was helpful to understand what restrictions different religious groups imposed. Doctors and nurses needed to be taught so many different things: how to assemble the facts; how to work with a team; how to respond to relatives; how to deal with stress; how to cope with different experiences; to name but a few. Understanding the fundamentals gave them a yardstick by which to measure reactions and developments. As was pointed out, the 'bare bones' could be taught in the classroom, it was the 'art' which was acquired through actual experience.

Some advocated multidisciplinary sessions which gave them opportunity to explore different perspectives and learn together. A single education bite, however, was not sufficient. Doctors and nurses required on-going opportunities to explore these issues, building on experience and knowledge. The enormity of the task of educating a huge workforce was acknowledged. As has been shown, many advocated targeting specific groups like junior house officers who were experiencing death for the first time and often feeling guilty about their own performance, inadequacies and possible failures. Others suggested limiting these efforts to specialists in intensive care who are the most likely people to encounter situations presenting these dilemmas.

Perhaps to describe these sessions as 'formal' is misleading since respondents suggested a variety of ways to make these events lively, relevant and powerful. The use of videos, bringing in actors, role play, debates, and the use of novels, were all recommended although some staff shuddered at the idea of role play.

It was important that these sessions were led by the right people, respondents said. They had to be convincing and touch people's feelings. Various suggestions were made: clinical experts, chaplains, bereaved parents, members of the Stillbirth and Neonatal Death Society (SANDS). Some advocated a panel of people to put different points of view. Feelings as well as practical tips for management needed to be covered and it was probably more likely that a balance would be achieved if there was input from the different groups involved.

> 'We run a symposium on death in paediatrics ... which really kicks things off ... I think it's good because it actually just exposes them to some of the reality, because one of the things that happens is usually a parent ... who has actually lost a baby, comes and describes their parenting experience from pregnancy, from looking forward to the baby, through to the baby being born, what happened, the death, how they coped with things afterwards. And it's probably the most chilling thing that I've ever seen – the most touching thing that I've ever seen. And there's no doubt the students find it emotionally touching. And in that respect I think it's good to give them an emotionally touching experience because they're totally detached from that sort of thing otherwise until they start working but even that just opens their eyes to the fact that these things are emotionally touching and difficult. And again, I say, the real time for education for this – for me – is right from the point of graduation when people start practising. That's when they should be supervised and are not.' (Senior Registrar, more than 5 years experience)

Discussion around clinical cases

Actual examples of families grappling with these momentous decisions provided the best basis from which to teach, many respondents claimed. This could be in the Unit or in the classroom. The inexperienced could learn from their seniors in day-to-day practice. Many junior staff spoke highly of the example shown by certain consultants. Some things could only be learned by watching an expert in action. In one Unit certain experienced sisters were referred to as 'ace communicators' and juniors watched and learned as these older women went about their daily business.

Ongoing discussion around cases could include students. Debriefing meetings which rehearsed the events after the death could offer valuable insights to the whole team and help junior staff to learn how best to handle situations. One person suggested that since too many people, especially the inexperienced, could be intrusive, it might be better to explore some system which allowed spectators to observe what was actually going on in discussion with parents, without actually being in the room. He did concede, however, that there were serious ethical issues to be addressed in any such development.

Teaching specific skills

A substantial number of people wanted more attention and time given to teaching specific skills. Those instanced included communication, counselling, and bereavement work. Furthermore, doctors and nurses needed to understand themselves and their emotions in order to help others. Appreciating why they personally adopted the position they did in relation to the acceptability of certain impairments could help them to argue their case more persuasively but could also make them more open to persuasion. As part of this framework, some advocated fostering a different approach by emphasizing the positive side of disability. Modern techniques of antenatal diagnosis and the easy availability of abortion have produced a society which is less accepting of impairment than cultures such as the Irish. A considerable number of respondents had experience of life in countries with more restrictive abortion laws and commented on the potentially damaging effect of a mentality which expects perfection in its children as a right.

Approach to students

The overall approach of a medical school or nursing college to its students could influence personal development in the field of ethical issues, respondents felt. Some suggested a radical approach of selecting only those students who demonstrated the right qualities to make them sensitive and intuitive practitioners.

One doctor advocated that all medical students should first get some experience of life, perhaps undertaking a course in a different discipline altogether, in order to broaden their horizons and mature them before they undertook their medical training. He had himself taken this route and compared his own development favourably against those who had gone from school straight into studying medicine. Monitoring students' progress in the finer art of caring sensitively was suggested as a way forward but it was acknowledged that attempting to do so would pose substantial logistical and ethical problems.

Medical training is especially intense and respondents recognized that students tended to be selective about what they embarked on. If sessions on ethics were add-on extras they could safely be skipped without detriment to the final degree. However, in some Units staff spoke warmly of the lively and enterprising programmes they had helped to develop in their faculties or had themselves experienced which encouraged students to participate and which were thoroughly enjoyed and helpful. A few respondents suggested that if the subject was made examinable it would be more attractive and acquire an air of acceptability and importance.

As has already been mentioned one doctor advocated a change of emphasis for students. They should be taught to think for themselves rather than being encouraged just to cram large amounts of factual information into their heads. Developing an enquiring mind and addressing situations from a broad base would be a healthier approach than the present fragmented and compartmentalized programme which dwelt on specific systems, specialties or diseases almost in isolation.

> 'I have very radical views on medical education ... You can't teach everything to medical students. It's impossible – a) they're too young, b) they want to have a good time, c) they have a passing dipping interest in every conceivable piece of medical sub-specialty you can care to mention. And every specialist he comes across – all will say, "Oh yes, if only we could teach medical students this, everything would be fine." That's a load of hooey! So there's only one thing to do with medical students – I have a very simple prescription. If you can teach them to think, they will be able to turn their hands to anything.' (Consultant, more than 10 years experience)

It was considered healthy to have the opportunity to see what happened elsewhere in practice. Doctors tended to move around and this gave them a broader perspective on normal practice. But many nurses did not have such opportunities once they had settled into the specialty of neonatal care. Large numbers were not in a position to move because of domestic commitments. In one Unit, for financial reasons they said, staff midwives were not even able to go to another Unit to obtain their neonatal qualification. Elsewhere there were difficulties in staff attending courses and study days outside their own area. It was quite evident that many nurses had no concept of the range of opinions prevailing across the country about the management of these cases where treatment was being withdrawn. They themselves lamented their enforced insular ideas.

Some respondents advocated a mentoring system. This theoretically allows juniors to be guided by one or more named seniors, and offers greater opportunities for supervised practice. In some Units such systems were said technically to be in place but many respondents criticized them as paper exercises with problems of lack of time and confidentiality. They simply did not work in the pressures of a busy Unit with serious understaffing.

One area where the approach to students could be usefully improved was in relation to the expectations set. A number of respondents from both disciplines remarked on the attitude fostered that it was unprofessional for staff to show emotion. These were profoundly moving matters and it helped if staff felt that it was permissible to show that they were personally affected by the events.

> 'Grief modifies the way people react. I wish I'd been told that it's normal for doctors to show that they are upset and things like that. I don't mean screaming at the top of your voice but [showing that you hurt too]. And also to be allowed to show that you care without implying that you are not a professional, competent doctor. Caring just means that you are a human being as well as a doctor – not some machine – and that you have sensitivities as well.' (Senior Registrar, more than 10 years experience)

Similarly protecting junior staff from these difficult cases was to some extent counterproductive since inevitably as they became more senior there came a time when necessity forced them to handle such a situation. They were then left regretting their inexperience even though they were now considered senior enough to deal with it.

> 'Even up to now, I've still been very shielded when there is life and death decisions to be made. It's always the senior midwife or the nurse in charge that are involved on the ward rounds. But you get on with the rest of the work – somebody's got to do the rest of the work. But you never seem to be actually involved in it. They don't say, "Maybe it's time you learned how to cope with these situations". You're just left until one of these days it happens that you've just got to get on and cope with it.' (Staff Midwife, less than 5 years experience)

Written material

A small number of respondents looked for a better literature on this topic. This should elaborate on the actual experience of people going through the trauma of deciding whether or not to withdraw treatment. It would be helpful to read how individuals felt, what had persuaded them, and how they had dealt with the situation. There was scope for parents as well as professionals to provide useful insights in this forum. But if the information was written rather than verbal, more people could benefit from it, it could be controlled by the writer, and there was less threat of others infringing his or her privacy or sensitivities.

Practical opportunities

One of the difficulties nurses experienced was not seeing sufficient babies or parents after discharge from hospital to really know what consequences followed decisions in the nursery. Their judgements were therefore potentially skewed. Some felt they would be more knowledgeable if they saw for themselves the outcomes of various conditions, the impact on families of different impairments, and the longer term effects of treatments or management decisions. One medical respondent had had many years experience as a community paediatrician and this had clearly influenced his views on what was acceptable and where lines should be drawn. Senior medical staff who saw families repeatedly at child welfare clinics, and neonatal sisters who went out into the community to support families after babies went home, were also able to appreciate more clearly what families were grappling with. To a limited extent other staff could gain a certain amount of understanding by attending follow-up clinics but it was appreciated that families in a hospital clinic are not the same as families at home. Actually dealing with parents and babies on an longer term basis gave staff insights into the consequences of events in the nursery which those staff who never went beyond that point could not readily acquire. These were important factors not just in forming their own opinions, but in guiding and supporting parents through the trauma of deciding which way to go.

Opportunities to sit in on the deliberations of an ethics committee was one suggestion. This might help a junior person better to appreciate the essential issues.

A wide-ranging combination of possible ways of helping staff to be more prepared for these difficult situations and better able to deal with them when they arose, were thus suggested. A special plea was registered by the night staff who said they often felt left out of things. They wanted to be included in educational events. Parents still had to be supported at night: babies died during the unsocial hours as well as during the day, decisions had to be made at 3am just as they were at 3pm. Staff around the clock require skills and sensitivities to help parents and team members through these traumatic experiences.

Discussion

Over the years a developing awareness of the questions related to values and moral choices has been growing within both the nursing profession[229] and the medical.[202] But teaching these subjects has not kept pace with recommendations. It is generally thought that nurses get more teaching than doctors on ethical matters relating to their professional roles[230] but the nurses themselves clearly think that even their current provision is inadequate.

To some extent it is both artificial and difficult to sift out ethics from the multiplicity of other topics to be considered. And moreover some wisdom in these matters can only be acquired with experience of life as well as of professional practice. Although efforts have been made to spell out the requirements for educating professionals in the skills required for ethical decision making,[231] a more important component seems to be obtaining insight into one's own opinions, values and prejudices and developing a personal capacity to think for oneself.

Whilst recognizing the burden of factual information imposed on its medical students, the General Medical Council, nevertheless recommended that '[l]earning though curiosity, the exploration of knowledge, and the critical evaluation of evidence should be promoted and should ensure a capacity for self-education.'[202] It advised that the emphasis on the 'uncritical acquisition of facts' should be reduced and more attention given to matters such as communication skills and appropriate attitudes of mind and behaviour. One of the specific attributes which are listed as desirable in an independent practitioner is the 'ability to recognize and analyse ethical problems so as to enable patients, their families, society and the doctor to have proper regard to such problems in reaching decisions.' This general statement covers knowledge of the legal responsibilities and ethical standards of the medical profession, understanding of the impact of medico-social legislation on practice, and recognition of the influence of the individual's own personality and values.

A similar picture has emerged in nursing. It has been suggested that nurses' education is traditionally scientifically based and that nurses have difficulty thinking in the abstract.[232] But ethics is based on both individual and societal morals, beliefs and values, and abstract thinking is required to grapple with the ethical issues relating to decisions on behalf of patients. There is encouraging evidence, however, that at least in some fields, the acquisition of analytical skills and insight are increasingly being advocated,[227] and nurse education is moving towards a model which encourages individual thought and expression. It is necessary for the nurse to understand her own value system and the origin of her own prejudices and moral stances, in order to distinguish the values and beliefs of the family or of colleagues, from her own.

> 'Who am I? Why do I do what I do? These are the questions that nurses need to ask themselves – and answer – before they can effectively support patients with ethical decision making.'[232]

For both disciplines then, the emphasis lies in the capacity for abstract thinking, and gaining insight into individual beliefs and values. Values play a central role in ethical decision making. An individual's values are the result of

> 'culturally learned beliefs and individually formed attitudes. The cultural belief component tends to be static and enduring, whereas the attitude component is open to change and refinement on the basis of life experiences and education.'[233]

Thus while some basic values remain fixed, others are dynamic, evolving as experience, knowledge and circumstances alter one's viewpoint. Maturity demands a recognition that values are often not absolutes even though they are originally taught as such. A child may be taught to be honest at all times; an adult may recognize times when half truths or even white lies are morally more acceptable than blatant honesty. But while perhaps not immutable, values are personal and subjective standards which serve as criteria by which to judge the rightness or wrongness of an action. They serve as orientation in a complex world and without them personal judgements would be arbitrary or whimsical. Understanding one's own values is a prerequisite to comprehending other people's standpoint when it comes to decision making in neonatology.

Preparation of practitioners

It is clear that most doctors and nurses in NICUs believe that the soundest lessons are learned through the fire of real life experience. Indelible impressions are left by traumatic encounters with families facing choices which all lead to tragic outcomes. But often junior staff are excluded from these most difficult cases and it can take years to learn this way. Even being involved only gives an individual limited experience and insight since every case has unique elements and it is dangerous to extrapolate too much from the extreme examples.

However, whilst the refinements are a matter of sensitivity to individual circumstances which only develops with practice, people can be taught the basics about what to do, or what not to say or do. It is still the case that people commit the classic blunders, saying tactless things like 'You can always have another one', or 'You've still got your other children', but some respondents felt that such comments are probably attributable more to the speaker's own stress and sense of insecurity and inadequacy than to a basic insensitivity. Giving them better insight into the effect their words and behaviours can have on the people for whom they care, can strengthen their sense of self and help them to greater thoughtfulness. One consultant referred to this kind of developing sensitivity to these situations as the 'art of care' as opposed to the 'science' which relates to the harder side of medicine. An awareness of the therapeutic use of the self is a necessary part of learning the art of caring.

But such preparation in the fundamentals only takes a person so far. To adopt the analogy of driving used by one nurse respondent: being a learner, being taught by a qualified driver, reading the highway code, prepares one for the basics. But once in the driving seat there are all sorts of experiences which have to be encountered and judgements made that no book or other person can actually teach one how to cope with. It is a matter of having a firm grounding of the essentials but having the intelligence, quick wittedness and ability to respond to external cues in order to interpret a situation wisely and behave appropriately and spontaneously.

Neither is there any suggestion that proper preparation and training will turn these momentous experiences into painless ones. To some extent it is right that staff should feel uncertain and tense about these situations. Indeed as one consultant put it, 'A little bit of autonomic dysfunction for doctors is a good thing!' The important thing is dealing healthily with the stress and powerful emotions generated and moving on in understanding, sensitivity and compassion.

'Finding for yourself a way of channelling this anguish and distress. And don't stop it – feel it. And let [other] people feel it – don't stop it. Experience it but then let it go in a nice way, I think. And just use your own experience to find a way through easing the pain and the anxiety and the distress for the family, the baby, your colleagues, your nurses, yourself.' (Consultant, more than 25 years experience)

Methods of teaching

The evidence that teaching strategies actually increase sensitivity to ethical issues is scant but recommendations have been made for educators to employ imaginative means of teaching to aid thinking about these matters.[228,234-236] Respondents in this study suggested a wide range of initiatives which might promote greater understanding. One feature which appeared often as a criticism about the methods currently employed was that they were boring. This threat did nothing to encourage participation. By contrast those who had had sessions which encouraged lively and vigorous peer debate found their interest stimulated and they valued the enforced learning which resulted from being so directly challenged.

An intensely powerful learning medium is listening to parents who have been through these experiences, a phenomenon found in other areas of clinical practice.[227] To hear first hand about the feelings of those most intimately affected by these momentous decisions is to be profoundly moved. And when the emotions are touched powerful lessons are learned.

But opportunities for such experiences are necessarily limited and very careful controls have to be kept on these demands to avoid adding unnecessarily to the heavy burdens already carried by parents. A less intrusive way of allowing people to enter into the traumatic lives of others is through fiction. There is considerable anecdotal and evaluative evidence that a novel written by one of the present authors[237] is being widely used to good effect in the teaching of the issues around withdrawing treatment from a neonate. A work of fiction allows greater freedom than real life cases do and if the plot is sufficiently powerful the reader can enter into the thinking and emotions of the different characters and come to understand something of their reasoning and actions.

Coverage of the subject

Attempts have been made to identify the essential components which should be included in educational programmes. These are seen to be:

1. stimulation of the moral imagination through the clarification of values
2. recognition of ethical issues, emphasizing the cognitive strategies involved in ethical reasoning and decision making
3. elicitation of a sense of moral obligation to become actively involved
4. development of analytical skills
5. toleration of disagreement and ambiguity and development of ways of dealing with conflict.[235]

In addition the need for the incorporation of both theoretical and practical ethics in medical education has been strongly advocated.[238] From the literature it is plain that there is a very real difference between the two and this distinction is important in any attempt to equip practitioners with the skills they require to deal effectively and sensitively in clinical practice. Situations are rarely as straightforward at the cotside as they seem from the armchair or lecture theatre.

Conclusions

These are painful and crucial decisions. There is strong reason for preparing doctors and nurses for the responsibility they must shoulder. Giving them a framework of knowledge of the law, of the ethical principles involved, of physiology and the science of medicine, can take them only so far. They must also understand themselves and the origin of their own beliefs and values. They must appreciate and respect the differing values and positions of other people. Only then will they be in a position to synthesise the facts, and be able to move flexibly and sensitively through the emotions and conflicting thoughts surrounding these difficult real-life decisions in order to reach a wise solution. Teaching in this area should capitalize on the wide range of approaches which best foster these qualities.

CHAPTER FIFTEEN

Some Concluding Thoughts

Even today when so much is possible, medicine has its limitations. Moreover it is widely accepted that medical interventions which cannot benefit the infant are inhumane.

Although the increasing knowledge and skill of neonatologists and neonatal nurses has meant a fall in perinatal mortality, a new and increasing dilemma has resulted. The fundamental question has changed from 'Can we?' to 'Should we?' In consequence, a greater proportion of deaths now result from non-treatment decisions. These situations have exercised the minds of ethicists and philosophers, lawyers and theologians, sociologists and psychologists as well as doctors and nurses. And the debates continue around the use of terms and the distinctions which may be drawn.[239] But it is quite evident that there is a fundamental difference between those who never see a terminally ill baby and who never face the distress of parents, and those people who do: the essential difference between theoretical ethics and real life ethics. It is infinitely easier to perceive these things in black and white if one is far removed from the reality of human tragedy in all its diversity.

As we have seen, real life practice is dogged by uncertainty, ambivalences and exceptions. Nevertheless there is every reason to feel reassured. It is clear that these decisions are treated with the utmost seriousness. Doctors and nurses in NICUs are immensely caring people and their commitment to the babies and families in their care is impressive to witness. They too grieve profoundly when things go wrong. They agonize deeply over the decisions which have to be made. Sometimes the personal cost is very high indeed and it was sobering to share burdens carried unseen for years, only uncovered by the opportunity to disclose doubts and pain in the strict confidence of private interviews. These burdens are usually shelved as the staff move on with the work of supporting and caring for the continuous stream of families who enter the NICU.

The babies concerned

It is evident that staff working with neonates feel strongly that each life is very precious, irrespective of gestation or age. Even those staff who confess to no particular religious beliefs, describe a certain sense of reverence for human life. It is not something to be readily disposed of. Some societies and groups believe that a period of time exists before a child is accepted as a member of a society, when it is acceptable to treat them more as a fetus than as a baby, but no respondent in the present study reported such a belief. In the literature, opinion spans the full range from at one end, the idea that all hours of life are of equal worth and death is no more of a tragedy at one point than at another, and at the other end, the idea that shortening a life by lethal injection is a humane and acceptable solution to the intractable problems created by modern medicine. A substantial part of this diversity is shared by the NICU teams who participated in this enquiry. But essentially, whilst they value life as something sacred, nevertheless staff do perceive differences between babies. Less trauma is attached to withdrawing treatment from a baby at the edge of viability, than to doing the same thing with a full term infant, or a premature infant who has been in the Unit a long time and has established himself as a unique little individual.

There are essentially three groups of infants for whom treatment may not be the preferred option: the congenitally malformed, the extremely immature and those who have suffered catastrophic irreversible damage. In the minds of clinicians there appears to be a fundamental distinction between infants who are living even where there is severe impairment, and those who are dying. But a particularly distressing phenomenon results when the quality of that continuing life is perceived as potentially worse than death. The loss of a child through death is final but a 'living death' is far more difficult to adjust to.[4] Babies with severe birth asphyxia, or those with severe mental impairment, or extremely premature infants who have survived multiple complications but with chronic problems from irreversibly damaged systems, fall into this category. But defining the line which marks out these babies is fraught with difficulty since it is open to so much individual interpretation. Probably the most basic criteria relate to an ability to communicate, and to the suffering of the child since the possession of these capacities is what begins to distinguish 'being alive' from 'having a life.'[240] Beyond that, what counts as a benefit or a burden is a largely subjective assessment complicated by the very discrepant approaches of different disciplines and specialists as well as amongst individuals. There is bound to be a certain amount of untidiness in these matters since every case is unique. When the determination hinges on quality of life decisions, these tend to be located in the value of human life as it is expressed in certain characteristics such as the capacity to think, communicate or act autonomously; in self awareness, in rationality, in the capacity to relate to others, in the ability to experience pleasurable states of consciousness and so on. Inevitably there is room for many shades of opinion. But it is an awesome responsibility to decide on behalf of an infant who has no history or formulated preferences to guide the discussion.

Furthermore a very real problem in such cases is knowing when to call a halt. The window of opportunity is sometimes only briefly open. Delays can mean that when equipment is removed the child is able to sustain life unaided; there is no longer an opportunity to withdraw treatment in order to allow death to intervene. Short of active measures to end that life or simply not resuscitating in an emergency there is no viable alternative to continued existence.

But in spite of this individual element, certain general factors do emerge. A widespread feeling exists that treatment withdrawal should, if anything, be carried out more frequently and sooner than it currently is. Ventilating and resuscitating 'anything and everything' as one respondent put it, is seen as a recipe for disaster. In the minds of clinicians, there is clearly a difference between not starting to treat and withdrawing treatment. And they do distinguish between killing and allowing to die, even though

ophical discriminations often appear to elude them. Intentions, opportunities,
ence between acts and omissions, and accepted practice are all open to
tion.[241] But whilst philosophers may well conclude that there is no moral
to be made, clinicians hold to a strong emotional difference. Although they
recognize the extremely difficult position in relation to those babies whose continuing
lives represent a fate worse than death, nevertheless the slippery slope remains a
source of real anxiety. It is easy to sympathize with their misgivings, and yet it could
be argued that in life we frequently make judgements about which slippery slopes we
will attempt to negotiate and which we will avoid. As long as our purpose is clear and
we know the limits of what we will allow, and provided we exercise proper control
and judgement, there is no reason to fear slippery slopes.[242]

What exactly constitutes euthanasia, however, remains a thorny question. Giving large
doses of analgesia, using paralysing agents for infants when ventilation is being
discontinued, and discontinuing feeding are all practices which raise doubts about the
legality and morality of what is done in the name of compassion, and challenge the
views of both society and the professionals.[243] But whilst most clinicians reject the
principle of changes to the law which would legalize euthanasia, when it comes to the
intractable problems in the nursery, they begin to doubt the value of a rigid opposition
to active measures to end lives which are not better than death.

The decision

Nowadays many decisions are made long before a baby presents in the NICU. Prenatal
deliberations between obstetricians and paediatricians in consultation with parents
tend to eliminate the necessity for more difficult choices after birth.

Once the babies are born, if decisions have to be made about which should be treated
and which not, there are no easy answers. Doctors are acting in what has been described
as 'an uncertain legal ambience',[143] and the risk of prosecution, though theoretically
small, is not the easiest companion for those at the sharp end of decision making,
required to combine compassion with science. Introducing new legislation to offer
greater security is fraught with complexities. It would need to be sufficiently clearly
defined as to be unambivalent in its meaning, whilst at the same time being sufficiently
flexible to take account of the fine nuances of individual circumstances and sufficiently
enabling to permit humane judgements to be made. It is apparent that there is little
support for a change in the law in Scotland since doctors feel that in general the courts
are in sympathy with their efforts. Rather would practitioners welcome guidelines
which offer an authoritative framework by which clinicians might measure their own
practice and through which they might defend their actions as those which reasonable
and competent colleagues would probably have adopted in similar circumstances.

The difficulty of setting arbitrary limits has been clearly recognized over the years.
There are many aspects of neonatology which engender powerful negative emotions,
but they in themselves should not be allowed to influence the decision to discontinue
treatment. Staff or parental despair, the 'ravages of chronic neonatal morbidity' reflected
in a baby's appearance, parental rejection – these are not adequate reasons for

withdrawal of life support.[244] Instead the concerns should be the extent of the baby's suffering, his chances of survival and the anticipated long term outcome. But so much uncertainty attaches to any assessment of long term prognosis that caution is inevitable and indeed desirable.

Acting in the best interests of the baby is an onerous responsibility but staff are rarely given an opportunity to gain insight into the multiplicity of factors which may be influencing them. This report has explored many of these factors. But ethical positions are not constant and static. Both personal and professional experiences exert profound influence and to some extent staff need repeatedly to revisit these issues if they are to remain insightful. Chiswick[244] recognized the potential for bias for doctors and advised paediatricians to analyse carefully their own motivations in order to recognize deceptive signals before suggesting treatment withdrawal. He suggested four questions to aid circumspection:

- Am I being driven by despair?
- Am I being unduly influenced by the external appearance of the baby?
- Would I think differently if the parents had been beside the cot every day?
- Are my predictions about outcome based on current scientific knowledge?

These questions could be equally applicable for nurses in considering their own positions.

The influence of resources on these decisions is a matter which concerns many. Most believe that the time has not yet come when lives are lost because the money is not there to provide the essential life-saving care, although shortages of staff necessarily limit the quality of the service provided. But some staff fear that the advent of Trust status and political pressures are bringing such a day closer. They recognize the difficulty of defending the use of huge sums of money on infants with an uncertain or objectively poor prognosis. It might well become increasingly difficult to allow 'softer', less quantifiable elements to influence choices, and some aspects of parental inclination and choice might become hard to uphold if quantitative parameters indicate that the child's future will be fraught with problems with massive financial implications.

The process

For the most part there is little dissent within teams about the decision itself, although isolated cases do crop up where a consultant apparently arbitrarily withdraws treatment from an infant leaving other staff dismayed and questioning. But there is room for improvement when it comes to the management of these difficult cases. Four issues particularly are singled out for closer scrutiny. Two relate to the decision and its implementation: the timing of events and the actual mechanics of the dying. Two relate to the team: involvement of the consultant and of the other team members, and communication.

The timing of events

As we have seen time and again in this report, the timing of events represents a major cause of tension and anxiety. Pacing things in line with the needs and wishes of the different players in this painful drama is fraught with perils since their understanding, emotional acceptance of the facts, and perceptions of roles differ greatly both in substance and in quality.

There is a sense in which these things are best managed at a fairly intuitive level. Patiently waiting until the bleak facts become apparent to all, gradually building up a picture of the hopelessness of this prognosis would seem to be a gentler and kinder approach than hitting people bluntly with the stark reality. They are more likely to accept the inevitability of the death if they have seen for themselves that things are deteriorating or at least not improving. But sometimes it is not possible to orchestrate things so sensitively, and at other times there is a price to be paid for the slow approach.

Babies are not predictable. On occasion they deteriorate rapidly and unexpectedly. Sometimes they collapse suddenly and die before there is opportunity to prepare the parents fully, even though there may have been some discussion about the wisdom of continued treatment. Staff worry at such times about whether parents will think something has been done to precipitate the death. They are intense in their desire to make the end a meaningful experience for the parents and a time of loving and comfort for the baby. Indeed sometimes they err on the side of resuscitating extremely aggressively to prolong a flickering life long enough to allow parents to get to the cotside and be present for the death itself. At other times, however, babies appear to be kept alive to avoid unpleasant publicity or to make the timing of the death more opportune. A few respondents spoke of deaths being postponed to keep the press from asking difficult questions; others commented that particular nurses sometimes grow so attached to babies they insist resuscitation continues while they are on duty.

Although many people referred to the necessity to take time over the decision to be sure it is as right as it can be for all concerned, there is sometimes a price to be paid for delays. Waiting for parents to feel the time is right can involve prolonged suffering for the baby himself. In extreme cases the delays can result in the child going on living but now with severe and irreparable damage, placing an even greater burden on the parents.

> 'I actually feel more often we should be withholding treatment from the start. Once you get started into treatment it can become almost impossible to stop. And by the time the parents realize how badly wrong things are going, you can be at a stage where withdrawing treatment might not actually result in the death of a very sick child, but merely in increasing problems, which will result in even further impairment in its future life.' (SHO, less than 1 year experience)

In general as we have seen, the nurses are more ready to withdraw treatment sooner than the consultants. The reasons for these differences relate principally to the respective curing and caring roles of the two disciplines and the locus of control in relation to the ultimate responsibility. Understanding these factors and gaining insight into the perceptions of other team members could go far towards removing this issue as a source of conflict.

The mechanics of the dying

Peculiar tensions surround the implementation of a decision to withdraw treatment. Whether it is because of the difficulty of providing privacy for the family or of deciding the means by which a severely birth asphyxiated baby will die, feelings run high. Staff are all too aware that parents pass this way only once. It is vital to get it right. Organizational and administrative constraints – insufficient staff, inadequate space, shift patterns – which limit the quality of the service they can provide frustrate them. But these things while sources of stress, are largely outside their control and do not hold a personal element of inadequacy even though the staff lament the effects on their opportunity to care well. More stressful are the factors which affect their caring more directly. Inflicting pain on dying infants, participating in starving a baby to death, concealing vital information from a parent – these are practices which compromise staff. In their aim to care well for terminally ill infants and their families, they are enormously distressed by any requirement which detracts from their capacity to provide comfort for the baby and support for the parents.

Involvement of the team

Two main features emerge from this study in relation to team effort. The consultant needs to be actively and closely involved throughout and the other team members need to have a role in both the decision making and the care and support of the baby and his family.

The consultant is clearly seen by all as the linchpin in these tragic cases. The whole wellbeing of the team, as well as of the family, hinges on his sensitivity. Unless he is actively participating in the case, staff believe he cannot know how to pace things, how to communicate well, how to manage developments wisely. He in turn depends on others for insight into various aspects of the decision making. Unless he is involved he will not be in a position to see and hear and feel the understanding which others can contribute. And the junior staff will be reluctant to feed him information if they do not perceive him to be engaged with this case.

But he is part of a team and there is a strong feeling that this should be a team effort. Whether it is a junior doctor who has been up all night and all weekend struggling to save this baby, or a nurse who has built up a relationship with the family, other people have an investment in this child. They too have an opinion about what ought to be decided. Nurses especially occupy a special place in the team. Their close involvement with the baby and the family gives them unique insights. But their emotional attachment makes them vulnerable to peculiar tensions when they are faced with the consequences of such decision making. It is hard enough to deal with the raw emotions of parents if they have been involved in the discussion and believe the course chosen is the right one. But if they have had no part in the decision itself, or worse still, disagree with it, the conflicts are strong indeed.

It is not to be wondered at that teams are sometimes less than harmonious. The team is made up of individuals each with his or her own strengths and weaknesses. Some are more robust than others. Some have special sensitivities where these life and death decisions are concerned. Most NICUs suffer from shortages of staff. They are consequently working under severe pressure much of the time. This produces tensions and irritability in itself. In a high powered environment there are always such tensions. When it comes to neonatology there are additional particular problems in recruiting and retaining staff of the right calibre, although some enlightened paediatricians have considered specific ways of enhancing and integrating the medical and nursing roles to offer more inducement to people to commit to this specialty.[245,246]

Working under these conditions tends to exacerbate underlying differences but it is important not to confuse the issues. It has often been argued that the inherent difficulties relate to gender and to conflict between the two disciplines: men and women have fundamentally different and incompatible moralities. These ideas stem largely from the work of Gilligan[166] who observed that the female approach to morality differs from that of the male. In the women's perspective, caring within personal relationships is given moral primacy, whereas respect for autonomy and justice tend to be the predominant moral concerns of men. Given the female dominance in nursing – and especially neonatal nursing – this is potentially a relevant consideration in NICUs. However, whilst much has been written on this subject, much has been misinterpreted. For Gilligan also points out that these differences are to be found in the starting perspectives of males and females and during the developmental process, but as they mature both men and women come to appreciate the importance of both perspectives. Thus with maturity comes a convergence of judgements. Neither is it relevant to equate these different perspectives with the fundamental differences between doctors and nurses. Apart from any other consideration large numbers of doctors are female. Furthermore, medicine has inculcated a sense of nurturing for the sick into its medical ethics teaching and there is eloquent testimony to the enhancement of medicine by the inclusion of emotions,[247] and nursing also concerns itself with issues of justice and respect for autonomy,[230] so these demarcations are mistaken. Far from being incompatible, these approaches are simply 'different voices'[166] all with an important contribution to make and complementary to each other.

But being tolerant of greyness and uncertainty is harder for some than for others. And such characteristics are to be found in abundance in ethical dilemmas. A rigid personality or someone who is personally very unsure of their ideas may crave the security of set policies. Lack of experience may limit knowledge of the possible options. It is vital that such people have the opportunity to benefit from wide consultation so that they are aware of the extent of the choices in general and the wisdom of this particular choice.

Powerful emotions are involved in these tragic choices but feelings, no matter how painful, should not become obstacles to good decision making. The emotional pain should be recognized but should be seen in its proper place – as a reminder of the human tragedy involved, part of the struggle with so many conflicting issues. Indeed an absence of strong emotion is a more worrying state of affairs than its existence.

These are profound decisions and the agony which accompanies such deliberations is part of the experience of making the best choice when all options carry a burden of exquisite pain and sorrow.

For ethical dilemmas,

> 'are truly difficult to resolve. They are likely to elicit doubt, anxiety and discomfort in the decision makers. This is a healthy sign. It is important to experience a certain amount of uncertainty and uneasiness when facing these decisions. To fail to do so might well be a sign of moral indifference or of self-protection. Decision makers need to be sure they have given careful consideration to all sides of the dilemma, have left "no stone unturned", and have struggled with the agonizing feeling that tough choices elicit.'[21]

Some staff encounter these difficult situations infrequently. They sometimes worry that they are too inexperienced to perfect their handling of them. Others have to deal with the pain more often. Frequent encounters with death, ethical dilemmas, poor support and staff shortages can lead to disillusionment and discouragement, with staff finding it difficult to maintain the clarity of thinking required for sound moral reasoning. Where their conflicts of conscience go unresolved or unnoticed they may well distance themselves from these situations and concentrate on the more mechanical tasks of neonatal care. It is important for senior staff to be vigilant for the effects of this kind of demoralization.

Communication

It is imperative that those involved in this process communicate effectively. More will be said later about this key issue but part of its effectiveness hinges on conveying appropriate messages. Decision making must be based on sound ethical principles, careful thought and reflection and not rely on intuition or pragmatic considerations alone. But ethical choices do not take place in a vacuum. Simply reflecting on one's own position is not enough. Others are involved and each participant has to be open to the ideas of others. It is possible to be 'locked in' to a certain option which has appeared the most appropriate choice and to be blind and deaf to other equally morally legitimate perspectives. Values, motivations, prejudices, emotions, as well as different levels of understanding and knowledge, all play a part in bringing individuals to a certain conclusion. Decision makers have not only to be conversant with their own values and beliefs but also receptive to and understanding of those of others. Only in this way will they make wise choices in individual cases. Although certain basic principles will apply universally, every case has its unique features and must be assessed on its own merits so there are no short cuts. The issues must be thoroughly thought through and discussed openly every time.

The success of this sharing of information depends in large measure on the qualities of each individual involved. A person with integrity uses existing rules, available theory and his or her own life experience together to make rational choices which can be carefully justified.[248] Indeed, having integrity involves integrating experience, virtues and moral rules.[249] When it comes to decision making, then, both nurses and doctors need to foster the skills of logical argument if they are to preserve their integrity. It is not enough simply to go with gut intuition or stick slavishly to theoretical principles. There must be an interweaving of all three aspects.

It is interesting to note that traditional bioethical principles are rarely invoked in practice in real life situations.[240] But given the vast scope for variation it is not surprising that attempts have been made to draw up decision models to guide practitioners.[250–252] As we have seen there are no commonly accepted tools and, as a result of this present in-depth enquiry, we are of the opinion that such frameworks are of limited value except in as much as they provide a pattern for thinking which ensures important elements are not ignored. Too rigid an application can turn them into straightjackets, limiting options. Such is the endless diversity of real life that it is impossible to capture all its complexity in one tool.

> 'We have no master key that will fit all cases [of moral decision]. The truth to which eyes and hearts are too fatally sealed [is] that moral judgements remain false and hollow unless they are checked and enlightened by a perpetual reference to the special circumstances that mark the individual lot [and] are informed by growing insight and sympathy.'[253]

There is more to these difficult decisions than simply a rational ticking of points on a checklist. Hearts as well as brains are involved. The decision makers themselves have an effect on each other. Human sympathy and understanding, common sense and compassion enter into the equation. Staff need to be flexible and accept some fluidity in these matters. It is neither possible nor desirable to have everything too buttoned up.

> 'The question of overtreatment of seriously compromised neonates with life prolonging hardware is, in the end, a weighing of values – a moral judgement. The most pressing issues of our time, it has been said, are not matters of engineering, but of human values.'[22]

And these values are changing constructs which vary between people and over time for a given individual. The experienced neonatologist, Silverman, found that as his social experience grew so did his moral ambiguity,[22] and many of the respondents in this present study could trace an emerging wisdom which had come with years of experience of human tragedy. Flexibility and sensitivity to individual matters are required and characterize a wise practitioner. Silverman summed it up with the words of Theognis of Megara, a Greek poet of the 6th century BC: 'Wisdom is supple, folly keeps to a groove.'

Influences on the staff

Most staff have experience of death in other specialties but they find that the death of a baby is a very different matter from that of an adult. Decision making is also different since adults have some past history and often expressed preferences to guide us. Neonates have none.

To some extent, all life's experiences potentially influence the decisions taken. But importantly they also impinge on the way those individuals manage these difficult situations, giving them more or less sensitivity. Many can trace a growing tolerance and understanding and this is especially apparent in those who enter neonatology with rigid religious stances of their own. They are often forced to work out an ethic of their own which takes account of the difficult situations which challenge fixed tenets. Many staff can trace a gradual change in where they draw their own lines. Those who come in with a rather naive belief that immature infants die can be so impressed by what is possible that they become convinced that everything should be attempted for all infants. Those who arrive with a picture gleaned from the media of miracle babies and cures can be sobered by the reality of modern iatrogenic problems and become much more cautious about the wisdom of treatment in certain circumstances. It is important to unpack the origins of each position as well as current thinking.

Another potential bias arises where staff do not see the effect of what they do. Remaining in the confines of the rarified NICU creates an artificial world. Staff need to be aware of the consequences of their decisions; not just the little they may glean from an occasional visit by the parent to the Unit, or even in the follow-up clinic where parents often sanitise their information. The guilt borne by families who decided their infant should die, the corrosive sorrow of coping with a severely impaired child – these are burdens which need to be experienced in all their rawness to be fully acknowledged. It is salutary for NICU staff to see at least an occasional glimpse of these realities if they are to increase in understanding.

Of course, experience does not always bring increasing wisdom and it is noteworthy that individuals' perceptions of their own skills and sensitivity were not always accurate. It is also the case that years in the service do not always reflect increase in exposure to these difficult decisions. Some very junior staff have dealt with many such cases; some long service staff have experienced very few. Information gleaned during fieldwork suggests that to some extent certain individuals are screened out. To a degree consultants can select those they wish to be involved and some do so. Senior nurses can manipulate staffing so that the nurses they want to be with a certain baby take responsibility for that room. And a few nurses determine the extent of their own involvement by volunteering for participation or absenting themselves by various means. It is certainly the case that those with deep religious scruples about the sanctity of human life are often excluded from these difficult decisions. But the external evidence seems to suggest that some at least of these nurses manage to co-exist harmoniously beside their colleagues who take an extra share of the burden.

Parents of infants who die in the NICU often have few memories and few people with whom they shared those experiences. Staff therefore occupy a significant place in their remembering.

The health care team intimately involved in the human experience of these families to some extent enter into the subjectivity of the situations. There is a poignant sort of agony in making these hard choices when one is so closely involved. But it is this very pain which offers a unique form of protection which cannot be conferred by any other group of people.

The experience is different for the two disciplines. While doctors tend to spend only short periods of time with the parents, nurses' exposure is long and intense. Doctors have other tasks to help them to keep things in perspective, nurses are usually employed to look after one or two such babies. In a sense there is more to gain and less to lose for nurses in these situations than for doctors. Being unable to save a child represents a kind of failure to many doctors who see their main role as one of curing. Once treatment has been embarked on, withdrawal becomes a very different concept from withholding from the outset. They have entered 'the vicious circle of commitment.'[45] And doctors do not find it easy to resist the impulse to rescue a patient in a crisis. But the responsibility of the nurses is to care and this they can do until the very end of a child's life, and can continue to do for the parents even beyond that point. Many gain great personal satisfaction in helping to orchestrate a 'good dying'. It is important to emphasize however, that this is not to imply that doctors do not care. They do, but emphasis in medical training is laid on therapeutic approaches to prolonging life, and it becomes difficult then to let the patient go, even though sometimes death is perceived as a greater good for the patient than prolonged existence.[249] No one doubts the value of intensive care. But used indiscriminately it can be unnecessary – because the same end could be achieved by simpler means; unsuccessful – because the condition is beyond influence; unsafe – because the risks outweigh the probable benefits; unkind – because the subsequent quality of life is unacceptable; and unwise – because resources are diverted from more beneficial activities.[45] It is important to counter the therapeutic imperative with this awareness.

It is now accepted that some staff will be upset when a baby suffers and dies. Indeed it seems to be the case that measures are sometimes adopted not so much for the sake of the baby's suffering but because of the staff's own discomfort with that suffering. But men and women in Western societies tend to grieve in different ways.[192] Women often will talk, cry, and endlessly rehearse the events. Men are more likely to wish to put the painful memories behind them and get on with present activities, not talking about the pain or their own emotions. These differences were seen amongst the respondents in this study, although many interpreted them as doctor-nurse differences rather than related to gender. The fact that the male respondents as well as the females shared their deep emotions at interview was a tribute to their generosity, although no men wept with the disclosures whilst many women did.

In the past doctors were taught to see beyond the patient, as a person, to the disease,[170] but in recent years, a more humanistic approach has gained acceptance which teaches students to value the experience of the patient him or herself. Clearly there is a balance to be struck. There are real dangers in becoming too intimately involved in the lives of patients; both psychological and practical complications can be a consequence of a lack of appropriate detachment. Doctors and nurses have to learn to deal with the emotional side of caring, to develop affective as well as cognitive skills, and to foster an attitude of 'detached concern.'[254] Success in this area can be expensive, however, because 'the skills utilized on the ward are not shed as easily as a white coat.'[170] In learning to protect themselves to some extent, at least from the pain and suffering in their working environments, they can become inured to the emotions of those encountered in their social lives. This is a well recognized phenomenon. Chekhov, himself a doctor, wove into his plays tales of doctors' struggles to remain connected to life and the temptation to distance themselves to protect their vulnerability. In a sense there is a 'professional self' and a 'personal self' – getting the balance between the two is a complex process which evolves and changes over time and with different situations.

But whilst open displays of emotion are more accepted than they used to be, it is clearly important to keep a balance in another way also. If parents witness such expressions of sadness, they can be comforted by the fact that their infant was loved and valued. As two mothers whose children died wrote:

'There was also the student nurse who cried with me when (my baby) was brought back for me to see next morning ... I don't know her name, but she gives me some of my most powerful, comforting memories. When no one else has seen your baby except your husband, yourself, and the medical staff, you need those people to react and share in the mourning. It is a further proof of his existence which you desperately need, and it can help to diminish your sense of feeling ridiculous.'[255]

'For families like ours the health professional's role is of the utmost importance. Their relationship with us needs to be empathic unless it is to be destructive. Their natural sense of impotency in such a situation must be overcome to form a positive, guiding, caring friendship, even at cost to their emotions. Sharing emotion is showing you *really* care. Being alongside should supersede any feeling of clinical failure. Therapeutic medicine may be just for the living, but the dying and their families are still in life and need just as much lovingly given expertise.'[256]

But a number of staff have found a danger in this sharing. For parents can also be left feeling that the child was the staff's baby rather than theirs. Mothers especially often already feel frustrated: their parental role has few outlets. For a variety of reasons they can sometimes find it difficult to feel strong attachment to this infant.[209] In most cases their right to grieve should take precedence and staff need to be aware of the dangers inherent in this situation.

'Something that I was once told, that really hit me hard and shocked me – it was a friend of a friend, and this was years ago, and she's got two normal children now, who are well on in their teens. But prior to that she had a neonatal death ... We were out one night – the three of us went out together, and she just happened to say, "Where do you work?" And [when I told her] the Special Care Baby Unit [she said,] "Oh I hate you!" "Thanks very much!" "No, not you personally, but I just don't like those places," she says, "I had a baby that died in a Unit and I feel guilty because I never grieved for that baby – because when he died the staff were so upset I never thought of him as my baby. He was theirs. They were so upset and I was the one that had to say, "There now, it's all right. He's better off. You've done all you could." *She* is feeling guilty because they never grieved. And that really hit hard. And I thought, "Are we really that harsh that we have to be supported by parents, parents are not supported by us?" And that left a very profound mark on my brain.' (Senior Sister, more than 20 years experience)

The parents' needs

The ultimate decisions about life and death are not simply medical decisions, they are ethical decisions too and the responsibility for assessment and consideration of the relevant values must be shared by the parents. Professionals may well err on the side of preserving life but it has to be remembered that they are not the ones to bear the burden of survival. It is clear that this burden is very great.[30,203,205] A parent could well ask the paediatrician advocating treatment, 'Where will you be when the child screams inconsolably for five hours through the night? Where will you be when he throws tantrums in the middle of a social event? Where will you be when he is forty and I am seventy and his nappy still needs changing?'

> 'A doctor cannot be obliged to act contrary to his or her own conscience but equally doctors should bear in mind that relatives also have consciences, and should not be forced to accept for their loved ones treatment that they consider to be unethical.'[161]

Most doctors do appear to recognize this fact. Indeed some commented about the awe they felt contemplating the resilience and stamina of parents whom they have known. One very experienced respondent used the analogy of mountain climbing to explain the challenge of having children who are seriously impaired.

> 'Well I never knew what awesome was really. People who climb Mount Everest have an awesome job on hand – but they do it because they *want* to do it. And there are people who come out in the press – I had a cutting of a lady in X holding a very handicapped boy well into his teens. And ... the headline was, "Don't let handicapped die," ... and I thought "There's someone who has climbed Mount Everest." ... I know that there *are* people who have an Everest ... Now whether they grow to that, attempt to climb Mount Everest after many many hills, or whether they have an issue in life which most of us wouldn't want [to cope with], I just wonder whether there are people who actually prepare themselves for that in some subtle, unknown but important way.' (Consultant, more than 20 years experience)

Often staff are aware of the conflict between parents' interests and the baby's, but there comes a point at which the parents' needs become paramount. While there is a chance of life for the baby, his interests come first. But when there is nothing more that can be done for him, many staff believe that parents' needs assume a greater importance. There is then a pressing need to make this as good an experience as it can be. To a large extent only the parents can say what they need. But staff participating in this enquiry provided a picture of what they thought parents wanted in order to help them to come to an appropriate decision and to cope with the dying.

Understanding

The point was well made by a few respondents that it is often easier for parents to acknowledge the problem if they can see it. If the child has a visible physical impairment, they can recognize that there is a need to make decisions on his behalf. If the problem is an invisible one, particularly if it involves probable mental impairment, they have to go by what they are told, most often without the benefit of personal experience of other babies in similar circumstances to guide them. Gaining understanding of the facts and the possible outcomes is difficult for the uninitiated. Staff need patience and perseverance to go over the information repeatedly, interpreting not only medical knowledge but parental cues.

Involvement

Having a baby in an incubator wired up to a battery of instruments and machines can frustrate the best endeavours of parents to be involved in their infant's care. They are often terrified that they will inadvertently harm him.[209] But it has been found that parents who have the opportunity to care for their terminally ill baby at home have a more positive and happier experience than those whose whole experience is in hospital.[257] Some Units have indeed attempted to transfer babies home to have intensive care withdrawn in the familiar security of the parents' own territory.[258] Being involved can give both present satisfaction and longer term memories. Within the constraints of the Unit environment, staff try to provide opportunities for parental involvement and it is clear from their stories that they are variously sensitive to needs. Small developments can make large impressions. It came as a surprise to one nurse that bathing a dead baby was the first 'normal' contact a particular mother had with her child, and she instantly regretted all the occasions when she had unthinkingly bathed other dead infants herself. A doctor made it a practice to let parents listen to their baby's heart beat before the child died once it had been brought to his attention that this created a precious and abiding memory for parents.

Communication

The breadth of what good communication involves was captured by one mother who, after a series of obstetric disasters, summed up what she looked for in her medical adviser:

> 'My consultant was wonderful, a knight in shining armour. He was an excellent communicator, and to me he communicated trust in his judgement and skill, reassurance, and a sense of partnership. His listening skills were excellent, and my fears (and probably neuroses) were never ridiculed. Everything was explained to me that I could possibly want explained, and I was always treated with dignity and respect. It helped more than anything could have done. I never felt that anything was happening to me that I could not control with him – very important in view of the lack of control and powerlessness that I experienced at the end of my first two pregnancies.'[255]

But this is a difficult goal to reach. More than one respondent echoed the misgivings of Stahlman[217,259] about the adequacy of communication with parents. Many have first hand experience of incomprehensible language being used, of conflicting information being supplied, of staff giving ambiguous messages through non-verbal cues. The right words might technically have been said but there is a real danger that they are heard selectively or interpreted by wishful thinking. They worry too that in a way they collude with the ideas promoted by the media which encourages parents to believe in miracles. Very few clinicians actually tell parents bluntly about the realities of the limits of what they can achieve, but many lament the impossible expectations they have helped to foster.

The way parents are given bad news remains with them so there is a real need for staff to pay careful attention to the way they communicate.

> 'You will never forget the words. For as long as you live, through the sad times and the happy times, those words will always come back to you. Those first words the doctor spoke to you, telling you there was a problem with your child. The way you accept and the way you begin to deal with the situation starts with those first words you hear.'[260]

And since a baby's life or death, his comfort and wellbeing, hang in the balance there is every reason to be diligent in seeking to improve the way parents are informed.

Information

Exactly what they are told, however, will depend on what cues a doctor or a nurse picks up from the parents' own behaviours and words. It is clear that they do tailor their information according to their own perceptions of the parents' knowledge, understanding and capacity to cope. Research has shown, however, that parents value direct and early information.[167,168,209] Sometimes, of course, situations change, and doctors are reluctant to divulge information prematurely which will raise doubts and fears in parents' minds if there is still a possibility that their own misgivings may be proved wrong. Doctors indeed sometimes regret nurses' compulsion to give parents all the information available. Nurses on the other hand feel compromised if they are in possession of grave news while parents are kept in ignorance for the time being. Trust is undermined. The hurt parents can show when they subsequently learn of the deception is in turn wounding for the nurses.

There is some evidence that to understand what the health care team are thinking does help families, and advance warning helps them to prepare themselves.[167,168] If they are kept so advised of developments, trust in the staff is enhanced. Some practising neonatologists, however, have cautioned against too open a sharing of medical thinking since early suggestions of brain involvement, for example, may be quickly ruled out by the health care team but may never be forgotten by the parents and indeed may affect how they react to and treat the child for years subsequently.[209,261]

Brewin has discussed sensitively the balance of information, truth and trust which should characterize the behaviour of doctors with patients.[262] Much has been said of paternalism and yet in a great many occupations trust that the expert will do the best job he can underpins contracts and professional responsibility. Most of us do not tell a car mechanic how to fix a leaking manifold on our ancient Rover; or an airline pilot how to get to Tasmania. And only a very insensitive person would adopt the position that what is right for one person must be right for another. Part of the skill of dealing empathically with families lies in assessing how much they can deal with and how much at various points in an experience they need protection from the full panoply of grim possibilities. As Brewin has argued, truth can sometimes create havoc. Unhelpful rhetoric about undermining autonomy is counterproductive. What is needed is better communication based on real understanding of a family's needs, fears and hopes. Then those who require to be told all the possibilities will get them, those who prefer to leave the secret worrying to the medical experts will be given this protection. Slavishly to apply blanket principles is to deny the reality of human variation. Common sense and compassion should soften rigid ideals.

Caring

As with adult patients in ICU,[167] so in NICUs, families greatly value small caring gestures and simple expressions of compassion and support. Distancing behaviours further isolate families already set apart from others in their grief and bewilderment.

Time

Parents have to understand the circumstances of their baby's condition, both intellectually and emotionally. They are often found to be some days behind the professional team in acceptance of the reality where the outlook is bleak. Some consultants deliberately refrain from informing parents about a poor prognosis until there is sufficient clear evidence for the parents to see for themselves that the child is deteriorating. They are then thought to be better prepared for and more receptive of bad news and thus more able to enter into meaningful discussions around which treatment option to pursue. King attributed the delays in parental acceptance of the situation in part to their failure to understand the *meaning* behind the information they were given.[150] She felt they were either not told or simply did not know how to ask for this enlightenment. But she was observing American practice. In the present study, the nurses believed that they filled this gap by ensuring the parents had opportunity to hear again and again what the situation was and to question them endlessly and repeatedly until the meaning did impinge on their understanding.

But in order to try to bridge this potential gap, a transparency model has been advocated.[150,263] In essence this technique makes the doctor's reasoning and current thinking transparent to the parents. That is not to say that all details are divulged immediately and indiscriminately. The process may well take time and occur over several encounters. But in this way the *meaning* of factual information is better understood.

However, the value of the time for parents to adjust and reflect must be weighed against the costs to the child, in terms of prolonged suffering, and to the service, in terms of the implications of continued resuscitating and treating infants with poor prognoses.[264] This does not mean that resources should influence the direction of the decision. There is a powerful argument to be made for keeping these decisions firmly in the domain of parents and their medical advisors. If outside agents were to take control, the risk of slipping along the moral slippery slope, and of too rigid an application of blanket policies could be great. For while the damage which may be done by a parent remains on a small scale, the State could do harm on a large scale. Nevertheless the cost of continuing futile treatment cannot be ignored.

Sometimes, in spite of the staff's best endeavours, parents continue to resist medical advice. Time and patience do not appear to bring understanding or acceptance. Those who baulk tend to be the articulate professional parents with high expectations for their children. They often leave an indelible impression on the staff involved and many negative feelings. But it is worth remembering that sometimes such aggressive and domineering parents are, below the surface, extremely frightened and disappointed people. And it is all too easy for staff to forget what a forbidding place the NICU can be.

The most difficult group to deal with are those with immovable religious scruples. No amount of time will influence some of them to see the baby's best interests in the way the staff do. This results in deep distress for all concerned, especially if the baby is suffering as a direct consequence of the delays in decision making. Staff, as well as parents, need on-going support and care to deal with these intractable cases sensitively and wisely. Involving outside agents can sometimes help but at other times merely inflames the situation and great care needs to be exercised.

The team

The conventional answer to the question, 'Who decides?' is: The parents and the medical team. But doctors, nurses and parents may assign different weightings to each of the moral values and contributory factors. Each may well arrive at a slightly different conclusion. All these end points may be morally defensible but they may be incompatible one with another. Much work has to be done to understand each other's position and to work towards a solution or at least an acceptable compromise.

In reality both health care professionals and parents often seek additional guidance. The doctors consult with their colleagues, outside specialists and sometimes even legal advisers. The parents talk to relatives, friends, social workers, ministers and other parents. So while the baby lies at the centre closely guarded by a select group, there are concentric circles of people drawn into the debate from the periphery. It is important too not to forget the impact of these awesome decisions on key figures such as grandparents and siblings. They may not physically sit in the room while the consultant neonatologist breaks the news of a poor prognosis but the effects of any decision have far reaching consequences for them too.

Consulting with other specialists is a practice widely adopted by paediatricians in NICUs. Increasingly some are talking to their obstetric colleagues before the birth. This development is significant since it has been found that obstetricians tend to underestimate the potential for survival of neonates[265] and potentially viable fetuses could be given less than optimal care if paediatricians are not involved early on in decision making. Indeed many respondents in the present study voiced strong opinions on this subject. They resented being called to attend deliveries where the delivery team had not made the welfare of the baby a priority. However it is important to note that paediatricians and neonatal nurses too have been found to overestimate morbidity and mortality in the NICU,[266] with many more neonatal nurses than paediatricians believing it to be unethical to save potentially severely disabled infants.[266] It is clearly important to listen to the views of a range of different people and keep the facts clearly in mind.

Although the parents are involved in almost every case where a decision is made about treatment withdrawal, the extent of their participation varies greatly. Some neonatologists present the facts and ask the parents to decide. More guide them in the direction they themselves think best. A very small number tell the parents what they have decided, seeking merely parental rubber stamping. In the judgement of the medical experts, parents cannot be given unlimited discretion. Indeed, because of their own specialized medical knowledge and prognostic skills, tolerance for medical uncertainty, considerable experience with other difficult cases, and personal ethical judgments, as well as their capacity to consult with appropriate experts and specialists, neonatologists can exert enormous influence on parents.[241] Given this powerful influence, it is right that there should be some vigilance maintained to ensure that abuses of power are detected. Where a consultant slips off to a quiet room with parents taking no one else with him, it is difficult for staff to feel confident that this is a team effort. Not only do other team members have difficulty knowing what to say to parents subsequently when they do not know what they have been told, but there is scope for misconceptions, misinformation and mistrust. Involvement of the wider team is probably the safest and most effective way that practice can be safeguarded. They are entitled to inside information, they know the details, they understand the issues, they are knowledgeable, they have opinions formulated on experience and understanding of the relevant facts and they bring different perspectives to bear. But to be effective the junior staff need to feel empowered to contribute honestly and openly. It was sobering to find so many Units where the nurses and junior doctors felt they could not directly challenge a decision. It was even more alarming to find experienced people going against their own better judgement rather than voicing their distress or opposition. Communication must be open and healthy, if the best interests of the baby and his family are to be protected, and tension and conflict are to be reduced to a minimum.

It is often suggested that nurses have a responsibility to represent the views of parents. Differences in attitudes between paediatricians, nurses and parents have been found[266] with nurses apparently less ready than the parents to save potentially damaged infants. But it is a reality that many staff working in NICUs believe that medical advances have outstripped common sense and compassion. There were of course, a few respondents who had severely damaged children and they were staunchly defensive: they could not have contemplated allowing their child to die and still say the same thing years later when they *do* know what the costs are. But for the majority who had not been tested in this way, their stated position was that they would not themselves want to bear the burden of a severely compromised infant, neither would they want their own child to go through weeks, months or even years of painful therapy when the benefits are so questionable. At least this was their theoretical position. Some wisely added that of course they might change their stance if they were actually confronted by the reality; the emotional ties to one's own infant are very strong and they had repeatedly seen the desire of parents to cling onto life and hope. But even though they believe they would not choose treatment, they were at pains to emphasize that they regret society's obsession with perfection. This has been a finding elsewhere too.[92] Their views reflect not an abhorrence of imperfection per se, but rather a rejection of pain and suffering for a baby of their own.

'I hate the way when you see these very tiny babies – or kids – who look as though they've got no hope, coming in here, they spend two days – the only two days – of their lives being stabbed and having blood taken and just kind of on machines and things like that. And that really distresses me. And in those situations I would rather we didn't do anything but at the same time, there's other times I've been wrong with these things. I've felt this baby looks as if it's a no-hoper and it's made some sort of recovery. So that worries me.' (Registrar, less than 5 years experience)

Believing that, it could be argued that it is not then right to inflict such a burden on others who are ignorant of the full ramifications of caring for such children relentlessly for years.

'I once said this to a paediatrician, "It wouldn't be good enough for your children, so why is it good enough for somebody else's?" I think actually he knew I was right, but he just didn't want to admit it. I think that's a good philosophy though, to keep in mind as a paediatrician: "Is this care good enough for your own children, and if not, why are you doing this?"' (SHO, less than 1 year experience)

It is important to remember, however, that when it comes to neonates, it is almost always able-bodied competent people who decide for them what constitutes a good quality of life. As we have seen, there are inherent dangers in such substituted judgements.[267] An impairment would have to be very severely burdensome before a disabled person would consistently rate death as preferable if he or she had never known a life without the impairment.

These are emotive issues. The language used can easily distort and colour perceptions. Thus paediatricians are understandably affronted and saddened by suggestions that they are life takers.[36] Nurses are indignant about accusations of becoming hardened to these things. Many of the staff themselves believe these difficult decisions do not get easier. Each one carries its own weight of pain and sorrow. They simply learn how to cope with the emotions. And where teams are strong, they support and comfort each other so that the devastation of the loss is kept in perspective and they are effective in the ongoing and endless work of caring for sick neonates and their families.

The need for support
The NICU is a strange rather unnatural world.

'As British people we're not particularly good because people'll say, "Are you OK?" and you go, "Yes, I'm fine," when underneath you're thinking, "This isn't normal." And often when I go home, I think, "It's *not* just been another day at the office. You have wrapped up a child which has died and put it in a box and you've spent the whole day with parents who've just lost somebody." And I think sometimes you have to really get [straight] with yourself and say, "Right, let's remember this isn't actually a normal day and … it's something quite momentous that's happened to these people. And how do *I* feel about what's happened to me today? What are *my* feelings about what's happened?" ... When you've lost somebody I can remember the biggest anger being, "Why does life go on? Why don't these people stop and realize?" I think that's the difficult thing here that life is just going on around these people all the time. And do they want to just yell, "Don't you realize what's happening here?" ... perhaps we give them enough confidence – I'm strong enough so that if you want to yell at somebody or swear at somebody or cry on somebody's shoulder, I can be there for you – you can have confidence that I can do that for you.' (Staff Midwife, less than 5 years experience)

The crucial nature of these events and their impact on all concerned should not be underestimated. Respondents at interview were grateful for an opportunity to unburden themselves of emotions which sometimes spanned a lifetime. They often wept remembering. But most then left the room and resumed their normal efficient practice with that day's quota of families (although one person volunteered that she was so shattered by the revelations that she needed to go away and cosset herself for the rest of the evening). It is important to recognize what is actually being done in an area where progress has acquired a momentum of its own. It is all too easy to get caught up in the excitement of developments and not pause to take stock of the human element. Just because people are functioning efficiently and competently and maintaining composure should not dull others to the effects of so much pain and anguish.

The problem of uncertainty
Perhaps the biggest single factor causing difficulty in decision making about treating sick neonates is that of uncertainty. From medical prognoses through to the coping capacity of parents, the whole process is fraught with imponderables.

> 'Medicine is a probabilistic discipline, and prognostic uncertainty is a fundamental characteristic of neonatology.'[21]

Even given the same syndrome or condition there is tremendous biological variability between babies. One consultant described each baby as like an unopened book: one cannot tell the story in advance. Treatments are variously effective. Group statistics are of limited value in individual prognostications. With the introduction of untried new treatments, the prediction of long term effects is impossible to state with any certainty. And it is within this hazy context that ethical decisions are made.

This very uncertainty makes it difficult to draw up guidelines or enshrine a framework in law. Indeed doctors and nurses are resistant to such changes simply because they do not take account of the immense variability involved. As has been said, rules mandate 'what one must do according to some predetermined precept or categorical imperative.'[50] They are a 'coercive, nondiscriminatory, doctrinaire or ideological method of deciding what is right.' On the other hand, situation ethics is 'flexible, and changeable according to variables (from which) the moral agent, the decision maker, judges what is best in the circumstances and in the view of foreseeable consequences.'

Even though they might wish some changes in the law, for example to allow euthanasia for severely damaged infants, staff nevertheless are fearful of certain potential consequences. A different kind of uncertainty attaches to such concerns. Will life be devalued? Will practitioners abuse their positions? Will health care professionals be brutalized by the practice? Again no one can give a categorical response. But to some degree medicine has to take risks. Slippery slopes notwithstanding, extremely difficult circumstances do arise in neonatology and medicine must accept some responsibility for the intolerable situations it produces. And after all, these matters are only part of an existing continuum.

> 'It is a characteristic of slopes, slippery or not, that their upper reaches are continuous with their lower reaches and that hence someone who steps onto a slippery slope half way down its length is just as likely to end up at the bottom as someone who steps on at the top.'[268]

In the world of adult medicine, advance directives and Dr Kevorkian's 'suicide machine' are two responses to the ethical issues posed by medical advances and technology. Neonatologists and neonatal nurses have to ask themselves, what are their responses to the ethical dilemmas their sophisticated treatments have produced? The issues relating to prolonging life or assisting death are complex and engender powerful feelings.

> 'We cannot resolve these moral tensions by making one side of the tension disappear. Instead we must learn to live with these tensions within a pluralistic society. This requires more reliance on negotiation, compromise, and practical reasoning, and less on abstract ethical theory.'[269]

It is not morally acceptable simply to walk away from the situations which medicine itself has created.

A personal viewpoint

It is the view of the authors of this report that a fundamental factor in all these difficult decisions relates to society's attitude to death. As the 'ultimate form of consumer resistance'[270] it has become something to be resisted at all costs. But, as has been said:

> 'If we can learn to view death from a different perspective, to reintroduce it into our lives so that it comes not as a dreaded stranger but as an expected companion to our life, then we can also learn to live our lives with meaning – with full appreciation of our finiteness, of the limits on our time here.'[270]

As far as much of medicine is concerned, at the moment, death is 'what happens when medicine fails', something which 'is kept beyond the borders of medicine, an unwelcome, unwanted, unexpected, and ultimately accidental intruder.'[272] Indeed medicine has been accused of such single-minded obsession with the longevity of life that it has both spawned new ethical dilemmas and become blinded to the other needs of society.[50] But death is not the greatest loss in life. It is a necessary and inevitable end point. If we begin our thinking with death as a reality, as a limit that cannot be overcome, rather than seeing death as the unwelcome end point or discordant note in our relentless search for health and wellbeing, then it would cease to be a scientific failure. The emphasis, the challenge, the questions would all change.

This is not a new concept.

> 'I suspect that the greatest injustice in some of these neonatal cases is done because we have lost sight of the fact that we must learn to love and care for our children as being destined for death. Our longing to protect our children from death has built neonatal units; yet the very presence of these units creates problems which remind us how we must learn again when it is time for our children to die. We should not under all conditions try to keep our children alive, but then neither should we kill some of our children because they do not conform to our ideal of "the good life".'[23]

But we believe it has been too little considered.

CHAPTER SIXTEEN

Recommendations

Withdrawing and withholding treatment from babies is 'accepted medical practice' amongst medical and nursing staff in the late 1990s. Some tension around these difficult decisions is both inevitable and desirable, but certain conflicts and stresses are avoidable and this study has uncovered particular areas where they could be reduced. It is important to emphasize that the study reports only the views of doctors and nurses. Without knowing what parents themselves think, some recommendations must be tentative. But given that caveat, we make suggestions in nine main areas.

Perspective

Withdrawing intensive therapy is not undertaken lightly and does not mean a withdrawal of care. Indeed the skilful provision of terminal care to ensure a baby 'dies well', and that the family gain solace and benefit from involvement in the dying process, is as much a successful outcome as ensuring the survival of an extremely sick infant. It is however, a demanding task: demanding in time, emotional reserves and physical resources.

We recommend that:

- **the care of infants from whom aggressive treatment is being withdrawn should be as highly valued as the management of infants receiving intensive care.**

Communication

As long as there are difficult cases in clinical practice it will be impossible to make totally objective and rational decisions. A vast amount of uncertainty renders these decisions both complex and agonizing. But what is lost by introducing an element of subjectivity and human emotion is made up for by the addition of human compassion. The success of each phase of the decision process hinges largely on the issue of communication. Communicating involves being perceptive to the cues of others as well as pacing and conveying information in a language and manner appropriate to the situation and needs of others.

In order to communicate effectively staff need to gain insight into their own values, beliefs and motives. They must then formulate a considered and logical argument based on the available evidence and experience of similar cases, which can be shared with colleagues. In addition they must each listen carefully and sensitively to the views of other team members and to parents. Each has a role to play. But the perspectives and understandings of the different groups are many and varied. Recognizing and respecting differing stances will go some way towards promoting healthy debate and resolving potential ethical dilemmas.

We recommend that:

- **each team member should try to develop critical awareness of his or her own values and beliefs, and should respect the views of those who hold divergent opinions;**

- **the team as a whole should foster a practice of open communication with a special responsibility to communicate sensitively resting with the consultant as team leader.**

Team effort

This aspect of neonatal care is not the exclusive domain of one individual. Although the consultant accepts the final responsibility, the rest of the team should be actively involved in the process of deciding. This not only ensures wide-ranging discussion, taking into account all interests and viewpoints, but it provides a safeguard against abuses of power. Teams need to work closely together complementing each other in the skills and services offered. The decision is painful enough without the addition of misunderstanding, guilt or criticism. Working together can reduce these additional burdens.

All grades of staff need to learn to listen well. This involves more than remaining in one place long enough physically to hear what someone says. It involves sensitively, picking up indicators of their true position and dealing carefully with doubts and fears. If all members understand the unique positions of their colleagues, this sharing will contribute substantially to a reduction of any unnecessary tension and conflict.

We recommend that:

- **consultants and senior nurses should encourage the active participation of those most closely involved with the baby in discussion about the decision, as well as in the management of the case.**

Staffing and resources

These are demanding cases. If the outcome is likely to be death, it is easy to relegate the needs of this baby to a lesser place. Managers have a special responsibility to ensure staffing is adequate for the provision of a high quality of care for every family experiencing one of the most profound and painful experiences known to mankind. Needs do not end at the door of the NICU and follow-up provision is considered an important part of the service required, although as yet the requirements of parents are not fully understood.

We recommend that:

- **where a decision is made to withdraw treatment, high priority should be given to ensuring sufficient staff are available to meet the needs of the baby and the family both during and after the dying process;**

- **where the decision is to treat but the outcome is a severely impaired baby, resources should be mobilized to support the family and to maximize the child's potential.**

Timing of events

Pacing discussion and events around treatment decisions requires great sensitivity, and the timing of the various happenings remains one of the single most stressful components of the whole process. Different people take varying amounts of time to accept the reality of these tragic situations. Consultants often delay longer than nurses and junior doctors think appropriate. As yet the perceptions of parents are unknown. Intuitive skills are relied on in order to work in tune with the understanding and emotional readiness of others, but sharing information and insights can help the decision makers to proceed sensitively.

We recommend that:

- **attention should be paid to the timing of events in any decision making, taking into account both the fact that delays cause distress and that people take varying amounts of time to accept the realities of a poor prognosis. The insights of different people involved should be capitalized on in order to work sensitively through the process.**

Continuity and consistency

Fragmentation of services and inconsistency in the management of cases are seen seriously to jeopardize the welfare of babies and families. Although it is recognized that the opinions of parents are vital to a true understanding of the best way to proceed, the staff concerned believe that a consistent and cohesive approach to care should be fostered both during the hospital experience and into the community. This does not mean one person taking on sole responsibility; it means rather a united approach based on agreed action and sound communication.

Until more detailed information is available from the parents, we recommend that:

- **consultant paediatricians/neonatologists should aim to be consistent in their approach, explaining to other team members as well as to parents deviations from an agreed plan. Close liaison with community staff should be fostered to ensure continuity between hospital and home.**

The management of specific cases

Especial difficulties surround certain practices. Differentiating between an abortion and a viable birth; knowing where treatment withdrawal ends and euthanasia begins; deciding how a baby will die who is severely compromised but no longer requires active treatment (e.g. a severely birth asphyxiated infant). These issues require continuing frank and honest debate. A forum should be offered through which thinking can develop and the protection of both babies and clinicians be safeguarded.

We recommend that:

• **for particularly difficult and sensitive cases for which there is no accepted practice (such as babies who are severely impaired but no longer dependent on intensive care) a forum should be created to bring the questions into the open and permit frank discussion of the issues. The nature of such a forum is best decided by the clinicians themselves.**

Support

These are immensely stressful experiences for staff as well as parents. Currently many staff feel that to admit a need for support is to suggest a degree of inadequacy and unsuitability for the job. But it is natural and inevitable that coping mechanisms will be strained by such powerful emotions.

We recommend that:

• **an ethos should be fostered which acknowledges that staff need support, that available sources of support, both formal and informal, be made generally known, but that choosing an appropriate type of support be left to the individual.**

Education

Both doctors and nurses should be given a thorough grounding in the legal, philosophical, medical and psychological framework within which these decisions are made. They should also be helped to gain insight into their own values and beliefs in order to equip them to think logically, but compassionately, through the issues relating to each case which presents for decision making.

We recommend that:

• **at undergraduate and postgraduate levels doctors and nurses should be helped to think for themselves, to gain insight into their values and opinions and themselves as therapeutic practitioners. Whilst all students and junior clinicians should be given a comprehensive framework which provides an accurate factual context of the law, ethics and medical**

knowledge against which to make sound scientific and moral judgements, detailed and on-going exploration of the specific issues relating to withdrawing treatment from neonates should be reserved for those clinicians who specialize in Neonatal Intensive Care. The issues need to be periodically revisited to take account of changes in attitudes and opinions which come with experience.

It can take time for society and for professionals to accept officially what has been recognized as desirable long before. At the beginning of this century the law in the USA declared birth control to be immoral and therefore illegal. However, Margaret Sanger recognized that the time had come for change – birth control was moral because its time had come irrespective of what the law said. In 1914 she wrote: 'Shall we look upon a piece of parchment as greater than human happiness, greater than human life?'[273] It took years for officialdom to recognize what she advocated: it was not until 1937 that doctors finally certified birth control as a legitimate medical service and not until 1973 that the laws were rescinded barring its legitimate practice.[50] Even now there are those who still oppose the practice.

More and more doctors are acknowledging that they do help suffering patients to die by a variety of means. And paediatricians and neonatal nurses are increasingly questioning the motivations behind their own actions.

'Shall we who respond to the throbbing pulse of human needs concern ourselves with indictments, courts, and judges, or shall we do our work first and settle with these evils after?'[273]

Are they to do what seems right for their patients or are they to consider the influence and weight of the law which is known to move more slowly than the advances in neonatology? Modern technology and medical expertise and understanding have produced new and complex dilemmas. Deciding when to withhold or withdraw treatment is one such dilemma. It may well take time for some enlightened views to gain acceptance. But in providing empirical evidence for what is current thinking and practice, this study moves the professional community one step further towards a compassionate response to dilemmas which involve some of life's most vulnerable people.

References

1. Habgood J. Searching for our moral roots. *British Medical Journal*, 1986; 293: 1600–1601.
2. Piccione JJ. This science is wrong way to create life. *USA Today*, 1989; August 1st, 6A.
3. Guillemin JH, Holmstrom LL. *Mixed Blessings: Intensive Care for Newborns*. New York: Oxford University Press, 1986.
4. Gustaitis R, Young EWD. *A Time to be Born, A Time to Die*. Mass.: Addison Wesley, 1986.
5. Anspach RR. *Deciding who Lives: Fateful Choices in the Intensive Care Nursery*. Berkeley: University of California Press, 1993.
6. Stinson R, Stinson P. *The Long Dying of Baby Andrew*. (Second printing) New York: Little Brown and Co, 1983.
7. Stinson R, Stinson P. On the death of a baby. *Journal of Medical Ethics*, 1981; 7, 1: 5-18.
8. Hill S. *Family*. London: Michael Joseph, 1989.
9. Ens-Dokkum MH, Johnson A, Schreider AM, Veen S, Wilkinson AR, Brand R, Ruys JH, Verloove-Vanhorick SP. Comparison of mortality and rates of cerebral palsy in two populations of very low birthweight infants. *Archives of Disease in Childhood*, 1994; 70: F96-100.
10. Hack M, Fanaroff AA. Outcomes of extremely immature infants - A perinatal dilemma. *New England Journal of Medicine*, 1993; 329, 22: 1649-1650.
11. Tew M. Infant statistics. In Crawford DA, Morris M (Eds) *Neonatal Nursing*. London: Chapman and Hall, 1994; pp. 346-371.
12. Saigal S, Feeny D, Furlong W, Rosenbaum P, Burrows E, Torrance G. Comparison of the health-related quality of life of extremely low birth weight children and a reference of children at age eight years. *Journal of Pediatrics*, 1994; 125, 3: 418-424.
13. Saigal S, Rosenbaum P, Stoskopf B, Hoult L, Furlong W, Feeny D, Burrows E, Torrance G. Comprehensive assessment of the health status of extremely low birth weight children at eight years of age: Comparison with a reference group. *Journal of Pediatrics*, 1994; 125, 3: 411-417.
14. Blank RH. International Symposium on critically ill newborns. An overview and introduction. *Journal of Legal Medicine*, 1995; 16, 2: 183-188.
15. Roberton NRC. Should we look after babies less than 800g? *Archives of Disease in Childhood*, 1993; 68: 326-329.
16. Tubman TRJ, Halliday HL, Norman C. Cost of surfactant treatment for severe neonatal respiratory distress syndrome. A randomised controlled trial. *British Medical Journal*, 1990; 301: 842-845.
17. Schwartz RM. What price prematurity? *Family Planning Perspectives*, 1989; 21, 4: 170-174.
18. Stevenson RC, McCabe CJ, Pharoah POD, Cooke RWI. Cost of care for a geographically determined population of low birthweight infants to age 8-9 years. 1. Children without disability. *Archives of Disease in Childhood*, 1996; 74, 2: F114-117.
19. Stevenson RC, Pharoah POD, Stevenson CJ, McCabe CJ, Cooke RWI. Cost of care for a geographically determined population of low birthweight infants to age 8-9 years. 2. Children with disability. *Archives of Disease in Childhood*, 1996; 74, 2: F118-121.
20. Field D, Hodges S, Mason E, Burton P. Survival and place of treatment after premature delivery. *Archives of Disease in Childhood*, 1991; 66: 408-411.

21. Rostain AL, Bhutani V. Ethical dilemmas of neonatal-perinatal surgery. *Clinics in Perinatology*, 1989; 16, 1: 275-302.
22. Silverman WA. Overtreatment of neonates? A personal retrospective. *Pediatrics*, 1992; 90: 971-976.
23. Hauerwas S, Bondi R, Burrell DB. *Truthfulness and Tragedy: Further Investigations into Christian Ethics.* (Second printing) Notre Dame: University of Notre Dame Press,1985.
24. Alderson P. *Choosing for Children: Parents' Consent to Surgery.* Oxford: Oxford University Press. 1990.
25. House of Lords Select Committee on Medical Ethics. *Volume 1. Report.* London: HMSO 1994.
26. Versluys Z, de Leeuw R. A Dutch report on the ethics of neonatal care. *Journal of Medical Ethics*, 1995; 21: 14-16.
27. House of Lords Judgement. *Airedale NHS Trust v Bland.* 1993.
28. Dyer C. GMC tempers justice with mercy in Cox case. *British Medical Journal*, 1992; 305: 1311.
29. Mason JK, Mulligan D. Euthanasia by stages. *Lancet*, 1996; 347: 810-811.
30. Kuhse H, Singer P. *Should the Baby Live? The Problem of Handicapped Infants.* (Reprinted) Gregg Revivals, 1994.
31. Lorber J. Spina bifida cystica. Results of treatment of 270 consecutive cases with criteria for selection for the future. *Archives of Disease in Childhood*, 1972; 47: 854.
32. Duff RS, Campbell AGM. Moral and ethical dilemmas in the special care nursery. *New England Journal of Medicine*, 1973; 289: 890-894.
33. Whitelaw A. Death as an option in neonatal intensive care. *Lancet*, 1986; 2: 328-331.
34. Campbell AGM, Lloyd DJ, Duffty P. Treatment dilemmas in neonatal care: Who should survive and who should decide? Biomedical Ethics: An Anglo-American Dialogue, *Annals of the New York Academy of Sciences*, 1988; 530: 92-103.
35. Rachels J. *The End of Life. Euthanasia and Morality.* Oxford: Oxford University Press, 1986.
36. Kohrman AF. Selective nontreatment of handicapped newborns: A critical essay. *Social Science and Medicine*, 1985; 20, 11: 1091-1095.
37. Sauer PJJ. Ethical decisions in neonatal intensive care units: The Dutch experience. *Pediatrics*, 1992; 90, 5: 729-732.
38. The Danish Council of Ethics. *7th Annual Report 1994. Debate Outline - Extreme Prematurity: Ethical Aspects.* Denmark: Thorup Grafik, 1995.
39. McMillan RC, Engelhardt HT Jr, Spicker SF. (Eds) *Euthanasia and the Newborn.* Holland: Reidel, 1987.
40. Keyserlingk EW. Against infanticide. *Law, Medicine and Health Care*, 1986; 14, 3-4: 154-157.
41. Robinson J. Euthanasia: The collision of theory and practice. *Law, Medicine and Health Care*, 1990; 18, 1-2: 105-107.
42. Rodney P. A nursing perspective on life-prolonging treatment. *Journal of Palliative Care*, 1994; 10, 2: 40-44.
43. Branthwaite M. Ethical aspects of intensive care. In Dunstan GR, Shinebourne EA. (Eds) *Doctors' Decisions: Ethical Conflicts in Medical Practice.* Oxford: Oxford University Press, 1989; pp. 177-186.
44. Jennett B. High technology medicine: Benefits and burdens. The Rock Carling Fellowship, 1093. *Nuffield Provincial Hospitals Trust*, 1984.
45. Jennett B. Inappropriate use of intensive care. *British Medical Journal*, 1984; 289: 1709-1711.
46. Doyal L, Wilsher D. Towards guidelines for withholding and withdrawing of life prolonging treatment in neonatal medicine. *Archives of Disease in Childhood*, 1994; 70, 1: F66-70.
47. Glover J. *Causing Death and Saving Life.* (Reprint) London: Penguin, 1990.

48. Fost N. Ethical issues in the treatment of critically ill newborns. *Pediatric Annals*, 1981; 10: 383-389.

49. Campbell AGM. The right to be allowed to die. *Journal of Medical Ethics*, 1983; 9: 136-140.

50. Kevorkian J. *Prescription: Medicide. The Goodness of Planned Death*. New York: Prometheus, 1991.

51. Dracup K, Raffin T. Withholding and withdrawing ventilation: Assessing quality of life. *American Review of Respiratory Disease*, 1989; 140: S44-46.

52. Campbell AGM. Some ethical issues in neonatal care. In Dunstan GR, Shinebourne EA. (Eds) *Doctors' Decisions: Ethical Conflicts in Medical Practice*. Oxford: Oxford University Press, 1989; pp 51-66.

53. Younger SJ. Who defines futility? *Journal of the American Medical Association*, 1988; 260, 14: 2094-2095.

54. Waisel DB, Truog RD. The cardiopulmonary resuscitation-not-indicated order: Futility revisited. *Annals of Internal Medicine*, 1995; 122, 4: 304-308.

55. World Health Organisation. *Definitions and Recommendations. International Classification of Disease*. 9th edition. Geneva: WHO, 1979.

56. Dunn PM, Stirrat GM. Capable of being born alive. *Lancet*, 1984; 553-555.

57. Feinsteen AR. An additional basic science for clinical medicine. The constraining fundamental paradigms. *Annals of Internal Medicine*, 1983; 99: 393-397.

58. Medawar P. *The Limits of Science*. Oxford: Oxford University Press, 1984.

59. Fisher MMcD, Raper RF. Withdrawing and withholding treatment in intensive care. Part 1. Social and ethical dimensions. *Medical Journal of Australia*, 1990; 153, 4: 217-220.

60. Salamy A, Davis S, Eldredge L, Wakeley A, Tooley WH. Neonatal status: An objective scoring method for identifying infants at risk for poor outcome. *Early Human Development*, 1988; 17: 233-243.

61. Pederson DR, Evans B, Chance GW, Bento S, Fox AM. Predictors of one-year developmental status in low birth weight infants. *Journal of Developmental and Behavioral Pediatrics*, 1988; 9, 5: 287-292.

62. Brazy JE, Eckerman CO, Oehler JM, Goldstein RF, O'Rand AM. Nursery neurobiologic risk score: Important factors in predicting outcome in very low birth weight infants. *Journal of Pediatrics*, 1991; 118: 783-792.

63. Scheiner AP, Sexton ME. Prediction of developmental outcome using a perinatal risk inventory. *Pediatrics*, 1991; 88, 6: 1135-1143.

64. Majnemer A, Rosenblatt B, Riley P. Predicting outcome in high-risk newborns with a neonatal neurobehavioral assessment. *American Journal of Occupational Health*, 1994; 48, 8: 723-732.

65. Richardson DK, Phibbs CS, Gray JE, McCormick MC, Workman-Daniels K, Goldmann DA. Birthweight and illness severity: Independent predictors of neonatal mortality. *Pediatrics*, 1993; 91, 5: 969-975.

66. Horbar JD, Onstad L, Wright E. Predicting mortality risk for infants weighing 501-1500 grams at birth: A National Institutes of Health Neonatal Research Network report. *Critical Care Medicine*, 1993; 21, 1: 12-18.

67. The International Neonatal Network. The CRIB (Clinical Risk Index for Babies) score: A tool for assessing initial neonatal risk and comparing performance of neonatal intensive care units. *Lancet*, 1993; 342: 193-198.

68. Lemeshow S, Klar J, Teres D. Outcome prediction for individual intensive care patients: Useful, misused, or abused? *Intensive Care Medicine*, 1995; 21: 770-776.

69. Martin A. A clinical model for decision making. *Journal of Medical Ethics*, 1978; 4: 200-206.

70. Siegler M. Decision making strategy for clinical-ethical problems in medicine. *Archives of Internal Medicine*, 1982; 142: 2178-2179.

71. Curtin L. No rush to judgement. In Curtin L, Flaherty MJ. (Eds) *Nursing Ethics: Theories and Pragmatics.* Maryland: Brady, 1982.

72. Candee D, Puka B. An analytic approach to resolving problems in medical ethics. *Journal of Medical Ethics*, 1983; 9, 10: 61-69.

73. Veatch RM. Limits of guardian treatment refusal: A reasonable-ness standard. *American Journal of Law and Medicine*, 1984; 9, 3: 427-468.

74. Pellegrino ED. The anatomy of clinical ethical judgments in perinatology and neonatology: A substantive and procedural framework. *Seminars in Perinatology,* 1987; 11: 202-209.

75. Seedhouse D. *Ethics: The Heart of Health Care.* Chichester: Wiley, 1988.

76. Weil MH, Weil CJ, Rackow EC. Guide to ethical decision-making for the critically ill: The three Rs and QC. *Critical Care Medicine*, 1988; 16, 6: 636-641.

77. Farrell PM, Fost NC. Long-term mechanical ventilation in pediatric respiratory failure: Medical and ethical considerations. *American Review of Respiratory Disease*, 1989; 140, 2: S36-40.

78. Dormire SL. Models for moral response in care of seriously ill children. *Image: The Journal of Nursing Scholarship*, 1989; 21, 2: 81-84.

79. Quinn JC. The nurse manager and ethical choices. *Journal of Post Anesthesia Nursing*, 1990; 5, 5: 365-366.

80. Grundstein-Amado R. An integrative model of clinical-ethical decision making. *Theoretical Medicine*, 1991; 12: 157-170.

81. Greipp ME. Greipp's model of ethical decision making. *Journal of Advanced Nursing*, 1992; 17: 734-738.

82. Rhoden NK. Treating Baby Doe: The ethics of uncertainty. *Hastings Center Report*, 1986; 16: 34-42.

83. Young EWD, Stevenson DF. Limiting treatment for extremely premature, low-birth-weight infants (500-750g). *American Journal of Diseases of Children*, 1990; 144: 549-552.

84. Editorial. The right to live and the right to die. *British Medical Journal*, 1981; 283, 6291: 569-570.

85. Miles MS. Helping adults mourn the death of a child. *Issues in Comprehensive Pediatric Nursing*, 1985; 8: 219-241.

86. Neidig JR, Dalgas-Pelish P. Parental grieving and perceptions of health care professionals' interventions. *Issues in Comprehensive Pediatric Nursing*, 1991; 14: 179-191.

87. Kohner N, Henley A. *When a Baby Dies. The Experience of Late Miscarriage, Stillbirth and Neonatal Death.* London: Pandora, 1991.

88. Kohner N, Leftwich A. *Pregnancy Loss and the Death of a Baby: A Training Pack for Professionals.* Cambridge: National Extension College, 1995.

89. Warman J, Fisher M. *Bereavement and Loss: A Skills Companion.* Cambridge: National Extension College, 1990.

90. Kohner N. *Pregnancy Loss and the Death of a Baby: Guidelines for Professionals.* London: Stillbirth and Neonatal Death Society, 1995.

91. Stewart A, Dent A. *At a Loss: Bereavement Care when a Baby Dies.* London: Balliere Tindall, 1994.

92. Harrison H. Neonatal intensive care: Parents' role in ethical decision making. *Birth*, 1986; 13, 3: 165-175.

93. Rue VM. Death by design of handicapped newborns: The family's role and response. *Issues in Law and Medicine*, 1985; 1, 3: 201-225.

94. Davis A. Informed dissent: The view of a disabled woman. *Journal of Medical Ethics*, 1986; 12: 75-76.

95. Jost KE, Haase JE. At the time of death: Help for the child's parents. *Children's Health Care*, 1989; 18, 3: 146-152.

96. Nursing Times. Euthanasia: What do you think? *Nursing Times*, 1988; 84, 33: 38-39.

97. Owen C, Tennant C, Levi J, Jones M. Suicide and euthanasia: Patient attitudes in the context of cancer. *Psycho-Oncology*, 1992; 1, 2: 79-88.

98. Huber R, Cox VM, Edelen WB. Right-to-die responses from a random sample of 200. *Hospice Journal*, 1992; 8, 3: 1-19.

99. Anonymous. The attitudes of GPs to voluntary euthanasia. *British Medical Journal*, 1987; 294: 1294.

100. Vincent JL. European attitudes towards ethical problems in intensive care medicine: Results of an ethical questionnaire. *Intensive Care Medicine*, 1990; 16, 256-264.

101. Suhl J, Simons P, Reedy T, Garrick T. Myth of substituted judgment. Surrogate decision making regarding life support is unreliable. *Archives of Internal Medicine*, 1994; 154, 1: 90-96.

102. Kuhse H, Singer P. Doctors' practices and attitudes regarding voluntary euthanasia. *Medical Journal of Australia*, 1988; 148, 12: 623-627.

103. Anderson JG, Caddell DP. Attitudes of medical professionals towards euthanasia. *Social Science and Medicine*, 1993; 37, 1: 105-114.

104. Cohen JS, Fihn SD, Boyko EJ, Jonsen AR, Wood RW. Attitudes toward assisted suicide and euthanasia among physicians in Washington State. *New England Journal of Medicine*, 1994; 331, 2: 89-94.

105. Shapiro RS, Derse AR, Gottlieb M, Schiedermayer D, Olson M. Willingness to perform euthanasia. A survey of physician attitudes. *Archives of Internal Medicine*, 1994; 154, 5: 575-584.

106. Caralis PV, Hammond JS. Attitudes of medical students, housestaff, and faculty physicians toward euthanasia and termination of life-sustaining treatment. *Critical Care Medicine*, 1992; 20, 5, 683-690.

107. Kinsella TD, Verhoef MJ. Alberta euthanasia survey: 1. Physicians' opinions about the morality and legalization of active euthanasia. *Canadian Medical Association Journal*, 1993; 148, 11: 1921-1926.

108. Baume P, O'Malley E. Euthanasia: Attitudes and practices of medical practitioners. *Medical Journal of Australia*, 1994: 137, 140: 142-144.

109. Ward BJ, Tate PA. Attitudes among NHS doctors to requests for euthanasia. *British Medical Journal*, 1994; 308, 6940: 1332-1334.

110. Genuis SJ, Genuis SK, Chang WC. Public attitudes toward the right to die. *Canadian Medical Association Journal*, 1994; 150, 5: 701-708.

111. Baume P, O'Malley E, Bauman A. Professed religious affiliation and the practice of euthanasia. *Journal of Medical Ethics*, 1995; 21: 49-54.

112. Berseth CL, Kenny JD, Durand R. Newborn ethical dilemmas: Intensive care and intermediate care nursing attitudes. *Critical Care Medicine*, 1984; 12, 6: 508-511.

113. Stevens CA, Hassan R. Management of death, dying and euthanasia: Attitudes and practices of medical practitioners in South Australia. *Journal of Medical Ethics*, 1994; 20, 1: 41-46.

114. Wilkes L, White K, Tolley N. Euthanasia: A comparison of the lived experience of Chinese and Australian palliative care nurses. *Journal of Advanced Nursing*, 1993; 18: 95-102.

115. Kuhse H, Singer P. Voluntary euthanasia and the nurse: An Australian survey. *International Journal of Nursing Studies*, 1993; 30, 4: 311-322.

116. Takeo K, Satoh K, Minamisawa H, Mitoh T. Healthworkers' attitudes toward euthanasia in Japan. *International Nursing Review*, 1991; 38, 2: 45-48.

117. Merriman A, Lau-Ting C. Reactions to death and dying by doctors, medical students and nurses in Singapore 1985-86. *Annals of the Academy of Medicine, Singapore*, 1987; 16, 1: 133-136.

118. Richardson DS. Oncology nurses' attitudes toward the legalization of voluntary active euthanasia. *Cancer Nursing*, 1994; 17, 4: 348-354.

119. McInerney F, Seibold C. Nurses' definitions of and attitudes towards euthanasia. *Journal of Advanced Nursing*, 1995; 22: 171-182.

120. Davis AJ, Slater PV. US and Australian nurses' attitudes and beliefs about the good death. *Image: The Journal of Nursing Scholarship*, 1989; 21, 2: 34-39.

121. Davis AJ, Davidson B, Hirschfield M, Lauri S, Lin JY, Norberg A, Phillips L, Pitman E, Shen CH, Vander Laan R et al. An international perspective of active euthanasia: Attitudes of nurses in seven countries. *International Journal of Nursing Studies*, 1993; 30, 4: 301-310.

122. Anderson JG, Caddell DP. Attitudes of medical professionals toward euthanasia. *Social Science and Medicine*, 1993; 37, 1: 105-114.

123. Verhoef MJ, Kinsella TD. Alberta euthanasia survey: 2. Physicians' opinions about the acceptance of active euthanasia as a medical act and the reporting of such practice. *Canadian Medical Association Journal*, 1993; 148, 11: 1929-1933.

124. National Hemlock Society. *1987 Survey of California Physicians regarding Voluntary Active Euthanasia for the Terminally Ill*. Los Angeles: Los Angeles Hemlock Society, 1988.

125. Center for Health Ethics and Policy. *Withholding and Withdrawing Life-sustaining Treatment: A Survey of Opinions and Experiences of Colorado Physicians*. Denver: University of Colorado Graduate School of Public Affairs, 1988.

126. Overmyer M. National survey: Physicians' views on the right to die. *Physicians Manage*, 1991; 31, 7: 40-45.

127. Kopelman LM, Irons TG, Kopelman AE. Neonatologists judge the 'Baby Doe' regulations. *New England Journal of Medicine*, 1988; 318: 677-683.

128. *The Neonatal Nurses Yearbook 1994*. Cambridge: CMA Medical Data, 1995.

129. Tourniet P. Foreword. In Powell J. *Why am I Afraid to Tell you Who I am?* London: Fount/Harper Collins, 1978; p1.

130. Powell J. *Why am I Afraid to Tell you Who I am?* London: Fount/Harper Collins, 1978.

131. Redshaw ME, Harris A, Ingram JC. *The Neonatal Unit as a Working Environment: A Survey of Neonatal Nursing. Executive Summary*. London: Department of Health, 1993.

132. Blank RH. Treatment of critically ill newborns in Australasia. *Journal of Legal Medicine*, 1995; 16, 2: 211-226.

133. Merrick JC. Critically ill newborns and the law: The American experience. *Journal of Legal Medicine*, 1995; 16, 2: 189-210.

134. Huibers AK. Beyond the threshold of life: Treating and non-treating of critically ill newborns in the Netherlands. *Journal of Legal Medicine*, 1995; 16, 2: 227-246.

135. Eidelman AI. Care of critically ill newborns: The Israeli experience. *Journal of Legal Medicine*, 1995; 16, 2: 247-262.

136. Siva Subramanian KN, Paul VK. Care of critically ill newborns in India: Legal and ethical issues. *Journal of Legal Medicine*, 1995; 16, 2: 265-275.

137. Campbell AGM, McHaffie HE. Prolonging life and allowing death: Infants. *Journal of Medical Ethics*, 1995; 21: 339-344.

138. *Re B* (a minor) (Wardship: medical treatment) 1981. 1WLR 1421.

139. Re C 1989. *NLJ Law reports*: 613.

140. Re J 1990. Court of Appeal Oct. 19. *Bulletin of Medical Ethics*, 1990; 63: 22-23.

141. Re J 1992. TLR 12-06-92. *Bulletin of Medical Ethics*, 1992; 79: 5-6.

142. Glantz LH. Withholding and withdrawing treatment: The role of the criminal law. *Law, Medicine and Health Care*, 1987-1988; 15, 4: 231-241.

143. Mason JK, Meyers DW. Parental choice and selective non-treatment of deformed newborns: A view from mid-Atlantic. *Journal of Medical Ethics*, 1986; 12: 67-71.

144. Marchwinski S. The dilemma of moral and ethical decision making in the intensive care nursery. *Neonatal Network*, 1988; 6, 5: 17-20.

145. Raphael DD. Handicapped infants: Medical ethics and the law. *Journal of Medical Ethics*, 1988; 14: 5-10.

146. *Government response to the report of the Select Committee on Medical Ethics.* Cm 2553. London: HMSO, 1994.

147. Harvard J. Legislation is likely to create more difficulties than it resolves. *Journal of Medical Ethics,* 1983; 9: 18-20.

148. Fenton AC, Field DJ, Mason E, Clarke M. Attitudes to viability of preterm infants and their effect on figures for perinatal mortality. *British Medical Journal,* 1990; 300: 434-436.

149. Campbell AGM. Baby Doe and forgoing life-sustaining treatment. Compassion, discrimination, or medical neglect? In Caplan AL, Blank RH, Merrick JC. (Eds) *Compelled Compassion: Government Intervention in the Treatment of Critically Ill Newborns.* Towota, New Jersey: Humana, 1992.

150. King NMP. Transparency in neonatal intensive care. *Hastings Center Report,* 1992; May-June, 18-25.

151. Cook DJ, Guyatt GH, Jaeschke R, Reeve J, Spanier A, King D, Molloy DW, Willan A, Streiner DL. Determinants in Canadian health care workers of the decision to withdraw life support from the critically ill. *Journal of the American Medical Association,* 1995; 273: 703-708.

152. Calabresi G, Bobbitt P. *Tragic Choices.* New York: Norton, 1978.

153. Walton DN, Donen N. Ethical decision making and the critical care team. *Critical Care Clinics,* 1986; 2, 1: 101-109.

154. Robertson JA. Legal aspects of withholding treatment from handicapped newborns: Substantive issues. *Journal of Health Politics, Policy & Law,* 1986; 11, 2: 215-230.

155. Wyatt J, Spencer J. *Survival of the Weakest: A Christian Approach to Extreme Prematurity.* London:Christian Medical Fellowship, 1992.

156. Geddes P, Pace N, Hallworth D. Selectively withholding treatment from newborn babies. *British Journal of Hospital Medicine,* 1992; 47, 4: 280-283.

157. Whitelaw A, Thoresen M. Ethical dilemmas around the time of birth. In Gillon R (Ed) *Principles of Health Care Ethics.* Chichester: Wiley, 1994: pp 617-627.

158. Redshaw ME, Harris A, Ingram JC. Nursing and medical staffing in neonatal units. *Journal of Nursing Management,* 1993; 1, 5: 221-228.

159. James N, Arthur T, Pittman A. *Nursing Quality Counts. A Case Study of Neonatal Services 1990-1992.* Department of Nursing and Midwifery Studies, University of Nottingham, 1993.

160. Martin DA. Nurses' involvement in ethical decision-making with severely ill newborns. *Issues in Comprehensive Pediatric Nursing,* 1989; 12, 6: 463-473.

161. Craig GM. On withholding nutrition and hydration in the terminally ill: Has palliative medicine gone too far? *Journal of Medical Ethics,* 1994; 20: 139-143.

162. Callahan D. The primacy of caring. *Commonweal,* 1990; February 23: 107-112.

163. Ramsey P. *Ethics at the edges of life.* New Haven: Yale University Press, 1978.

164. Stanley JM (Ed) The Appleton International Conference: Developing guidelines for decisions to forgo life-prolonging medical treatment. [Also] Decisions involving neonates and other patients who have never achieved decision-making capacity. *Journal of Medical Ethics,* 1992; 18, supplement: 3-5 and 13-15 respectively.

165. Dunstan GR, Shinebourne EA. (Eds) *Doctors' Decisions: Ethical Conflicts in Medical Practice.* Oxford: Oxford University Press, 1989.

166. Gilligan C. *In a Different Voice. Psychological Theory and Women's Development.* London: Harvard University Press, 1982.

167. Tilden VP, Tolle SW, Garland MJ, Nelson CA. Decisions about life-sustaining treatment. Impact of physicians' behaviors on the family. *Archives of Internal Medicine,* 1995; 155: 633-638.

168. McHaffie HE. *A Study of Support for Families with a Very Low Birthweight Baby.* Nursing Research Unit Report, Department of Nursing Studies, University of Edinburgh, 1991.

169. Bernal EW. The nurse as patient advocate. *Hastings Center Report,* 1992; 22, 4: 18-23.

170. Landis DA. Physician distinguish thyself: Conflict and covenant in a physician's moral development. *Perspectives in Biology and Medicine*, 1993; 36, 4: 628-641.

171. Kemp VH. The role of critical care nurses in the ethical decision-making process. *Dimensions of Critical Care Nursing*, 1985; 4, 6: 354-359.

172. Miya PA. Imperiled infants: Nurses' roles in ethical decision-making. *Issues in Comprehensive Pediatric Nursing*, 1989; 12, 6: 413-422.

173. Martin D. Withholding treatment from severely handicapped newborns: Ethical-legal issues. *Nursing Administration Quarterly*, 1985; 9, 4: 47-56.

174. Elizondo AP. Nurse participation in ethical decision making in the neonatal intensive care unit. *Neonatal Network*, 1991; 10, 2: 55-59.

175. Erlen JA, Frost B. Nurses' perceptions of powerlessness in influencing ethical decisions. *Western Journal of Nursing Research*, 1991; 13, 3: 397-407.

176. Baggs JG. Collaborative interdisciplinary bioethical decision making in intensive care units. *Nursing Outlook*, 1993; 41, 3: 108-112.

177. Raines DA. Values influencing neonatal nurses' perceptions and choices. *Western Journal of Nursing Research*, 1994; 16, 6: 675-691.

178. Wilson-Barnett J. Ethical dilemmas in nursing. *Journal of Medical Ethics*, 1986; 12: 123-126, 135.

179. Bertolini CL. Ethical decision-making in intensive care: A nurse's perspective. *Intensive and Critical Care Nursing*, 1994; 10, 1: 58-63.

180. Haddad AM. The nurse/physician relationship and ethical decision-making. *Association of Operating Room Nurses Journal*, 1991; 53, 1: 151-154, 156.

181. Cassidy VR. Ethical responsibilities in nursing: Research findings and issues. *Journal of Professional Nursing*, 1991; 7, 2: 112-118.

182. Duckett L, Rowan-Boyer M, Ryden MB, Crisham P, Savik K, Rest JR. Challenging misperceptions about nurses' moral reasoning. *Nursing Research*, 1992; 41, 6: 324-331.

183. Yarling RR, McElmurry BJ. The moral foundation of nursing. *Advances in Nursing Science*, 1986; 8, 2: 63-73.

184. Berseth CL, Kenny JD, Durand R. Newborn ethical dilemmas: Intensive care and intermediate care nursing attitudes. *Critical Care Medicine*, 1984; 12, 6: 508-511.

185. Lantos JD, Tyson JE, Allen A, Frader J, Hack M, Korones S, Merenstein G, Paneth N, Poland RL, Saigal S, Stevenson D, Truog RD, van Marter LJ. Withholding and withdrawing life sustaining treatment in neonatal intensive care: Issues for the 1990s. *Archives of Disease in Childhood*, 1994; 71: F218-223.

186. Phillips DF. Pastoral care: Finding a niche in ethical decision-making. *Cambridge Quarterly of Healthcare Ethics*, 1993; 2, 1: 99-106.

187. Leikin S. Children's hospital ethics committees. A first estimate. *American Journal of Diseases in Children*. 1987; 141, 9: 954-958.

188. Savage TA. The nurse's role on ethics committees and as an ethics consultant. *Seminars for Nurse Managers*, 1994; 2, 1: 41-47.

189. Edens MJ, Eyler FD, Wagner JT, Eitzman DV. Neonatal ethics: Development of a consultative group. *Pediatrics*, 1990; 86, 6: 944-949.

190. La Puma J, Schiedermayer DL. The clinical ethicist at the bedside. *Theoretical Medicine*, 1991; 12, 2: 141-149.

191. Meslin E. Personal communication.

192. Newman LR, Willms J. The family physician's role following a neonatal death. *Journal of Family Practice*, 1989; 29, 5: 521-525.

193. Downey V, Bengiamin M, Heuer L, Juhl N. Dying babies and associated stress in NICU nurses. *Neonatal Network*, 1995; 14, 1: 41-45.

194. Grundstein-Amado R. Ethical decision-making processes used by healthcare providers. *Journal of Advanced Nursing*, 1993; 18: 1701-1709.

195. Uden G, Norberg A, Lindseth A, Marhaug V. Ethical reasoning in nurses' and physicians' stories about care episodes. *Journal of Advanced Nursing*, 1992; 17: 1028-1034.

196. Watts DT, McCaulley BL, Priefer BA. Physician-nurse conflict: Lessons from a clinical experience. *Journal of American Geriatrics Society*, 1990; 38: 1151-1152.

197. Prescott PA, Bowen SA. Physician-nurse relationships. *Annals of Internal Medicine*, 1985; 103, 1: 127-133.

198. Frampton MW, Mayewski RJ. Physicians' and nurses' attitudes toward withholding treatment in a community hospital. *Journal of General Internal Medicine*, 1987; 2, 6: 394-399.

199. Holly CM. The ethical quandries of acute care nursing practice. *Journal of Professional Nursing*, 1993; 9, 2: 110-115.

200. Valentine PEB. Management of conflict: Do nurses/women handle it differently? *Journal of Advanced Nursing*, 1995; 22: 142-149.

201. Theis EC. Ethical issues. A nursing perspective. *New England Journal of Medicine*, 1986; 19: 1222-1224.

202. General Medical Council. *Tomorrow's Doctors*. London: General Medical Council, 1993.

203. Hannam C. *Parents and Mentally Handicapped Children*. Second edition. Harmondsworth: Penguin, 1980.

204. Strong C. Defective infants and their impact on families: Ethical and legal considerations. *Law, Medicine and Health Care*, 1983; 11, 4: 168-172, 181.

205. Simms M. Severely handicapped infants: A discussion document. *New Humanist*, 1983; 98, 2: pp 15-22.

206. Shepperdson B. Abortion and euthanasia of Down's Syndrome children -The parents' views. *Journal of Medical Ethics*, 1983; 9: 152-157.

207. Tolstoy L. *Anna Karenina*, Oxford: Oxford University Press, 1918.

208. Duff RS. Counselling families and deciding care of severely defective children: A way of coping with 'medical Vietnam.' *Pediatrics*, 1981; 67, 3: 315-320.

209. McHaffie HE. *A Prospective Study to Identify Critical Factors which Indicate Mothers' Readiness to Care for their Very Low Birthweight Baby at Home*. Unpublished PhD thesis, University of Edinburgh, 1988.

210. Pinch WJ, Spielman ML. The parents' perspective: Ethical decision-making in neonatal intensive care. *Journal of Advanced Nursing*, 1990; 15: 712-719.

211. Shaw NJ, Dear PRF. How do parents of babies interpret qualitative expressions of probability? *Archives of Disease in Childhood*, 1990; 65: 520-523.

212. Thomas JE, Latimer EJ. When families cannot 'let go': Ethical decision-making at the bedside. *Canadian Medical Association Journal*, 1989; 141, 5: 389-391.

213. Woolley H, Stein A, Forrest GC, Baum JD. Imparting the diagnosis of life threatening illness in children. *British Medical Journal*, 1989; 298: 1623-1626.

214. Eikner S. Dealing with long term problems: A parent's perspective. *Parent Care Inc.* 1987; January: 2-5.

215. Dowling ED. Breaking the news: Parents' perceptions of professionals. *Health Visitor*, 1995; 68, 6: 242-243.

216. Reid M, Lloyd D, Campbell G, Murray K, Porter M. Scottish neonatal intensive care units: A study of staff and parental attitudes. *Health Bulletin*, 1995; 53, 5: 314-325.

217. Stahlman M. Withholding and withdrawing therapy and actively hastening death. In Goldworth A, Silverman W, Stevenson DK, Young EWD. (Eds) *Ethics and Perinatology.* New York: Oxford Medical Publications, 1995: pp 163-171.

218. Campbell AGM. Quality of life as a decision-making criterion. In Goldworth A, Silverman W, Stevenson DK, Young EWD. (Eds) *Ethics and Perinatology.* New York: Oxford Medical Publications, 1995: pp 82-104.

219. Astbury J, Yu VYH. Determinants of stress for staff in a neonatal intensive care unit. *Archives of Disease in Childhood*, 1982; 57: 108-111.

220. Walker CHM. Neonatal intensive care and stress. *Archives of Disease in Childhood*, 1982; 57: 85-88.

221. Sheldon W. *Report of the Expert Group on Special Care for Babies.* Reports on Public Health and Medical Subjects No 127. London: HMSO, 1971.

222. Oppe TE. *Report of the Working Party on the Prevention of Early Neonatal Mortality and Morbidity.* London: DHSS, 1975.

223. Court SDM. *Fit for the Future. Report of the Committee on Child Health Services.* Cmnd 6684. Vol I and II. London: HMSO, 1976.

224. Walker J. *Report of the Joint Working Party on Standards of Perinatal Care in Scotland.* National Medical Consultative Committee. Edinburgh: Scottish Home and Health Department, 1980.

225. Short R. *Perinatal and Neonatal Morbidity. Second Report from the Social Services Committee 979-80.* London: HMSO, 1980.

226. Boyle A, Grap MJ, Younger J, Thornby D. Personality hardiness, ways of coping, social support and burnout in critical care nurses. *Journal of Advanced Nursing,* 1991; 16: 850-857.

227. McHaffie HE. *The Care of Patients with HIV and AIDS: A Survey of Nurse Education in the UK.* Institute of Medical Ethics Report, Department of Medicine, University of Edinburgh, 1993.

228. National Association for Staff Support. *A Charter for Staff Support.* London: NASS/RCN, 1992

229. Gallagher U, Boyd KM. (Eds) *Teaching and Learning Nursing Ethics.* Harrow: Scutari Press, 1991.

230. Gillon R. Caring, men and women, nurses and doctors, and health care ethics. *Journal of Medical Ethics,* 1992; 18: 171-172.

231. American Board of Pediatrics Medical Ethics Subcommittee. Teaching and evaluation of interpersonal skills and ethical decision making in pediatrics. *Pediatrics,* 1987; 79, 5: 829-834.

232. Seroka AM. Values clarification and ethical decision making. *Seminars for Nurse Managers,* 1994; 2, 1: 8-15.

233. Raines DA. Values: A guiding force. *AWHONNS Clinical Issues in Perinatal and Women's Health Nursing,* 1993; 4, 4: 533-541.

234. Pederson C, Duckett L, Maruyama G, Ryden M. Using structured controversy to promote ethical decision making. *Journal of Nursing Education,* 1990; 29, 4: 150-157 (with published erratum in Vol 5: p 240).

235. Holly CM, Lyons M. Ethical practice in acute care nursing: Are we there yet? *Journal of the New York State Nurses Association,* 1992; 23, 4: 4-7.

236. Sofaer B. Teaching health care ethics: Enhancng humanistic skills: An experiential approach to learning about ethical issues in health care. *Journal of Medical Ethics,* 1995; 21: 31-34.

237. McHaffie HE. *Holding on?* Cheshire: Books for Midwives Press, 1994.

238. Byrne PJ. Tyebkhan JM, Laing LM. Ethical decision-making and neonatal resuscitation. *Seminars in Perinatology,* 1994; 18, 1: 36-41.

239. Goldworth A, Silverman W, Stevenson DK, Young EWD. (Eds) *Ethics and Perinatology.* New York: Oxford Medical Publications, 1995.

240. Loewy EH. Suffering as a consideration in ethical decision making. *Cambridge Quarterly of Healthcare Ethics,* 1992; 1, 2: 135-146.

241. Weir R. Withholding and withdrawing therapy and actively hastening death. In Goldworth A, Silverman W, Stevenson DK, Young EWD. (Eds) *Ethics and Perinatology.* New York: Oxford Medical Publications, 1995; pp172-183.

242. Gorovitz S. (Contributor to) Appendix: *HEW support of research involving human in vitro fertilization and embryo transfer.* Washington DC: US Government Printing Office, 1979.

243. Banja JD. Nutritional discontinuance: Active or passive euthanasia? *Journal of Neuroscience Nursing,* 1990; 22, 2: 117-120.

244. Chiswick ML. Withdrawal of life support in babies: Deceptive signals. *Archives of Disease in Childhood*, 1990; 65: 1096-1097.

245. Chiswick ML, Roberton N. Doctors and nurses in neonatal care: Towards integration. *Archives of Disease in Childhood*, 1987; 62: 653-655.

246. Dunn PM. Medical and nurse staffing for the newborn. *Archives of Disease in Childhood*, 1988; 63: 98-99.

247. Connelly JE. Emotions and the process of ethical decision making. *Journal - South Carolina Medical Association*, 1990; 86, 12: 621-623.

248. Hadley J. Nurse advocacy, ethics, and health care reform. *Journal of Post Anesthesia Nursing*, 1994; 9, 1: 55-56.

249. Thomasma DC. The ethics of letting go. *Journal of Critical Care*, 1993; 8, 3: 170-176.

250. Brody H. *Ethical Decisions in Medicine*. Michigan: Michigan State University Press, 1976.

251. Payton RJ. Pluralistic ethical decision making. In *Clinical and Scientific Sessions*, Kansas City, Missouri: American Nurses' Association, 1979; pp 9-16.

252. Thompson JE, Thompson O. Ethical decision making: Process and models. *Neonatal Network*, 1990; 9, 1: 69-70.

253. Eliot G. *The Mill on the Floss*. New York: Signet, New York, 1965.

254. Fox RC. *The Sociology of Medicine: A Participant Observers' View*. New Jersey: Prentice Hall, Englewood Cliffs, 1989.

255. Darbyshire M. Our baby. In Cooper A, Harpin V (Eds) *This is Our Child: How Parents Experience the Medical World*. Oxford: Oxford University Press, 1991; pp 1-9.

256. Cooper A , Cooper A. Hamish. In Cooper A, Harpin V (Eds) *This is Our Child: How Parents Experience the Medical World*. Oxford: Oxford University Press, 1991; pp 132-143.

257. Delight E, Goodall J. Babies with spina bifida treated without surgery. *British Medical Journal*, 1988; 297: 1230-1233.

258. Hawdon JM, Williams S, Weindling AM. Withdrawal of neonatal intensive care in the home. *Archives of Disease in Childhood*, 1994; 71: F142-144.

259. Stahlman MT. Ethical issues in the nursery: Priorities versus limits. *Journal of Pediatrics*, 1990; 116, 2: 167-170.

260. Swirydczuk K. Natalia. In Cooper A, Harpin V (Eds) *This is Our Child: How Parents Experience the Medical World*. Oxford: Oxford University Press, 1991; pp34-43.

261. Klaus MH. Ethical decision making in neonatal intensive care. Commentary: Communicating with parents. *Birth*, 1986; 13, 3: 175.

262. Brewin TB. Truth, trust and paternalism. *Lancet*, 1985; August 31: 490-492.

263. Brody H. Transparency: Informed consent in primary care. *Hastings Center Report*, 1989; 19, 5: 5-9.

264. Bohin S, Draper ES, Field DJ. Impact of extremely immature infants on neonatal services. *Archives of Disease in Childhood*, 1996; 74, 2: F110-113.

265. Goldenberg RL, Nelson KG, Dyer RL, Wayne J. The variability of viability: The effect of physicians' perceptions of viability on the survival of very low-birth weight infants. *American Journal of Obstetrics and Gynaecology*, 1982; 143: 678-684.

266. Lee Shoo K, Penner PL, Cox M. Comparison of the attitudes of health care professionals and parents toward active treatment of very low birth weight infants. *Pediatrics*, 1991; (88,1:) 110-114.

267. Graner JL. Thoughts and ethics. The place for thought in medical ethical decision-making. *Lancet*, 1989; 2, 8655: 150.

268. Fairbairn GJ. Kuhse, Singer and slippery slopes. *Journal of Medical Ethics*, 1988; 14: 132-134.

269. Brody H. Assisted death - A compassionate response to a medical failure. *New England Journal of Medicine*. 1992; 327, 19: 1384-1389.

270. Illich I. *Limits to Medicine. Medical Nemesis: The Expropriation of Health*. Harmondsworth: Penguin, 1977.

271. Kubler-Ross E. *Death: The Final Stage of Growth.* New Jersey: Englewood Cliffs, 1975.
272. Callahan D. Pursuing a peaceful death. *Hastings Center Report,* 1993; 23, 4: 33-38.
273. Sanger M. *My Fight for Birth Control.* New York: Farrar & Rinehart, 1931.

Index

Introducing another title from
Hochland & Hochland Limited
by Marianne Hancock

JUST CAROLE
The True Story of Carole Baker

'How strange life was. One day everything can be fine, life plodding along in its normal, predictable routine – and then another day something totally unexpected can suddenly happen to throw it all completely off course, never to be the same again.'

It is 1980 and Carole Baker, housewife and mother, is living in Tanzania with her two children and husband Nick, who is completing an overseas contract.

Carole's world is turned upside down the day she finds lumps in her neck leading to the diagnosis of Hodgkin's Disease. To add to Carole's trauma, she discovers Nick is having an affair.

The odds are stacked against her. Can she beat this life threatening disease? Can she win her husband back?

This moving novel takes you through the emotions and experiences of a woman searching to find the strength to survive.

About the author
Marianne Hancock, a close friend of Carole Baker, is a freelance writer from Leicester and has had several articles published in magazines and the local press.

Price: £9.95

To order your copy, call our Credit Card Hotline now on
(0161) 929 0190

Introducing another title by Hazel McHaffie from
Hochland & Hochland Limited

HOLDING ON?

Should Peter Flanaghan, a pre-term baby on the edge of viability, be kept alive on life support? Set in a busy, regional Neonatal Unit, this novel traces the agony of staff and parents in trying to decide Peter's fate. Each of the individuals involved brings something of their own, personal life experience to their attempt of answering this question – experience with severely abnormal children, with infertility, with incapacitating illness. Personalities, religious convictions and childhood trauma all influence the way each of them feels and responds to the issue. Can so divertgent a group of individuals reach a consensus? Resolving the dilemma is urgent. A decision cannot be put off. The hours tick by inexorably. The reader is held in suspense to the last page.

This book will touch the hearts of parents and all those who have experienced the tragedy that the birth of a 'less than perfect' baby can bring to a family. It will also open the eyes of health professionals to the living reality that can surround the care of premature or severely abnormal infants and pose the ethical dilemmas that this novel illustrates so poignantly.

In writing her novel, Hazel McHaffie, a Research Fellow in the Institute of Medical Ethics in Edinburgh, has drawn upon a wealth of experience. In her professional life she worked in a variety of settings as a nurse and midwife, before embarking on her career in research. She holds a PhD for her work on the care of premature infants. Well known in professional circles for her extensive research in this specialty, she has also carried out work in the field of HIV and AIDS, much of it used in the training of doctors and nurses.

Price: £9.95

To order your copy, call our Credit Card Hotline now on (0161) 929 0190